communicating

in the health sciences

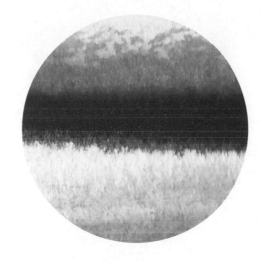

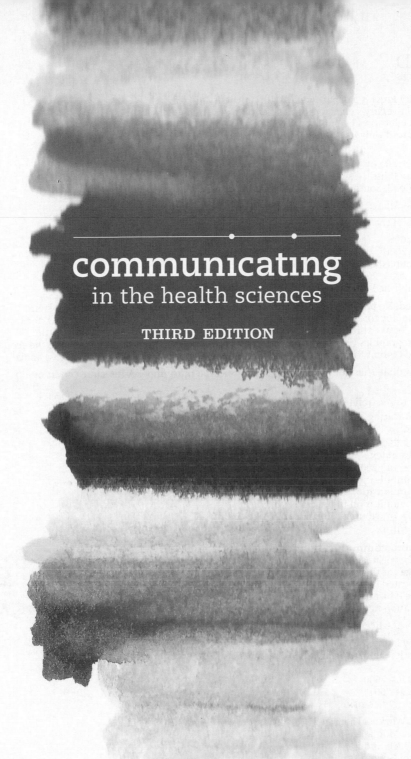

communicating
in the health sciences

THIRD EDITION

JOY **HIGGS** | ROLA **AJJAWI** | LINDY **McALLISTER** | FRANZISKA **TREDE** | STEPHEN **LOFTUS**

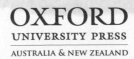

OXFORD
UNIVERSITY PRESS
AUSTRALIA & NEW ZEALAND

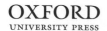

OXFORD
UNIVERSITY PRESS

Oxford University Press is a department of the University of Oxford.
It furthers the University's objective of excellence in research,
scholarship and education by publishing worldwide. Oxford is a registered
trademark of Oxford University Press in the UK and in certain other
countries.

Published in Australia by
Oxford University Press
253 Normanby Road, South Melbourne, Victoria 3205, Australia

First published 2005
Reprinted 2005, 2006
Second edition published 2008
Reprinted 2008, 2009, 2010 (twice), 2011
Third edition published 2012

National Library of Australia Cataloguing-in-Publication entry

   Title: Communicating in the health sciences / Joy Higgs ... [et al.].
   Edition: 3rd ed.
   ISBN: 9780195579048 (pbk.)
   Notes: Includes index.
             Previous ed.: 2008.
   Subjects: Communication in medicine.
             Communication in the social sciences.
             Communication in human services.
   Other Authors/Contributors: Higgs, Joy.
Dewey Number: 610.14

Reproduction and communication for educational purposes

Cover image: YouWorkForThem
Edited by Amanda Morgan
Typeset by diacriTech, India
Proofread by Carol Goudie
Indexed by Jeanne Rudd
Printed by Sheck Wah Tong Printing Press Ltd.

contents

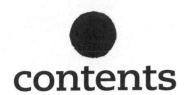

PART
01

Understanding
communication
pg.3

PART
02

Learning to
communicate
pg.45

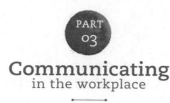

PART
03

Communicating
in the workplace
·
pg.173

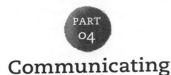

list of figures

list of tables

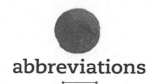

abbreviations

AAC	Augmentative or alternative communication
ABS	Australian Bureau of Statistics
APA	American Psychological Association
Apps	Applications
BP	Blood Pressure
CLR	Commonwealth Legal Reports
CVP	Central Venous Pressure
DOAJ	Directory of Open Access Journals
GPs	General practitioners
ID	Identity
IM	Instant messaging
IMRAD	Introduction, method, results and discussion
IT	Information Technology
LMS	Learning Management System
MMSE	Mini Mental State Evaluation
Mobile apps	Mobile phone applications
NHMRC	National Health and Medical Research Council
PBL	Problem-based learning
PLE	Personal Learning Environment
SMS	Short message service
TBI	Traumatic brain injury
TM	Trademark

contributors

Rebecca ACHESON
Rebecca Acheson BA (English/Sociology), B Teach (Secondary), Educational Designer, Division of Learning and Teaching Services, Charles Sturt University, Australia

Rola AJJAWI
Dr Rola Ajjawi BAppSc(Physiotherapy) Hons, PhD, Senior Lecturer in Medical Education, Centre for Medical Education, University of Dundee, Scotland UK, Adjunct Senior Lecturer, The Education For Practice Institute, Charles Sturt University, Australia

Ros ALLUM
Ros Allum DipT Syd, GradCertEd Monash, GradCertTESOL NSW, Publications Officer, The Education For Practice Institute, Charles Sturt University, Australia

Fiona BOGOSSIAN
Associate Professor Fiona Bogossian PhD, MPH, BAppSci (N), DipAppSci (NEd), RM,RN, School of Nursing and Midwifery, Director of Research, The University of Queensland, Australia

Wendy BOWLES
Associate Professor Wendy Bowles BSW(Hons), PhD NSW, School of Humanities and Social Sciences, Charles Sturt University, Australia

Julia COYLE
Associate Professor Julia Coyle PhD, MManipPhty, GradDipManipPhty, GCertUniTL MCSP, GAICD: Head, School of Community Health, Charles Sturt University, Australia

Anne CROKER
Dr Anne Croker BAppSc(Physio), GradDipPublicHealth, PhD, Adjunct Research Associate, The Education For Practice Institute, Charles Sturt University, Australia

Claudio DIONIGI
Claudio Dionigi MAppSci, GDipEd, BA(Hons), Faculty Liaison Librarian, Charles Sturt University Library, Charles Sturt University, Australia

Elizabeth ELLIS
Dr Elizabeth Ellis PhD, MHL, GradDipPhty, Honorary Senior Lecturer, Faculty of Health Sciences, The University of Sydney, Australia

Alison GATES
Dr Alison Gates PhD, Practice-Based Education Projects Coordinator, The Education For Practice Institute, Charles Sturt University, Australia

Iain HAY
Professor Iain Hay PhD, MA, GradCertTertEd, BSc(Hons), Professor of Human Geography and ALTC Discipline Scholar for the Arts, Social Sciences and Humanities, Flinders University, Australia

Charles **HIGGS**
> Charles Higgs MAppSci(SocEcol), MEd (ITET), GradDipEd(Tech), BSurv, Key Performance Consulting, Wollongong, Research Associate, The Education For Practice Institute, Charles Sturt University, Australia

Joy **HIGGS**
> Professor Joy Higgs AM, PhD, MHPEd, BSc, Director, The Education For Practice Institute, Charles Sturt University, Australia

Barbara **HILL**
> Dr Barbara Hill PhD, MA, BA, Indigenous Curriculum and Pedagogy Coordinator, Division of Learning and Teaching Services, Charles Sturt University, Australia

Jill **HUMMELL**
> Dr Jill Hummell DipOT (USyd), BA (Macq), MA (Macq), PhD (USyd), Manager, Community Integration Program, Westmead Brain Injury Rehabilitation Service, Sydney, Adjunct Research Associate, The Education For Practice Institute, Charles Sturt University, Australia

Sarah **HYDE**
> Dr Sarah Hyde BA (Psych) (Hons), PhD, Lecturer in Problem Based Learning, Member of The Research Institute for Professional Practice, Learning & Education, Charles Sturt University, Australia

Sue **JONES**
> Associate Professor Sue Jones BSc(Physio), GDipPubSectMgmt, Dean, Teaching & Learning, Curtin University, Australia

Stephen **LOFTUS**
> Dr Stephen Loftus BDS Sheff, MSc Wales, PhD, Senior Lecturer, The Education For Practice Institute, Charles Sturt University, Australia

Mary Jane **MAHONEY**
> Dr Mary Jane Mahony PhD, MS, GradDipDistEd, DipEd, BS, Honorary Senior Lecturer and Affiliate, Centre for Research on Computer Supported Learning and Cognition, Faculty of Education and Social Work, University of Sydney, Australia

Lindy **M^cALLISTER**
> Professor Lindy McAllister PhD, MA(SpPath), BSpThy, Professor and Associate Dean of Work Integrated Learning, Faculty of Health Sciences, The University of Sydney, Australia, Adjunct Professor, Charles Sturt University, Australia

Sandra **MACKEY**
> Dr Sandra Mackey PhD, BN (Hons) RN, Senior Lecturer, School of Nursing and Midwifery, University of Western Sydney.

Tony **MᶜKENZIE**
> Tony McKenzie BA, DipEd, MSc(Hons), Adjunct Research Fellow, The Education For Practice Institute, Charles Sturt University, Australia

Peter **MILLS**
> Peter Mills MScAgric, Lecturer in Horticulture, School of Agricultural and Wine Sciences, Charles Sturt University, Australia

Shazia **NASER-UD-DIN**
> Dr Shazia Naser-ud-Din PhD, MSc, BDS, DPHDent, FICCDE, DCPSP-HPE, Senior Lecturer & Discipline Lead, Orthodontics, School of Dentistry, The University of Queensland, Australia

Marissa **OLSEN**
> Marissa Olsen MSc (Nutr/Diet), APD, PhD Candidate, Lecturer in Nutrition & Dietetics, School of Dentistry and Health Sciences, Charles Sturt University, Australia

Narelle **PATTON**
> Narelle Patton BAppSc(Phty), MHSc, PhD Candidate, Lecturer in Physiotherapy, School of Community Health, Charles Sturt University, Australia

Linda **PORTSMOUTH**
> Linda Portsmouth MHlthComm, PGradDipHlthProm, BA, BAppSc, PhD, Lecturer & Researcher School of Public Health, Curtin University, Australia

Charlotte **REES**
> Professor Charlotte Rees BSc(Hons), MEd, PhD, CPsychol, Director of the Centre for Medical Education, University of Dundee, Scotland, UK

Joan **ROSENTHAL**
> Joan Rosenthal MA, BA, LACST, Research Associate, The Education For Practice Institute, Charles Sturt University, Australia

Jennifer **SCHAFER**
> Dr Jennifer Schafer MBBS DRANZCOG FRACGP, Director MBBS Program, School of Medicine, The University of Queensland, Australia

Susie **SCHOFIELD**
> Dr Susie Schofield BSc (Hons), PGCE, MSc, PhD, Lecturer in Medical Education, University of Dundee, Scotland, UK

Stephanie **SEDDON**
> Dr Stephanie Seddon BSc. Syd (Hons) JCU PhD Syd, PhD Adel, Higher Degree Research Coordinator, The Education For Practice Institute, Charles Sturt University, Australia

Ann **SEFTON**

> Emeritus Professor Ann Sefton PhD, DSc, MB, BS, BSc(Med), The University of Sydney, Australia

Lucie **SHANAHAN**

> Lucie Shanahan BSpPath, PGDipRuralHealth, CPSP, The Kids' Team, South West Brain Injury Rehabilitation Service, Murrumbidgee Local Health District, Albury, NSW, Australia

Maree **SIMPSON**

> Associate Professor Maree Donna Simpson B Pharm, BSc (Hons), PhD, MPS, Grad Cert Univ Teach & Learn, Charles Sturt University, Australia

Megan **SMITH**

> Associate Professor Megan Smith, PhD, MAppSc (CardiopulmPhysio), GradCertUT&L, BAppSc(Physio), School of Community Health, Charles Sturt University, Australia

Annette **STREET**

> Professor Annette Street PhD, BEd(Hons), Professor & Director, Research Education and Development (RED) Unit, La Trobe University, Australia

Diane **TASKER**

> Diane Tasker B(Phty), PhD Candidate, Charles Sturt University, Australia; Mountain Mobile Physiotherapy Service, Blue Mountains, Australia; Research Associate, The Education For Practice Institute, Charles Sturt University, Australia

Franziska **TREDE**

> Associate Professor Franziska Trede PhD, MHPEd, DipPhys, Deputy Director, The Education For Practice Institute, Charles Sturt University, Australia

Lyndal **TREVENA**

> Associate Professor Lyndal Trevena PhD, MPhilPH, MBBS(Hons), Associate Dean (International), School of Public Health, The University of Sydney, Australia

Philip **UYS**

> Associate Professor Philip Uys, PhD, Grad.Cert Univ.L&T., B.Comm.Hons., B.Comm., Adv. Dip. Tertiary Teaching, Director, Strategic Learning and Teaching Innovation, Division of Learning and Teaching Services, Charles Sturt University

Helen **WOZNIAK**

> Associate Professor Helen Wozniak MHlthScEd, DipAppSc(Orth), Elearning Coordinator, Northern Territory Medical Program, FlindersNT, Flinders University

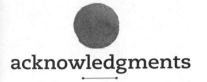

acknowledgments

The Editors wish to acknowledge the exceptional work of Ros Allum in coordinating the production and scheduling of the manuscript and the invaluable contribution of Joan Rosenthal for her excellent document checking and professional advice on the manuscript. Our thanks to the OUP team for their support and great work in the book's production.

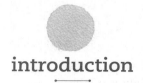

introduction

In this *third* edition of Communicating in the Health Sciences we extend our exploration of the nature of communication, and the communication issues facing teachers, students and professionals in the health sciences. We examine many aspects of communication as a key dimension of the pursuit of sound person-centred practice and the provision of quality services to people and communities.

The third edition builds on the success of the second edition. All chapters have been reviewed, with major updates in areas where significant recent changes have occurred in technology and practice. The structure of the book has been revised into five updated sections: Understanding Communication, Learning to Communicate, Communicating in the Workplace, Communicating in Teams and Doing Advanced Communication.

Joy **HIGGS**

Understanding
communication

Communication in the health sciences

Joy **HIGGS** | Lindy **M^cALLISTER** | Ann **SEFTON**

key topics

This chapter covers the following topics:

- what are the health sciences?

- what is communication?

- why is communication important in the health sciences?

key terms

HEALTH SCIENCES

COMMUNICATION

PROFESSIONALISM

Introduction

This is a book about the nature and importance of communication in the **health sciences**. Communication plays an important role in the daily activities of all these people and professions as they work with others. This book is also relevant for workers in the social sciences; for example in social work, psychology and welfare studies. Similarly, communication is a key aspect of the work of other service-related disciplines and professions, such as economics, law and veterinary science.

Why is communication important in the health sciences?

The key role played by writing, speaking and other communication skills in the work of health professionals is emphasised by a number of authors (see The Healthcare Communication Group, 2001). Quality client service requires good communication. A person-centred approach to health service requires practitioners to understand clients' needs and expectations in relation to their personal healthcare and wellbeing. Practitioners need to communicate clearly with clients and their families in setting up shared goals and priorities for healthcare. Good communication among health professionals is the basis of the effective teamwork necessary for efficient delivery of healthcare services. Also, sound communication skills are essential for meeting the legal requirements related to documenting encounters, assessments, investigations, management plans and treatment outcomes, and communicating about them with relevant team members.

Liptak, Leutenberg, Sippola and Brodsky (2008) stress the importance of learning to communicate and recognising that, in this learning process, people need to realise that they are making choices. These choices, they argue, need to be informed choices so that, like any other action, communication can encompass the possibility of change for the better, and for the enrichment of our lives and the lives of others.

Another key factor in learning to communicate well is to understand how the world (both the global community and local worlds such as workplaces and people's life-worlds) is constantly changing. O'Connell and Groom (2010) remind us of the importance of connecting, communicating and collaborating as we learn in this changing world.

Communication

To say that you have *communicated* means that a message has passed between you and another person or persons. **Communication** is effective when what people intended to say has been heard, and the people involved have reached a point of shared meaning. Effective communication (whether oral or textual) requires:

- an intention to share information
- a desire to reach common understanding
- active listening (or reading) by the receiver
- an understanding by both parties of the person they are communicating with (including relevant aspects of background and culture)

/ HEALTH SCIENCES /
The term health sciences refers to the variety of professional groups that provide healthcare services to people in community settings or healthcare facilities. These professions include medicine, dentistry, nursing, physiotherapy, occupational therapy, radiography, speech pathology, dietetics, emergency care work, podiatry, pharmacy, health education and public health.

/ COMMUNICATION /
Communication is conferring through speech, writing or non-verbal means (including body language) to create a shared meaning. It is a two-way process: whereas talking, listening, writing and reading can be one-sided; communicating involves two or more people sharing information.

- a commitment by the sender to use language that the receiver can understand and to communicate in a manner that is appropriate to the abilities and needs of the receiver (such as a client and family)
- a mutual willingness to understand the other person's point of view.

Types of communication

Health and social professionals need to be proficient at communicating in a variety of styles and across a range of media (such as oral, written and electronic forms). Later chapters in this book discuss these different types of communication in more detail.

Communication can also be categorised as either *formal* or *informal*.

Formal communication is often associated with systems and organisations in which information is distributed about the way the system operates (such as exam schedules, referral procedures, and institutional rules and regulations). People who receive such information use it to operate within that system (e.g. students read exam timetables and attend the right exams at the right time, and health professionals refer patients to the appropriate people). Such messages are explicit and 'official'. Presentations at conferences and in lectures of clinical and scientific work, generally supported by evidence, are also instances of formal communication. The language of such communication can be called formal, scholarly, scientific, academic or professional. Much of what is called communication in organisations or via mass communication is simply the one-way dissemination of information (such as mass electronic mail-outs, television and noticeboard bulletins). In these cases, information is indeed sent. But is it received and understood as intended?

Informal communication is more spontaneous; it occurs in groups, among friends and colleagues, and between practitioners and their clients during professional interactions. The language used is commonly more casual, informal and colloquial. People talking informally, or sending notes, SMS texts (short messages via phone) or emails often use incomplete sentences, commonly understood language or jargon, abbreviations and examples, rather than detailed evidence. In communicating with patients or clients, practitioners usually need to 'de-jargon' their messages and adapt their language to each client's circumstances (considering the client's language, culture, age, educational background, wellness and comprehension skills). When we speak of *effective* or *good* interpersonal communication, we are referring mainly to informal communication that considers the relevant circumstantial factors and addresses them effectively.

Issues and skills in communication

Each professional is expected to attain competence in a range of discipline-specific and generic areas of performance. Throughout this book, a number of key issues and competencies are examined in relation to the practical aspects of helping health students (and practitioners) to learn and use oral and written communication skills. These issues are shown in Figure 1.1, and are discussed in this chapter.

Being person-centred

Communication should, first and foremost, be conducted in a spirit of humanity. As well as helping provide high-quality professional services for individuals and the community, interpersonal skills are important in demonstrating respect for all people, whether in the classroom or in professional practice.

handy hint 1.1

BEING PERSON-CENTRED

Being person-centred rather than task-centred involves using skills such as active listening or reading, empathic understanding and cultural competence. The goal here is to genuinely hear and understand the sender's message and to acknowledge both the message and the person.

FIGURE 1.1 | ISSUES IN COMMUNICATION IN THE HEALTH SCIENCES

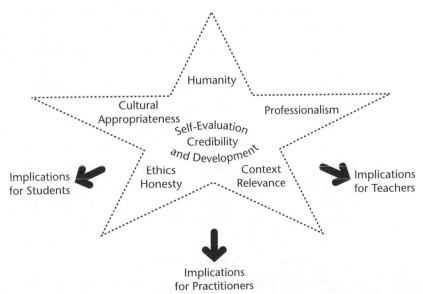

Active listening to oral communication and *active reading* of text (written or electronic) involves paying attention to the sender and to what he or she is trying to say or ask. It includes conveying interest, concern and attention, and demonstrating that you want to hear what the person has to say. In face-to-face oral communication, body language plays a large part in showing interest. In other verbal communication (such as telephoning), interest can be shown by your tone of voice. In interactive text communication (such as SMS, email or electronic bulletin boards), the style of language, the words used and the order of content of your message can show how well you are attending to the other person's messages. For instance, you can show interest by acknowledging or commenting on the other person's message before sending your own.

Empathy is 'the ability to enter the perceptual world of the other person, to see the world as they see it. It also suggests an ability to convey this perception to other people' (Burnard, 1997, p. 172). Empathy is not about feeling sorry for other people, but about demonstrating a willingness to explore their concerns and point of view, allowing and encouraging the other person to express him- or herself fully and to have communication needs met. Fundamentally, health professionals seek to foster the health and wellbeing of people and communities. This is achieved in part through supportive communication. Carlopio and colleagues (1997) detail eight attributes of supportive communication—see Handy Hint 1.2.

BEING SUPPORTIVE IN COMMUNICATION

Supportive communication is:

- problem-oriented, not person-oriented; asking 'How can we solve this problem?'

- congruent, not incongruent; communicating real effects, not pretending; for example, 'Your behaviour really upset me.'

- descriptive, not evaluative; describing, not blaming or criticising; for example, 'This is what I think happened and what I suggest we do.'

- validating, not invalidating; for example, 'I have some ideas, and I'd like to hear your suggestions too.'

- specific, not global; for example, 'You interrupted me three times just then', rather than 'You always take over the conversation.'

- conjunctive, not disjunctive; relating your input to what is being discussed; for example, 'In relation to that point, I'd like to suggest …'

- owned, not disowned; for example, 'I would like to pick up your idea about this case because …'

- supportive listening, not one-way listening; for example, 'What do you think would solve this problem?'

Source: Based on Carlopio, Andrewartha, & Armstrong 1997, p. 224.

Cultural appropriateness

Professionals are expected to practise with integrity and personal tolerance, and to communicate effectively across language, cultural and situational barriers (see Warren & Fassett, 2011). Fitzgerald (2001, p. 153) defines *culture* as 'the learned and shared patterns of perceiving and adapting or responding to the world [that is] characteristic of a society or population'. For example, culture is reflected in a society's learned shared beliefs, values, attitudes and behaviours. Although culture is dynamic and ever-changing, it maintains a sense of coherence. *Intercultural communication* refers to interactions between peoples of different cultures who differ from each other in terms of shared knowledge or language. Such communication is a core part of interacting with people (patients, clients, colleagues and carers) in the health sciences. To be culturally competent requires going beyond token gestures in acknowledging another person's culture, beyond the use of stereotypical images and responses to cultural differences. Cultural competence involves seeking a clearer understanding of what it means to belong to the culture of the person with whom you are interacting, and adapting your manner of interaction as well as your professional services to that person's needs and background.

Professionalism

The notion of **professionalism** encompasses not only issues of standards, codes of behaviour and humanity, as listed above, but also includes appropriate manners and styles of behaviour. Relevant behaviours include showing respect for others, recognising the rights of others, demonstrating a duty of care, respecting the cultural backgrounds of others, and being responsible for the quality and appropriateness of one's practice and behaviour. Professionalism in oral and written communications includes addressing the requirements of the task, demonstrating respect for individuals, meeting deadlines and understanding best practice.

Students and practitioners are bound by workplace and university rules, and the expectations that govern the performance of individuals and teams, and indicate the conduct expected of them. These expectations can include 'unwritten rules', formal established ward protocols, and institutional regulations and expectations. Underpinning all these workplace codes is the principle that health professionals are accountable for their practice. Members of different professions have codes of ethics that guide their behaviour. Related to ethical and workplace standards are the legal requirements of professional practice: written and oral communication must operate within requirements such as duty of care. Poor communication between clients and health professionals is a major source of complaints to ethics boards (Body & McAllister, 2009). Poor communication between health professionals is a major risk to client care and can lead to markedly adverse outcomes for clients (Australian Commission on Safety and Quality in Health Care, 2011).

/ **PROFESSIONALISM** /

'Professional behaviour (or professionalism) comprises those actions, standards and considerations of ethical and humanistic conduct expected by society and by professional associations from members of professions' (Higgs, Hummell, & Roe-Shaw, 2009, p. 58).

Chapter 4 highlights the issue of academic honesty as a central concern of communicating for university students. Academic honesty is particularly important in professional education, because the same honesty students learn to demonstrate is required of graduates throughout their professional practice, teaching and research.

The relevance of context

Students are learners and novice professionals, and they need to understand the context of each learning and professional practice task. What are the expectations of educators, patients, clients and colleagues? More and more, the community expects healthcare services to be individualised, relevant and timely. To achieve this, professionals must elicit and share information that helps them understand and address their clients' needs. Listening carefully to clients is critically important.

Moreover, students and professionals need to understand their audience to ensure that communication is appropriate. Different aspects of effective professional communication (such as formality of language, use of gestures or jargon, and strategies for negotiation and conflict resolution) should be tailored to the audience.

BEING PROFESSIONAL IN CONTEXT

Communicating professionally includes showing respect for people, providing sound evidence or arguments to support your proposed or actual actions, and working within the relevant ethical and legal parameters of professional healthcare practice. It also means choosing the appropriate mode of address and means of communication for the given context. For example, a speech pathology student communicating with a Principal at a school where she is working should not send an SMS message to the Principal, especially not one ending 'c u later'. Instead, she should send a more formally written email or letter.

Credibility

Whether people see you as a credible professional depends on how you address many of the above issues. Do people (fellow professionals as well as clients) think you demonstrate the professional practices and standards expected of your group? Are you responsive to your clients and colleagues? Do you consider and adapt to the age, background and culture of the people with whom you are communicating? Do you keep good records? (See Chapter 22.) Your standing as a professional depends also on whether you can credibly justify your professional behaviour.

Can you provide sound evidence to support your decisions? Do you keep your professional knowledge and skills up-to-date? Do you undertake research or evaluate the quality of your practice?

Self-reflection and self-evaluation

Finally, as a professional, you need to reflect upon and critically evaluate your professional performance, your knowledge and your skills. This evaluation also involves seeking feedback about your practice from supervisors, peers and colleagues. On the basis of your self-evaluation, you can develop and implement strategies to improve your performance (e.g. by independently studying certain topics, practising skills you need to master and participating in professional development activities). Developing the skill of honest self-evaluation as a student is an excellent preparation for professional life.

Learning to communicate

Understanding the topic or message to be communicated

Being an effective communicator involves learning about the topic you want to communicate and understanding it well. Sometimes this understanding comes during the communication process, such as in a dialogue with others. Understanding the topic often means being able to look at it from multiple perspectives; for instance, looking at the pros and cons, and looking at the issue from different angles.

Explaining well

Having understood your topic well, you must frame your message, identify the key points you need to explain and communicate them clearly to your co-communicator(s). When you are trying to explain something, it is often helpful to cover the following points: What do you want to communicate? Who is involved? Where and when is it occurring? How is it done or how does it work? Why is it important?

In written communication, such as patients' notes, student essays and journal papers, explaining can take the form of clearly documenting the client's history or treatment, setting out the rationale for a proposed treatment regime or education program, referring a client to another professional, presenting an argument or reporting on research. Such communication needs to be clear, relevant and appropriate in length, content and style. For example, medical prescriptions and requests for investigations must be correct and unambiguous, and clinical notes need to contain clear and relevant information to facilitate communication between care providers and to meet legal and ethical standards.

Self-monitoring

As with any complex skill, effective communication needs you to be aware of how and how well you are doing it. This involves learning to observe your own behaviour and its effects on other people, and developing strategies to see if others have understood your messages, as well as you understanding theirs. You could 'sum up' the key points made, check next steps or deadlines, or ask if the other person wants to add any points to the discussion. Being open to feedback from others is often a key to success in self-monitoring.

Communication and advances in technology

In the current digital age we have access to and are challenged by an ever-increasing range of information, communication technologies and situations. In choosing our spaces and tools for communication we need to consider the accessibility, cost (to purchase, use, and take time to learn) and suitability of these tools for our purpose. There are times when social networking communication, e-meetings, or video and teleconferences are ideal for our group communication purposes, when one-to-one (or group) communication can be enhanced through mobile communication devices (e.g. smart phones) and when individuals remotely accessing system information (e.g. web databases, university schedules and lectures) can greatly facilitate students' access to learning and enrolment information. Keppell, Souter and Riddle (2011) provide an in-depth look at how we can create a range of physical and virtual spaces for learning. Care needs to be taken in all communication; this is particularly so when professional communication occurs through email and social media, where the tone and intent of the communication may be open to misinterpretation.

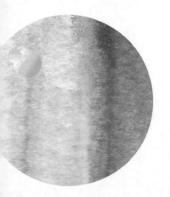

conclusion

Professional communication in the health sciences is both challenging and rewarding. Effective communication is an essential aspect of sound professional practice. Professionals need to be adept at using a range of communication methods and adapting their communication to the context, culture and people involved. Our professionalism is judged in part on our competence as communicators. Communication competence involves being able to achieve your goals in communication while allowing others in the communication process to achieve theirs, as well as supporting the relationship that frames the communication. Understanding and learning the skills for effective communication is an important part of your socialisation into the health professions. Communication can be enhanced through self-evaluation and practising the skills involved. In the chapters that follow, many aspects and skills of oral, embodied, written and electronic communication are examined, along with guidelines and handy hints to help you become a competent communicator.

references

Australian Commission on Safety and Quality in Health Care. (2011). *OSSIE guide to clinical handover improvement*. Available from http://www.safetyandquality.gov.au/internet/safety/publishing.nsf/content/PriorityProgram-05_OssieGuide.

Body, R., & McAllister L. (2009). *Ethics in speech and language therapy*. Chichester, UK: Wiley & Sons.

Burnard, P. (1997). *Effective communication skills for health professionals* (2nd edn). Cheltenham, UK: Stanley Thornes.

Carlopio, J., Andrewartha, G., & Armstrong, H. (1997). *Developing management skills in Australia*. Melbourne: Longman.

Fitzgerald, M. H. (2001). Gaining knowledge of culture during professional education. In J. Higgs & A. Titchen (Eds.), *Practice knowledge and expertise in the health professions* (pp. 149–56). Oxford: Butterworth-Heinemann.

Higgs, J., Hummell, J., & Roe-Shaw, M. (2009). Becoming a member of a health profession: A journey of socialisation. In J. Higgs, M. Smith, G. Webb, M. Skinner & A. Croker (Eds.), *Contexts of physiotherapy practice* (pp. 58–71). Melbourne: Elsevier Australia.

Keppell, M., Souter, K., & Riddle, M. (2011). *Physical and virtual learning spaces in higher education: Concepts for the modern learning environment*. Hershey, PA: IGI Global.

Liptak, J. J., Leutenberg, E., Sippola, C., & Brodsky, A. L. (2008). *The communication skills workbook*. Duluth, MN: Whole Person Associates.

O'Connell, J., & Groom, D. (2010). *Connect, communicate, collaborate (Learning in a changing world)*. Camberwell, VIC: ACER Press.

The Health Care Communication Group. (2001). *Writing, speaking, & communication skills for health professionals*. New Haven, CT: Yale University Press.

Warren, J. T., & Fassett, D. L. (2011). *Communication: A critical/cultural introduction*. Thousand Oaks, CA: Sage.

further reading

Adler, R. B., & Rodman, G. (2003). *Understanding human communication* (8th edn). New York: Oxford University Press.

Baker, E., Barrett, M., & Roberts, L. (2002). *Working communication*. Milton, Qld: John Wiley & Sons.

DeVito, J. A. (2001). *Human communication: The basic course* (9th edn). New York: Longman.

Griffin, E. A. (2012). *A first look at communication theory* (8th edn). Boston: McGraw-Hill Higher Education.

Perkins, P. S., & Brown, L. (2008). *The art and science of communication: Tools for effective communication in the workplace*. Hoboken, NJ: John Wiley & Sons.

Tyler, S., Kossen, C., & Ryan, C. (2002). *Communication: A foundation course* (2nd edn). Sydney: Prentice Hall Australia.

Theories of communication

Rola AJJAWI | Charlotte REES

key topics

This chapter covers the following topics:

- communication and language
- models of communication
- contextual features of communication
- recommendations for effective communication

key terms

TRANSACTIONAL MODEL OF COMMUNICATION

PARALANGUAGE

NON-VERBAL COMMUNICATION

Introduction

> We are a long way from a unified theory of communication and it seems unlikely that we will ever achieve that (Thompson, 2003, p. 20).

Communication and language are the essential ingredients through which human beings understand and transform the realities in which they live. Communication is not just about two or more people exchanging information; it is concerned with the negotiation of relationships and all the complexities inherent in those relationships, such as identity, power and culture. In this chapter, we begin by summarising two models of communication, the linear and the transactional models. We then explore in more detail important contextual influences on face-to-face communication at three different levels: the personal, the cultural and the structural. We end the chapter with an attempt to bridge the theory–practice gap by providing some brief recommendations about effective face-to-face communication within healthcare settings.

Models of communication

The most basic model of communication is the *linear model* (also referred to as the transmission view, or the Shannon–Weaver model, after the authors who first described it in 1949). This mathematical model involves a *sender* (source) formulating and sending a message to a *receiver* (destination), who interprets the message. The sender is responsible for the choice of code (that is, the form the message takes, such as the type of language) and the channel used (that is, the medium through which the message is sent, such as oral or visual channels). In this linear model, the notion of *codes* suggests that the sender 'encodes' the message and the receiver 'decodes' it, in order to make sense of it (Tyler, Kossen, & Ryan, 2002).

An important feature of this linear model is the concept of *noise*, which refers to factors that influence or disturb the message while it is being transferred along the channel from the source to the destination. There are various types of noise in healthcare communication. Noise can be physical (such as external sound or poor lighting), physiological (such as a hearing or visual impairment), psychological (individual factors such as mood and emotion), and/or semantic (e.g. differences in understanding the meaning of certain words related to previous experiences). Although the linear model may be relevant for some channels of communication, such as written communication, it is generally inadequate for describing face-to-face communication. Not only does it fail to account for the interactive nature of communication as a dialogue rather than a monologue, and to factor in the communicators' experiences, but it also suggests that messages are always encoded by the sender; whereas, in reality, we often convey messages to others that we did not wish to send (Adler & Rodman, 2003). An example would be the way in which **non-verbal communication**, such as looking away and not smiling, can communicate distance between practitioners and their clients (Ambady, Koo, Rosenthal, & Winograd, 2002).

The second model, referred to as the **transactional model of communication** (De Vito, 2001; Tyler et al., 2002; Adler & Rodman, 2003), presents a more sophisticated explanation of person-to-person communication than the linear model (see Figure 2.1, Higgs, McAllister, & Sefton, 2005). It suggests that communication is a dynamic process in which individuals receive and send

/ NON-VERBAL COMMUNICATION /

Non-verbal communication includes aspects such as eye contact, posture, facial expression, fine and gross movements, and artefacts such as clothing (Thompson, 2003).

/ TRANSACTIONAL MODEL /

The transactional model of communication suggests that communication is a dynamic process in which individuals receive and send information simultaneously.

information simultaneously. The concept of *feedback* is therefore central to this model. In contrast to the passive role in the linear model, the receiver in the transactional model plays an active role in communicating by responding to the sender's message with verbal (such as 'What do you mean?'), paralinguistic (such as laughter) and non-verbal actions (such as frowning or nodding in agreement). Such feedback communicates to the sender how the message is being received and understood.

FIGURE 2.1 | A TRANSACTIONAL MODEL OF COMMUNICATION

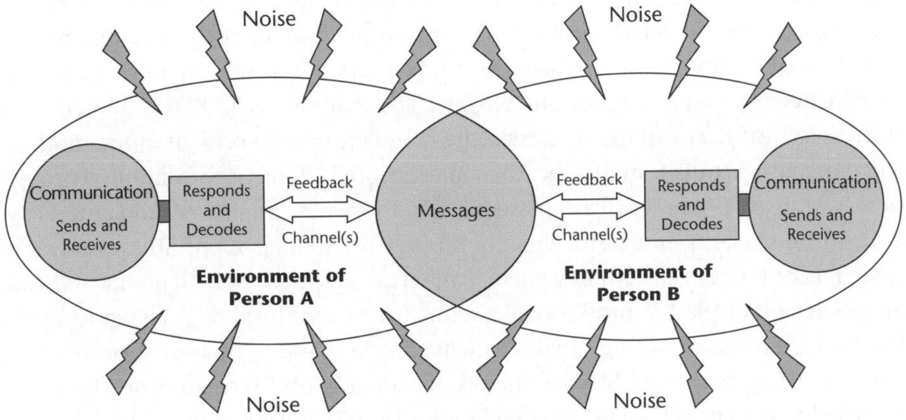

In the transactional model, communication is seen as ongoing evolving dialogue, such that understanding and interpretation are informed by previous communicative interactions. Meaning is negotiated between individuals, taking into account their respective ideas, feelings and points of view. Indeed, the experiences of both participants (their frames of reference) influence the way the message is formed and interpreted. Situational, temporal, historical and socio-cultural dimensions of context are all relevant for effective interpersonal communication. The transactional model emphasises that communication is based on dynamic and evolving processes involving relationships between participants with individual and overlapping frames of reference that are context-dependent.

Contextual influences in communication

All parties involved in a conversation share a degree of responsibility for constructing the meaning within that verbal encounter (Thompson, 2003).

As detailed earlier in this chapter, meaning emerges through social interaction. Although the relationship between meaning and context is complex, communication theorists have attempted to simplify it by focusing on three distinct but related levels: personal, cultural and structural (Thompson, 2003). In this section, we briefly discuss the roles of identity (personal), culture (cultural), and power and gender (structural) in shaping face-to-face communication in healthcare settings.

Identity

A sense of identity, that sense of who we are as healthcare students and practitioners, is fluid rather than static. Our sense of identity is created through social interaction with teachers, peers, other healthcare professionals and clients (Thompson, 2003). Health professional education is about the development of a professional identity and language, and talk plays a key role in how identity is constructed in social interaction. Lingard and colleagues (2003) explored how third year healthcare students learned the language of case presentation, and how this language acquisition shaped their professional identity formation. Through observation of 19 student case presentations to faculty members (and interviews with those students and staff), they found that the management and portrayal of uncertainty was a recurrent key theme. Whereas teachers modelled what Lingard and colleagues called a 'professional rhetoric of uncertainty' (e.g. recognising the limits of scientific knowledge, of the patient's account and of their own knowledge), students demonstrated a 'novice rhetoric of uncertainty' (centring on their own knowledge deficits). Lingard and colleagues (2003) found that by learning the language of case presentation, some students shifted from this novice rhetoric towards the professional rhetoric of uncertainty, and in doing so shaped their professional identities. Indeed, learning the language (or jargon) of their healthcare profession not only helps shape students' professional identities but also gives them access to the profession and legitimises their participation within it.

Another example of how identities are constructed and co-constructed through talk is communication in multi-professional teams, which require the construction of identities that demonstrate acceptance and trust (Monrouxe, 2010). Rees and Monrouxe (2010) found that the use of laughter within medical workplace learning settings can help to construct gendered identities.

Culture

To every communicative act we bring assumptions and rules based on our own culture. *Culture* has been defined as a 'set of shared meanings, assumptions and understandings which have developed historically in a given community' (Thompson, 2003, p. 109). It may be understood as the lens through which we interpret meaning, language and situations. We tend to view the world from the standpoint of our own culture. We are often unaware of the assumptions, values and lenses that influence our actions and communication, but talking with people who subscribe to a different set of assumptions, rules and meanings can bring our assumptions to a conscious level. Meeuwesen, Harmsen, Bernsen, and Bruijnzeels (2006) studied intercultural communication in consultations between Dutch general practitioners (GPs) and their non-Western immigrant and Dutch patients. Although the GPs spent more time trying to understand their non-Western immigrant patients, they spent more time being empathic and involved with their Dutch patients. Dutch patients were more assertive: they talked more, disagreed with their GPs more and exchanged more information than did immigrant patients. Not only was this verbal asymmetry attributable to language barriers between the Dutch GPs and their immigrant patients, it was also possibly attributable to the immigrant patients' acceptance of greater power differentials between doctors and patients (Meeuwesen et al., 2006). From an alternative perspective, this research evidence represents inequality in access to healthcare services and problematic issues of language and self-presentation rather than culture-specific health beliefs. Indeed, *culture* is a much contested concept, with some scholars arguing that each one of us constructs his or her own culture, rather than 'belonging' to a cultural group (Piller, 2007). See also Chapter 20.

Power

> Medical discourse not only reflects the power of the medical profession but actively contributes to constructing, re-enacting and thus perpetuating such power (Thompson, 2001, p. 32).

A fundamental criticism of the linear model of communication is that this 'monologue' privileges professional over lay expertise (Gravois Lee & Garvin, 2003). Indeed, health professionals communicate their power within the professional–patient relationship through their use of profession-specific jargon, which serves as a barrier to communication and underscores their expert status and the subordinate status of their patients (Gravois Lee & Garvin, 2003). Relevant here is Bourdieu's concept (1991, cited by Thompson, 2003) of *habitus*, which reflects the rules governing who can speak, and when and whether people will listen to and value what is being said. However, patients can (and do) resist this power hierarchy through their questioning, challenging and resisting of information provided to them by healthcare practitioners (Gravois Lee & Garvin, 2003; Rees & Monrouxe, 2010).

Kettunen and colleagues (2002) explored how patients reduced the power asymmetry in their interactions with nurses. Through conversational analysis of 38 nurse–patient health counselling sessions in a Finnish hospital, Kettunen and colleagues discovered that power was jointly constructed by nurses and patients within these counselling sessions. They found that patients used various strategies, including question-asking, interruption and extensive disclosure of information, to control the flow of the dialogue. The use of pronouns is another strategy that can lead to power asymmetry; for example, referring to a patient in the third person when the patient is present (such as when presenting the patient to your supervisor) can disempower and exclude the patient from the interaction (Rees & Monrouxe, 2008). Traditionally, these linguistic and paralinguistic strategies have been associated with professionals who want to emphasise their power in health professional–patient interaction. Indeed, the expertise that patients (and their caregivers) bring to the relationship should be valued, and the potential for power asymmetry to have an adverse impact on professional–patient communication should never be underestimated.

Gender

Linked to the concept of power in healthcare communication is the issue of gender. According to feminist theory, women are frequently excluded from arenas of power, and when they do have access they are often ignored (Thompson, 2003). The effects of gender on communication have been explored in various disciplines in the health sciences. Roter and colleagues (2002) conducted a meta-analytic review of 23 observational studies exploring the effect of gender on the communication of physicians at various levels of training and from numerous specialties, including general practice, paediatrics, obstetrics and gynaecology. They found that female physicians had more discussion with their patients about psychosocial issues than did male physicians. Female physicians also used more positive verbal and non-verbal communication behaviours, and actively facilitated patient participation in the medical encounter by assuming a less dominant stance. The authors concluded that female physicians engaged in more communication that could be considered patient-centred, by addressing psychosocial issues through questioning and counselling, and through their greater use of emotional and positive talk, and more active partnership-building. The gender aspect emphasises that transactional communication is influenced by socialisation to language and is therefore socially constructed in interaction. We stress, however, that communication can be improved through heightened self-awareness and education to reduce such gender differences.

Bridging the theory–practice gap: recommendations for effective communication

Communication is effective when what is intended to be said is heard and the communicants reach a shared understanding. There are a number of ways in which you can improve your face-to-face communication with others: with your teachers, peers, other healthcare professionals and clients. Although some of these recommendations may seem obvious, they can easily be taken for granted.

Our list of recommendations is not exhaustive, but those we present should help you reflect critically on different aspects of your face-to-face communication (see Handy Hint 2.1).

The key recommendation is to consider all the factors that can have an impact on communication, such as noise, context, audience, and the process and outcomes of communication. For example, practitioners can reduce semantic 'noise' (and power asymmetry) by avoiding the use of jargon and abbreviations when communicating with patients, their relatives and carers. Practitioners need to adapt their communication to suit their patients' frames of reference (language, educational background, culture, age, level of wellness and life situation). Being mindful of the different assumptions, rules and meanings that you and others might bring to communication is essential to effective communication. Also, practitioners must be mindful of patients' psychological states, including their mood and emotion, as anxiety and fear can interfere with their capacity to take in what the practitioner is saying and interpret intended messages. It is always important to tailor your message to suit the needs of others. Seeking feedback and regularly checking to see that your messages are understood as intended is valuable.

Our final recommendations for effective communication in healthcare relate to **paralanguage** and non-verbal communication.

These are features that help you better understand what a person is saying, and can also help you identify, for example, the speaker's emotions. *Non-verbal communication* is also powerful; if non-verbal messages conflict with verbal messages, we are more likely to believe the non-verbal.

An example of this would be that clothing can suggest socio-economic class, status, gender, age and subculture, such as people's interests in music (Thompson, 2003). But it is also important to avoid stereotyping patients and assuming you know their healthcare needs on the basis of visual cues. Such assumptions can lead to mismatched communication between health professionals and patients, with patients' personal needs not being met (Hordern & Street, 2007). Try to achieve open and respectful communication with patients, seeking negotiation of goals and expectations to reach a shared understanding.

/ PARALANGUAGE /
Paralanguage includes communicative aspects such as speed, tone, volume, pitch and intonation of the voice (Thompson, 2003).

IMPROVING YOUR COMMUNICATION

- Consider all the factors that affect your communication in a particular situation.
- Adapt your communication to suit your co-communicators' frames of reference.
- Be mindful of assumptions in communication, avoid stereotyping.

- Be aware of non-verbal and paralanguage aspects of communication.
- Be open, flexible and reflexive—observe a video of yourself communicating with others.
- Seek feedback from your educators, peers and patients. ●

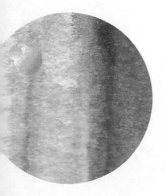

conclusion

Communication is a complex and context-dependent process. As suggested by the transactional model, it is not a simple act of information exchange, but involves the creation of meaning and relationships. Inherent in those relationships are complex issues of power, gender and culture. Your identity as a healthcare practitioner is shaped by your communication with patients, teachers, peers and other healthcare practitioners. Because communication is context-dependent, it is difficult to draw up an exhaustive list of recommendations about effective communication: what is effective in one situation might not be effective in another. The key to developing your communication skills is to be open, flexible and reflexive, not only about your communication skills but also about your relationships with others.

references

Adler, R. B., & Rodman, G. (2003). *Understanding human communication* (8th edn). New York: Oxford University Press.

Ambady, N., Koo, J., Rosenthal, R., & Winograd, C. H. (2002). Physical therapists' nonverbal communication predicts geriatric patients' health outcomes. *Psychology and Aging, 17*(3), 443–52.

De Vito, J. A. (2001). *Human communication: The basic course* (9th edn). New York: Longman.

Gravois Lee, R., & Garvin, T. (2003). Moving from information transfer to information exchange in health and health care. *Social Science and Medicine, 56*, 449–64.

Higgs, J., McAllister, L., & Sefton, A. (2005). Communicating in the health and social sciences. In J. Higgs, A. Sefton, A. Street, L. McAllister & I. Hay (Eds.), *Communicating in the health and social sciences* (pp. 3–12). Melbourne: Oxford University Press.

Hordern, A. J., & Street, A. F. (2007). Communicating about patient sexuality and intimacy after cancer: Mismatched expectations and unmet needs. *Medical Journal of Australia, 186*(5), 224–7.

Kettunen, T., Poskiparta, M., & Gerlander, M. (2002). Nurse–patient power relationship: Preliminary evidence of patients' power messages. *Patient Education and Counseling, 47,* 101–13.

Lingard, L., Garwood, K., Schryer, C. F., & Spafford, M. M. (2003). A certain art of uncertainty: Case presentation and the development of professional identity. *Social Science and Medicine, 56,* 603–16.

Meeuwesen, L., Harmsen, J. A. M., Bernsen, R. M. D., & Bruijnzeels, M. A. (2006). Do Dutch doctors communicate differently with immigrant patients than with Dutch patients? *Social Science and Medicine, 63,* 2407–17.

Monrouxe, L. V. (2010). Identity, identification and medical education: Why should we care? *Medical Education, 44,* 40–49.

Piller, I. (2007). Linguistics and intercultural communication. *Language and Linguistic Compass, 1*(3), 208–26.

Rees, C. E., & Monrouxe, L. V. (2008). 'Is it alright if I-um-we unbutton your pyjama top now?' Pronominal use in bedside teaching encounters. *Communication & Medicine, 5,* 171–82.

Rees, C. E., & Monrouxe, L. V. (2010). 'I should be lucky ha ha ha ha': The construction of power, identity and gender through laughter within medical workplace learning encounters. *Journal of Pragmatics, 42,* 3384–99.

Roter, D. L., Hall, J. A., & Aoki, Y. (2002). Physician gender effects in medical communication: A meta-analytic review, *Journal of the American Medical Association, 288*(6), 756–64.

Shannon, C., & Weaver, W. (1949). *The mathematical theory of communication.* Champaign, IL: University of Illinois Press.

Thompson, N. (2001). *Anti-discriminatory practice* (3rd edn). Basingstoke: Palgrave Macmillan.

Thompson, N. (2003). *Communication and language: A handbook of theory and practice.* Basingstoke: Palgrave Macmillan.

Tyler, S., Kossen, C., & Ryan, C. (2002). *Communication: A foundation course* (2nd edn). Sydney: Prentice Hall.

Communication and duty of care

Franziska **TREDE** | Elizabeth **ELLIS** | Sue **JONES**

key topics

This chapter covers the following topics:

- duty of care

- obligations to inform

- effective communication

- valid consent

key terms

DUTY OF CARE

Introduction

In this chapter we discuss duty of care and good communication practices from an ethical and legal perspective, to highlight our obligation to inform clients of the risks and benefits associated with our interventions. Clients may be individuals, groups, families, organisations or communities and, consequently, the type and style of communication needs to be adapted to meet client needs. Responding to clients' questions and non-verbal cues, and checking they have understood what you have said are good communication practices that help increase client safety, prevent adverse events, and reduce the risk of negligence claims or complaints.

Duty of care

Duty of care is a professional's responsibility to take reasonable care and ensure no harm is done to patients and clients. Practitioners have ethical and legal obligations to adhere to a reasonable standard of care for people who come for services or interventions. One of the most fundamental ethical principles is 'first, do no harm' (Kerridge et al., 2005). Failure to adhere to a reasonable standard of care may result in an adverse event leading to a complaint or a negligence case. It has been claimed that communication is the main factor determining whether an event will result in a complaint or court case (Tito Report, 1995).

Professionals are considered to be legally negligent if *injury* occurs to a person to whom they owe a *duty of care*, and if that injury arises *as a result* of a *breach of professional standards*.

> You must take reasonable care to avoid acts or omissions which you can reasonably foresee would be likely to injure … persons who are so closely and directly affected by my act that I ought reasonably to have them in contemplation (*Donoghue v Stevenson* [1932] AC 562).

Usually, it is not difficult to determine to whom we have a duty of care, because of the direct and close interaction in most therapist–client relationships. However, it is more ambiguous if, for example, someone is referred to a practitioner for care; the person waits in the waiting room for so long that he or she cannot wait any longer, and the symptoms become exacerbated as a result of the practitioner's failure to attend or at least keep the person informed. Sometimes health practitioners are employed to manage all relevant clients within a unit or facility. This can complicate duty of care, as some clients may not come to the attention of the practitioner and may then experience an adverse outcome. Frequent causes of breaches of care are listed in Handy Hint 3.1.

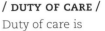

/ DUTY OF CARE /
Duty of care is a professional's responsibility to take reasonable care and ensure no harm is done to patients and clients.

BREACHES OF CARE

Types of breaches of standards of care which might come about by failure to communicate effectively include:

- inadequate or poor advice on self-management
- failure to prevent preventable complications
- failure to disclose risks of intervention
- failure to obtain valid consent to intervention
- failure to maintain client confidentiality
- failure to communicate with other relevant professionals to provide a reasonable standard of client care
- failure to warn authorities when in the public interest.

irrational or ill-considered (Wallace, 1995). The moral purpose behind this principle is the protection of human dignity and respect for the individual's autonomy, both of which are fundamental ethical principles for healthcare practice.

To deliver healthcare services without valid consent can be considered assault. In many instances, consent is implied and not in writing. There must, however, be a clear agreement between the practitioner and the client about the nature of action. A client may put out her arm for a routine pulse or blood pressure measurement, but she is not necessarily agreeing by that action to having blood taken. If there is any danger of misunderstanding, the practitioner should make the intention explicit.

Practitioners cannot assume that, merely because clients have turned up for some intervention, they consent to anything. Sometimes practitioners assume that clients consent to an intervention until they refuse a procedure. It is probably more appropriate to assume that a person does not want an intervention unless it is specifically agreed to.

The criteria for valid consent include: that consent should be voluntary, that it should be informed, and that the person giving the consent should be competent to give it (Kerridge et al., 2005). Voluntary consent implies that consent has not been given under duress or on the basis of misinformation. Consent is considered valid only if clients have been informed of the nature of the procedure to which they are agreeing. It has been held that this information needs to be a broad description of the procedure; however, it must be sufficiently specific for there to be no doubt as to the nature of the procedure. For example, it is not good enough to have consented to having spinal mobilisation and then receive cervical manipulation. In this example there is a fundamental difference between the intervention that is given (and the associated risks) and that consented to.

An important point to consider is that, although a client may have given consent for a procedure, they may also withdraw that consent at any time during the procedure. The less comfortable a client feels about a procedure, the greater the likelihood of withdrawing consent, and therefore the greater need to ensure that informed consent is obtained.

Open disclosure

Worldwide, there are standards for disclosure. For example, the National Standard for Disclosure in Australia (Australian Commission for Safety and Quality in Health Care, 2008) provides a set of principles for open disclosure and considers the needs of consumers, healthcare professionals, managers and organisations. The key principles include that information be communicated in an open and timely way, with acknowledgment of any adverse incidents to the consumer and the family/carers, and with an expression of regret for any harm which might have been caused. An expression of regret need only address your regret that the incident occurred and need not necessarily be an admission of liability. The principles also indicate that practitioners should recognise the reasonable expectations of the client for supportive or corrective action. There is an onus on healthcare organisations to create an environment where staff can recognise and report adverse events and be supported through an open disclosure process. Confidentiality should be offered if required by the situation.

Failure to maintain client confidentiality

It is worldwide ethical practice to maintain confidentiality. In Australia, for example, practitioners must not divulge any information about their clients without their permission, unless required to by law (*Privacy Act 1998* (Cwlth)). Practitioners should continue to respect client privacy, even within multidisciplinary teams when exchanging client information that might be in the client's best interest. If the general public cannot trust health practitioners to respect their right to confidentiality, they might not come for treatment or might avoid disclosing sensitive information that could be important, and this is not in anyone's interest.

Reporting to authorities

In some special circumstances, clients can reveal something about themselves within a consultation that a practitioner feels strongly would be in the public interest to report. Under these circumstances, the practitioner must weigh up which is greater in the particular circumstances: the public interest served by confidentiality or the public interest to report. Under most circumstances, reporting should be confined to the appropriate authority only, observing the minimal requirements for disclosure. A client may reveal, for example, that she is continuing to drive even though she is subject to blackouts. In this example, most people would judge that there is a need to report. The appropriate authority here would usually be the government authority responsible for road safety.

Alternatively, there may be information which is not revealed by the client, but which health professionals suspect during the course of their intervention, and which should be reported to the relevant government authority, as illustrated in the case study below.

CASE STUDY 3.2
CHILD ABUSE

A mother who has recently separated brings her 4-year-old child, who has moderate physical and intellectual disabilities, for outpatient services twice weekly. Over a period of time, the occupational therapist notices that the child is becoming more withdrawn and has now become faecally incontinent. During recent sessions the therapist observed that the child had bruising on her arms and legs. The therapist did not raise this with the mother or any of her colleagues, who were also providing services for the child. Mandatory reporting to the relevant authority is required by some professionals where there is reasonable suspicion of abuse or harm, and is most often associated with people who are vulnerable; for example, children, the elderly or those with severe disabilities. Mandatory reporting legislation overrides any professional code of conduct or ethical guidelines that may apply to your particular profession (Australian Institute of Family Studies, 2009).

Getting the message across verbally

Providing clients with opportunities to ask questions or to reframe their understanding of the situation helps practitioners to appreciate what clients have understood. Asking clients to tell you if you have communicated clearly to ensure safety and consent reduces misunderstandings. Providing additional written information, especially when instructions are complex, is a useful way to enhance understanding. Such a reciprocal approach to communication builds rapport, and also enables clients to say honestly what they feel and think. Make sure that clients are not interrupted, and give them time—even if you do not have much time available. This can save you trouble in the longer term, ensure better quality care, and help avoid complaints of negligence. Handy Hint 3.2 is a checklist of effective communication skills that enhance mutual understanding.

COMMUNICATION SKILLS THAT ENHANCE MUTUAL UNDERSTANDING

- Make sure you know what your clients' biggest concerns are.
- Keep clients informed at all times during your consultation.
- Tell clients what they can expect, in terms of physical reactions, pain and other effects, because of an intervention.
- Give clients your full attention.
- Do not interrupt.
- Respect clients' privacy and honour their dignity.
- Adapt your communication style in recognition of different cultural requirements, to create a safe environment.
- If the client does not speak English well, use a registered interpreter.

- Involve clients in decision-making.
- Follow up with clients who are angry or in distress.
- Allow time for information to be absorbed.
- Enhance communication by providing written information sheets.
- Ensure explanations are in plain English.
- Check with clients what they have understood.

An important and often neglected aspect of communication is *non-verbal communication*. Check your eye contact and physical distance to others, and observe clients' body language. Do not assume clients' consent from their body language alone, but check your assumptions and interpretations of their body language with them. Another related aspect of communication is silence. When we are busy and feel rushed it can be difficult to allow time for silences. However, silences say a lot, and they allow time for absorbing what has been said and digesting what is happening. Further, sensitive communicators engage in dialogues, not monologues, and they start communication by accepting and respecting perspectives other than their own, and establishing clients' expectations. They negotiate treatment or intervention plans without coercion. They are aware that clients have diverse expectations: some want to be told what to do, prefer explanations, and are happy to grant the health professional expert status; some want lots of information from multiple sources and prefer to be actively involved in the decision-making process; some seek specific answers to specific questions; others like to express their concerns and want you to listen to them.

Clients who are not proficient in English have a right to an interpreter. If a client requests an interpreter it is your legal requirement to organise one (see also Chapter 20).

Recording communication

As a general rule of thumb, the greater the risk of injury or invasiveness of a procedure, the more important it is to have a formal means of establishing consent and to have that consent documented.

When courts weigh the value of a client's recollection versus a practitioner's recollection of what was said, the courts tend to give the client the benefit of the doubt (Kerridge et al., 2005). This is based on the principle that for the client it was a relatively isolated incident, therefore more likely to have significance and stand out more strongly in memory. The practitioner is held to have had many such interactions in one day, and the details of each one are less likely to be clearly remembered. The courts will therefore seek evidence that the practitioner actually did seek consent, such as a notation in records, or better, that there is a consent form signed and witnessed.

CONSENT FORMS

Consent forms must:

- specify the procedure, not use a blanket phrase (such as 'manual techniques' if you mean *manipulation*)
- include the name and full identity of the client and practitioner
- avoid ambiguous expressions such as 'informed of risks'
- include the date and time of consent noted
- be written in lay language.

Written client records

There is a well-established understanding in medico-legal circles:

- If there are poor records, there is poor defence.
- If there are good records, there is a good defence.

It is recommended that when practitioners obtain informed consent they record that information was given, consent was obtained, and that the client had an opportunity for questions to be answered. The best defence is written consent from the client.

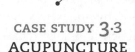

CASE STUDY **3·3**
ACUPUNCTURE

Consent was given for acupuncture to be applied to the shoulder and neck, but the practitioner moved the needling to the thoracic area. The client experienced a pneumothorax, and claimed that he had not consented to a thoracic treatment, and would not have given consent if he had known that there was any risk of a pneumothorax. There was no consent recorded after the first treatment to the shoulder.

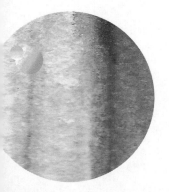

conclusion

In this chapter we have discussed the importance of communication and our duty of care. Social and health professionals have the best interests of their clients at the forefront of their decision-making, and most practitioners are devastated when a client experiences an adverse outcome. Good communication skills and diligence ensure that professionals do not make decisions based on erroneous assumptions, and that their efforts to communicate have been effective. The result should benefit both clients and professionals.

references

Australian Commission for Safety and Quality in Health Care. (2008). *Open disclosure standard: A national standard for open communication in public and private hospitals, following an adverse event in health care*. Retrieved from www.safetyandquality.gov.au/internet/safety/publishing.nsf/Content/compub-OD-Standard-2008

Australian Institute for Family Studies. (2009). Mandatory reporting of child abuse and neglect. Retrieved from www.secasa.com.au/infosheet/aifs_rs3.pdf

Bolam v Frien Hospital Management Committee [1957] 1 WLR 582.

Commonwealth of Australia. *Privacy Act 1988*, Information Privacy Principles.

Donoghue v Stevenson [1932] AC 562.

Kerridge, I., Lowe, M., & McPhee, J. (2005). *Ethics and law for the health professions* (2nd edn). Annandale, NSW: Federation Press.

Kirby, M. (1995). Patients' rights: Why the Australian courts have rejected 'Bolam', *Journal of Medical Ethics, 21*(1), 5–8.

NSW Health. (2005). *Consent to medical treatment: Patient information*, PD2005_406, retrieved from www.health.nsw.gov.au/policies/PD/2005/PD2005_406.html

Rogers v Whitaker [1992] 175 CLR 479.

(*Tito Report*) Commonwealth Department of Human Services and Health. (1995). *Compensation and professional indemnity in health care: Final report*. Canberra: AGPS.

Wallace, M. (1995). *Health care and the law* (2nd edn). Sydney: The Law Book Company.

useful web resources

For a comprehensive outline of the legal aspects of duty of care, see www.chp.org.au/homepages_accr/items/174538-upload-00001.pdf

Academic integrity and honesty

Ann **SEFTON** | Iain **HAY** | Wendy **BOWLES**

key topics

This chapter covers the following topics:

- understanding academic honesty
- practising academic integrity
- understanding ethical communication

key terms

ACADEMIC HONESTY

ACADEMIC INTEGRITY

COPYRIGHT

ETHICAL RESEARCH

HONESTY

INTELLECTUAL PROPERTY

Academic honesty and integrity

This chapter introduces **academic honesty** and **academic integrity** and explains why they are important at university and in professional practice settings. Behaving ethically is at the heart of professionalism. Learning to become a professional is a foundation for all university courses and professional practices in the health sciences.

Academic honesty, integrity and ethical communication are related but different concepts. The term *academic integrity* encompasses academic honesty, ethical communication and other values. It is one of the core qualities required for good scholarship. This term is increasingly used in Australia, Europe and North America.

'Explaining academic integrity [is] ... harder than it looks', according to Stephen Matchett (2012), reporting on a large national study of Australian university students and integrity policies by Tracey Bretag et al. (2011). Matchett (2012) reported that only two-thirds of 15,000 university students surveyed in Australia were confident that they understood what the term academic integrity meant. If you want to be proud of your work as a student and, later, as a professional, you need to be in the group that understands this term.

Honesty is about being truthful (a positive element) and not being deceitful; for example, by telling lies or omitting relevant information (negative elements). An example of how both these elements come together in the concept of honesty is the pledge used in various forms in courts in Western justice systems: 'I swear to tell the truth, the whole truth and nothing but the truth'. Some universities require students to sign honour pledges as part of examination procedures, citing research that finds that signing such pledges reduces the incidence of academic cheating (see e.g. Colorado State University, 2010).

According to the *Macquarie Dictionary* (Macquarie Library, 1985, p. 838), honesty involves 'uprightness, probity or integrity', being truthful, sincere or frank and being free 'from deceit or fraud'. Thus, honesty and integrity are closely related. You need to develop courage and insight into your own behaviour if you are to learn to act honestly.

There are five values to which you must be committed in order to practise academic integrity. These are: honesty, trust, fairness, respect and responsibility (Bretag et al., 2011; Center for Academic Integrity, 2010). Of these, academic honesty is central, as illustrated in the definition adopted by Bretag et al. (2011, p. 49) in their wide-ranging study of academic integrity in Australian universities. This national project preferred the University of Tasmania's (2010) broad definition of academic integrity, which also highlights the importance of honesty:

> Academic integrity is about mastering the art of scholarship. Scholarship involves researching, understanding and building upon the work of others and requires that you give credit where

/ ACADEMIC INTEGRITY AND HONESTY /
The term academic integrity encompasses academic honesty, ethical communication and other values. It is one of the core qualities required for good scholarship.

/ HONESTY /
Honesty is about being truthful (a positive element) and not being deceitful by for example, telling lies or omitting relevant information (negative elements).

it is due and acknowledge the contributions of others to your own intellectual efforts. At its core, academic integrity requires honesty. This involves being responsible for ethical scholarship and for knowing what academic dishonesty is and how to avoid it.

Academic dishonesty

Several commentators mention that it is easier to define what academic integrity and honesty are not, rather than what they are (see e.g. Bretag et al., 2011; Staats, Hupp, & Hagley, 2008). Plagiarism is the most common form of academic dishonesty. According to Schofield and Ajjawi in Chapter 17, *Avoiding Plagiarism*, of this book, 'there are two parts to plagiarism: theft (of a thought or words) and fraud (presenting them as our own)'. Because plagiarism is so important, it has its own chapter in this book (Chapter 17). So, we will not discuss it here, other than to emphasise that it is critical to understand what the term means and how to avoid being accused of plagiarism. Remember that ignorance is no excuse. Read carefully Chapter 17, *Avoiding Plagiarism*.

Besides plagiarism, there are many other forms of academic dishonesty. Bretag et al. (2011, p. 49) list some of these as:

> cheating in exams or assignments, collusion, theft of other students' work, paying a third party for assignments, downloading whole or part of assignments from the Internet, falsification of data, misrepresentation of records, fraudulent publishing practices or any other action that undermines the integrity of scholarship and research.

Behaving with academic honesty and integrity has to be learned; it is not something that people have or do not have. Sometimes students do not realise they are behaving dishonestly (again, see also Chapter 17). It takes courage to resist the pressure to cheat, especially when work, family or other pressures start to compete with the time you set aside for study. In recognising the increasing pressures to cheat, along with the accessibility of the internet, with its various resources for dishonest practice, Staats et al. (2008) describe students who stand up to those pressures and behave with integrity as 'everyday heroes'.

Everyday heroes are the students who resist academic dishonesty. Staats et al. (2008) described how dishonest students can 'neutralise' feelings of guilt with excuses that minimise the seriousness of academic dishonesty. These excuses can include denying responsibility (blaming someone else), denying the harm caused to others and to the system by the dishonesty, denying that there are victims (people who suffer from the cheating, either because their work was copied, or because the dishonesty of others disadvantaged the honest people), and condemning authorities as unjust (Staats et al., 2008, p. 358). Please refer to Handy Hint 4.1. The rest of this chapter looks at some of the key areas in university life in which issues of academic integrity and honesty can arise.

HOW TO BE AN 'EVERYDAY HERO'

- Search your university's website using the terms academic integrity and academic honesty.
- Download any guides or policies about academic honesty and integrity.
- Make sure you understand what is expected of you and how to demonstrate academic honesty and integrity.
- Remember: ignorance is no excuse—take responsibility for your behaviour.
- If you are uncertain, seek advice or help.
- Watch out for 'neutralisation' tendencies in yourself and your colleagues.

Key areas of academic integrity and honesty

Intellectual property

An important aspect of academic honesty relates to **intellectual property**, which is the 'research, words and ideas generated by an author' (see Baker, Barrett, & Roberts, 2002, p. 164). When a member of staff, a student or a team makes an original discovery or offers a reinterpretation of ideas, it becomes the intellectual property of that individual or team. It is their right to publish the discovery or, through the university, to pursue the possibility of developing it and/or selling the rights, or patenting it. For further information, see the Australian Government Intellectual Property website (listed in the 'further reading and useful websites' section at the end of this chapter).

/ INTELLECTUAL PROPERTY /
Intellectual property is the 'research, words and ideas generated by an author'.

Copyright

When an author's work is published, it becomes subject to **copyright**, which means it may not be reproduced except with the author's permission. You can also copyright your own original unpublished work by adding your name and the copyright symbol © after the title. It is generally accepted that you may photocopy a journal paper, a key diagram or small sections from a book for your own study.

/ COPYRIGHT /
Copyright means something may not be reproduced except with the author's permission.

Copying large sections or several chapters, however, breaches copyright. If you want to include a published diagram or illustration in an essay or paper, you must acknowledge the source. Some universities expect you to redraw the material yourself. You need to check the precise requirements of your institution.

Ethical research work

/ **ETHICAL RESEARCH** /
Integrity and the five values it encompasses are central features of ethical research. For research to be ethical there are also related principles, including respecting the privacy and confidentiality of participants and others involved, which researchers must follow.

In many programs you are encouraged to participate in research. Integrity and the five values it encompasses are central features of **ethical research**. For research to be ethical there are also related principles, including respecting the privacy and confidentiality of participants and others involved, which researchers must follow. There are specific guidelines for research with Indigenous communities. See 'Further reading and useful websites' at the end of this chapter for more information on how to communicate ethically when undertaking research.

Research findings are ethical when the data is accurate, critically analysed and honestly reported. Conclusions must be carefully drawn on the basis of rigorous, trustworthy analysis and interpretation. Rigorous standards of honesty are expected, regardless of the duration of the research and the research mode (e.g. whether it is based on reviewing texts or web-based material, or conducting laboratory, practice or community work). All universities have detailed processes you must complete to ensure your research is ethical.

Ethical group work

There are considerable benefits from learning cooperatively in academic and practice teams and groups. In general, the most effective learning in groups comes when all members participate actively and complete required tasks. For a group project, it is important that the group determines roles and responsibilities from the outset, but be prepared to be flexible. Honesty in group interactions is essential. You must be prepared to both offer and accept help, but never take advantage of other members. It is clearly unfair to the rest of the group if someone fails to turn up and contribute, or does not complete agreed tasks on time. If the group is not working well, confront the problems collectively and resolve them before the situation deteriorates.

Particular difficulties can arise in collaborative work when the group is assessed collectively and given a single mark or grade. Group members who do not participate or contribute equitably are unfairly or dishonestly taking advantage of their colleagues. The group needs to discuss the issue openly. If lack of participation is a result of personal or health-related difficulties, fellow students are usually tolerant and willing to help. If it represents an unwillingness or inability to cooperate, the group needs to confront the issue. If it persists, the problem may need to be discussed with staff. We provide some handy hints for ethical group work.

ETHICAL GROUP WORK

Group project

Imagine that groups of five students are required to prepare and present a poster on an aspect of smoking and community health in 6 weeks. The following guidelines will help the groups achieve these goals collaboratively and fairly.

Assessment

- Check that everyone in the group is clear about the assessment expectations.
- Are students being assessed as a group or individually?
- Work out what this means for the expected contributions of each member.

Brainstorming (immediately)

- What knowledge and skills do we have (such as access to specific information, skills in IT, data analysis and design)?
- What is the most interesting aspect of the subject to research and present?
- Agree on a broad direction, an outline and a method of presentation.
- Divide responsibilities, focusing first on gathering information and data.
- Set a realistic timetable for individual preparation and meetings.
- Agree on the expected contributions of each member—keep a written record of your agreement.
- Decide in advance how the group will deal with conflict and what the group will do if any members do not keep to the agreement about their contribution. Include this in your written agreement.

Ongoing meetings

- Review the data elements as they are contributed.
- Modify the tasks in the light of experience.
- Agree on a broad framework and design after data is collected.
- Settle on a 'message', layout and means of preparation.
- Assemble the elements and finalise them well before the deadline.
- Review the group's progress, including how it has handled any difficulties.

Many students find it helpful to learn in an informal, self-selected group. It is important, however, to establish what is legitimate cooperation for tasks that will be individually assessed. As you prepare an assignment, it is time-efficient

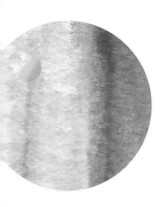

conclusion

Communicating ethically is a prerequisite for academic honesty and integrity. Ethical communication and academic honesty are dealt with in many chapters in this book. For instance, each chapter in Part 1 has something to say about ethical communication. As you read the book, keep an eye out for discussions relating to academic honesty, integrity and ethical communication. Clearly, these ideas are central for teaching you to be a genuine professional.

All professions within the fields of health sciences demand consistently honest and ethical behaviour from practitioners. It is important to develop, demonstrate and refine the high standards required of you as a student in practice situations. You should make sure that you understand the expectations that your university and future profession hold regarding honesty, integrity and legitimate collaboration, but you must also be aware that *you* are ultimately responsible for your ethical behaviour.

references

Baker, E., Barrett, M., & Roberts, L. (2002). *Working communication*. Milton, Qld: John Wiley & Sons.

Bretag, T., Mahmud, S., East, J., Green, M., James, C., McGowan, U., et al. (2011). Academic integrity standards: A preliminary analysis of the academic integrity policies at Australian universities. In Australian Universities Quality Agency (AUQA) *Proceedings of AuQF2011 Demonstrating Quality*, AUQA Occasional Publications no. 24, Melbourne: Australian Universities Quality Agency, pp. 48–53. Available: http://www.auqa.edu.au/files/publications/auqf_proceedings_2011.pdf

Center for Academic Integrity. (2010). *Fundamental values project*. Available: http://www.academicintegrity.org/fundamental_values_project/index.php

Colorado State University (2010). *Does using an honor pledge make a difference?* Available: http://tilt.colostate.edu/integrity/honorpledge/doesUsing.cfm

Matchett, S. (2012, February 13). Explaining academic integrity: It's harder than it looks. *The Australian*, retrieved from: http://www.theaustralian.com.au/higher-education/explaining-academic-integrity-its-harder-than-it-looks/story-e6frgcjx-1226268119986

Macquarie Library. (1985). *The Macquarie dictionary* (rev. edn). New South Wales: Macquarie Library.

Staats, S., Hupp, J. M., & Hagley, A. M. (2008). Honesty and heroes: A positive psychology view of heroism and academic honesty. *Journal of Psychology*, *142*(4), 357–72.

University of Tasmania. (2010). *Academic integrity*. Available: http://www.academicintegrity.utas.edu.au/

further reading and useful web resources

Search your university or educational institution's website for guides and instructions about academic integrity and academic honesty (see Handy Hint 4.1).

For guidance on ethical research visit the Australian National Health and Medical Research Council's (NHMRC) website: http://www.nhmrc.gov.au/

For guidelines on research with Indigenous peoples see:

Australian Government, National Medical Health and Research Council. (2006). *Keeping research on track, a guide for Aboriginal and Torres Strait Islander peoples about health research ethics*, Australian Government, http://www.nhmrc. gov.au/_files_nhmrc/publications/attachments/e65.pdf

Australian Government Intellectual Property website: IPAustralia: http://www. ipaustralia.gov.au/

Learning to
communicate

Getting organised for effective study

Tony M^cKENZIE | Rebecca ACHESON | Iain HAY | Ann SEFTON

key topics

This chapter covers the following topics:

- preparing for study
- finding time for study
- getting even more organised
- getting involved

key terms

TIME BUDGET

TASK MANAGEMENT

WORK–LIFE BALANCE

Introduction

Constantly plugged in and on the go, jumping from one task to another with punctuated attention, simultaneously navigating streams of data, we're cultivating a split-focus culture of distraction and detachment, intellectual fragmentation and sensory overload. Addicted to instant-click access, we expect knowledge to come in quick fixes and easily digestible info-bits, trading depth and nuance for bullet points and sound bites … and swapping sustained thought and close attention for the shallow skimming and skipping encouraged by our online reading habits (Herschbach, 2009).

You may not see yourself in Herschbach's word picture, but to some extent, some of your classmates may identify with that world. Such is the cultural shift we witness around us. Such is the context in which we ask you to seriously consider how you will learn to study effectively.

Effective study skills are a foundation for learning success. In this chapter we set out some vital elements of successful study. Key concerns in plannng your study include working to achieve a work–life balance, learning to budget your time and developing skills in time management. Many of the ideas outlined in this chapter, particularly those to do with effective time management, will serve you well in study and in the workplace. Probably the most important key to successful study at university is careful time and **task management**. Another key is finding somewhere suitable to study.

/ **TASK MANAGEMENT** /
Understanding the job, planning what to do, getting it done, evaluating the outcome, then asking 'what now?'.

Preparing for study

Enjoying a positive and productive headspace is an important element of successful study. Your mood can affect the way that you study and the value of your learning. To establish good study practices and routines, it is important to find an appropriate place to study that minimises distractions and ensures that the time you spend studying is productive and leads to good retention of knowledge.

Creating a space for study

Look for a place that is pleasant, quiet and well-lit, a place where you will be able to work relatively undisturbed. If you can, avoid working on the dining-room table or in front of the television. Try to make your study space (such as an office or part of your bedroom) somewhere dedicated to that task, because it helps if you are able to get up and walk away from your study for periods of rest and relaxation. If you can't find an appropriate place at home you might be able to use a desk or carrel in the university library or your local library, where you can work comfortably without being interrupted.

Also, consider any specific equipment you may need to ensure that you can complete all your study activities and eliminate barriers to effective study. Many subjects and courses have online elements that you will need to incorporate into your study routine and take into consideration when choosing your study space. To allow for full participation in online activities, you need to incorporate a computer and internet access into your study place. Not being able to use a computer to complete online aspects of your study will cause you to skip elements or put things off. When you come back to the task later you may have lost your train of thought.

Minimising distractions

We began this chapter with Herschbach's picture of today's switched-on world. You may find that having computers and access to the internet in your study place can lead to distractions and unproductive behaviour. Make sure that you are using your study time effectively, not straying onto social media websites or playing games. An effective way to ensure that you are not tempted to procrastinate is to lock your internet browser from visiting certain sites by downloading an extension for the internet browser Google Chrome. This application allows you to set the time you can spend on certain sites; after that set time, the site will time out. This is a useful way to manage misuse of the internet during study time.

TAKE CONTROL OF YOUR STUDY TIME

Another common distraction during study can be mobile phones. Try to make sure that you leave your phone outside of the study area. It may even be worthwhile to set it to silent. Make the commitment to your study; inform friends, family and others who contact you regularly that you are not available during these times. Minimising distractions is just as important as finding an appropriate place to study.

Having a pleasant and productive place for study, with all the equipment you need, is a very important part of a successful study routine. It is also important to assess potential distractions and to take steps to remove them or minimise their impact.

Finding time for study

Task assessment

At the beginning of each semester, teaching staff should provide you with a fairly clear indication of all class times, clinical placements and assessment requirements. This will include such details as due dates and assignment values. Plot all the placements and assignment due dates on a calendar or year planner. You will probably find pile-ups of assignments due just before and after the mid-semester break, and shortly before exams begin at the end of the semester. To avoid the stresses of trying to complete all these assignments at the same time, you need to plan your work.

Look at your calendar of due dates and consider the work required to complete each piece of assessment. How much time do you think you need to finish each assignment? Be realistic. For instance, a good 2000-word essay is more likely to take two weeks to write than two days. Think about the time you will need to find relevant references, gather material, read and take notes, and write, type and edit. You might then consider doubling the amount of time you expect a task will take, to get a more accurate assessment of how long it really will take! Make sure you keep a back-up copy of your work to avoid wasting time rewriting if your computer crashes.

You have now completed the first part of a successful time-management plan. You know what tasks you have and, roughly, how long they will take. The next part of the plan is to work out how much time you actually have to work on projects and exactly when you will work on them.

Budgeting your time

To know how much time you have and when you can complete tasks, try drawing up a timetable, broken into one-hour intervals. Start by adding your regular commitments, such as a part-time job or sporting activities. Then add your lecture, clinical and other class times, to generate a time-management template for your week. You can now use this as the basis for planning study and other activities for each day or week of the semester.

Consider creating your time-management template in software such as Microsoft Excel™. This has the advantage of allowing you to use search functions to find specific events within your semester's timetable. Or use timetabling software such as Microsoft Outlook™. Google Calendar™ is a great web tool and a good way to ensure you have access to your schedule at all times. There are a number of online calendars and mobile applications (apps) that are useful and easy to use. The trick is to find a scheduling program that works for you; one that you want to use and refer to regularly. Having a time-management planner that is easy to access will encourage you to use it regularly to organise yourself.

If you make your study time regular and constant throughout the semester, you will go a long way toward avoiding the need for panic-stricken cramming at exam time and less-than-useful 2 a.m. essay-writing sessions the night before each paper is due. Note that a part-time student would spend proportionately less time studying. A half-time student might spend about 20 hours each week at lectures, reading and attending practical classes.

ALLOW FOR THE UNEXPECTED

Leave a little extra time each week to cope with unplanned events. A friend from overseas might arrive unexpectedly, or your housemate might have a family emergency to deal with. Allow for the unforeseen by building spare time into your diary. If you overfill your timetable you are likely to become frustrated because you can't complete things.

/ **WORK–LIFE BALANCE** /
Taking care of yourself
by seeking to balance
the important parts of
your day.

/ **TIME BUDGET** /
Your estimate of time
to be allocated to your
various study tasks. The
way you apportion your
total study time for
optimal results.

Now that you have worked out your timetable, do you actually have enough time for study, work and leisure, sometimes called the **work–life balance**? This chapter is about helping you to use your study time effectively, but if you don't live a balanced life—if you don't sleep properly or have a personal life—your study-time productivity will probably be affected. If you have concerns, you might need to reconsider your **time budget**, amend your enrolment, or seek advice from a study counsellor.

Sticking to your timetable

The final and critical part of successful time management is sticking to the timetable you have so carefully created. Tasks tend to expand to fill the time available so, where possible, give yourself a realistic agenda for study periods, then be sure to use allocated times for allocated tasks. If you find that your work isn't good enough, try to maintain a positive attitude, take a break, and look forward to things falling in place in your next session.

Time management of the sort set out here may *seem* regimented and restrictive, but it allows you to exercise control over your work and study, rather than have it control you. A firm timetable can actually make you feel freer because you know when you are relaxing that you have the right to do so. You will also feel a sense of achievement for having your work and study under control. In later employment, you will find that good time-management skills developed during study will stand you in good stead.

Getting even more organised

The third key to successful study is organisation. If you have good time-management and task-management skills, you have gone a long way down this path. To capitalise on your skills in these areas, it is useful to be organised in other ways.

In your studies, you will be trying to digest and organise texts from a range of sources. You will want to be able to locate particular ideas in your expanding collection of data. You need a logical way of organising your data and an efficient way of managing the publication details of these texts. It is possible to use reference-management software to integrate your expanding referencing information with the texts themselves. Software such as EndNote™, ProCite™, or Microsoft Word's built-in citation tool allows you to record bibliographic and other details of material you have read, and also produce correctly formatted reference lists for essays and other written reports. Some of these products also allow you to embed a link within a publication record to your locally stored electronic copy of that item. *Wikipedia's* entry on reference-management software lists the various products available, or you could check whether your institution will provide you with a copy—see also Chapter 9.

SAFEGUARDING YOUR NOTES AND FILES

Whenever you can, avoid carrying an entire semester's notes with you or leaving them in your car. Every year, lecturers meet with distraught students whose notes—and often the cars containing their notes—have been stolen. Likewise, always back up your electronic files, perhaps keeping a copy of materials on a memory stick, but never use memory sticks to store the only copy, the master copy, of your work! ●

Getting involved

The final important study skill is simply *getting involved in learning*. You need to actively engage in your studies to gain the most out of them. You can do this in a variety of ways.

First, if you have a choice of subjects, study things you are interested in, not necessarily those things your friends and relatives say you should enrol in. Your teachers will offer advice on appropriate options.

Second, when you are in class, listen to understand. If there is something you don't follow, ask! It can sometimes be a little intimidating to put your hand up in a large lecture class, but take comfort in knowing that if you don't understand something, there is a strong chance others do not either. If you are too shy to speak out in class, see the lecturer afterwards or send an email. Most lecturers and tutors will be willing to help.

Third, when you are reading books and articles, be sure you are reading to comprehend. It is often helpful to write two or three sentences summarising the key points of an article or book. When you challenge your mind to encapsulate the message of a large work you will know whether you have understood it. Try sharing your summary with someone else, or discussing it with your lecturer or tutor to confirm your interpretation. The summaries you produce can be useful additions to the notes you make about books and articles in reference-management software.

Finally, consider working in an informal study group. Many students find that their learning is enhanced through discussion. 'Engaged learners … are able to see themselves and ideas as others see them, can articulate their ideas to others, have empathy for others, and are fair-minded in dealing with contradictory or conflicting views' (Jones et al., 1994). But do take care to ensure that study group times are focused on learning and not on distractions.

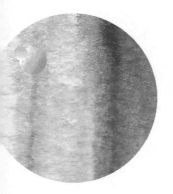

conclusion

Intelligence, good communication skills and innate flair for a subject are certainly helpful for success at university study, but good study skills are absolutely vital. If you want to do well at university, and do so with relatively little anguish, it is critical to develop time-management skills, get organised, and get involved in your learning. You can also take heart in knowing that many of the time and organisational skills you practise and refine at university will be useful for any professional role.

references

Herschbach, E. (2009). Review of *Distracted: The erosion of attention and the coming dark age* by Maggie Jackson. Metapsychology Online Reviews, *13*(2). Retrieved from http://metapsychology.mentalhelp.net/poc/view_doc.php?type=book&id=4658&cn=159

Jones, B. F., Valdez, G., Nowakowski, J. & Rasmussen, C. (1994). *Designing learning and technology for educational reform*, North Central Regional Educational Laboratory. Extract on engaged learning retrieved from http://www.ncrel.org/sdrs/areas/issues/content/cntareas/math/ma2lindi.htm

further reading

Burns, T. & Sinfield, S. (2003). *Essential study skills: The complete guide to success at university.* London: Sage.

Hay, I., Bochner, D., & Dungey, C. (2006). *Making the grade: A guide to successful communication and study* (3rd edn). Melbourne: Oxford University Press (see especially Chapter 2).

Marshall, L., & Rowland, F. (2006). *A guide to learning independently* (4th edn). Sydney: Pearson Education Australia.

McIlroy, D. (2003). *Studying at university: How to be a successful student.* London: Sage.

Wong, L. (2007). *Essential study skills* (7th edn). Boston, MA: Wadsworth.

useful web resources

For checklists and activity sheets on aspects of time and study management which form part of the Learning Skills Program at the University of Victoria (Canada), see www.coun.uvic.ca/learn/LearningSkillsPrograms. html

For time management challenges ~ prioritising ~ scheduling ~ concentrating ~ goal-setting ~ self-motivation, see www.mindtools.com/pages/main/ newMN_HTE.htm

For advice and activities to help you make the most of what you've got, of every available minute, see www.time-management-guide.com/index.html

For tips on self-motivation for effective study, see www.self-improvement-mentor.com/study-motivation.html

For guides on many aspects of effective study refer to this 'international, learner-centric, educational public service' website: www.studygs.net/timman.htm

For tools to help you discover how you learn, and what your preferences, strengths and weaknesses are, see *Skills audit* from the University of Manchester: www.humanities.manchester.ac.uk/studyskills/essentials/ start/index.html

For online workshops offered to *TUNE up your study skills*, see the University of New England website: www.une.edu.au/tlc/aso/aso-online/

Learning to do academic writing

Joy **HIGGS** | Lindy **M**c**ALLISTER** | JOAN ROSENTHAL

key topics

This chapter covers the following topics:

- what is scholarly or academic writing?

- what are the purposes and types of academic writing?

- what are the characteristics of academic writing?

- what are the grammatical conventions of academic writing?

key terms

ACADEMIC WRITING

GRAMMAR

Introduction

Students enrolled in tertiary education programs need to learn many skills of professional communication. One of these skills is writing in an academic or scholarly style. This is the style used for writing essays, assignments, journal papers, research reports and theses. **Academic writing** is a genre. It differs from the more colloquial language of a letter or a magazine article, the more colourful language and discursive style of a novel, and the more abbreviated style of lecture notes.

/ ACADEMIC WRITING /
Academic writing presents a scholarly argument clearly.

Academic or scholarly writing is of particular importance to students and professionals in the health sciences. Writing is an important skill for a range of reasons: it allows you to communicate your knowledge to colleagues, lecturers and members of the public; it helps you achieve satisfactory results in the classroom and practical settings; and it enhances your credibility as an emerging professional.

Characteristics of academic writing

Conventions of the academic writing genre include writing clearly and with correct **grammar**, punctuating according to the format required, using words precisely, avoiding long complex sentences, being consistent (with spelling, tenses—past, present and future—and active and passive voice), explaining and minimising jargon, limiting slang and colloquial language, and avoiding ambiguity. The level of formality of your writing varies with your audience. Following these conventions will help you get your message across, engage your readers and avoid confusion. Readers should be able to focus on your message.

/ **GRAMMAR** /
Grammar refers to the structural rules of language.

As well as being clear, academic writing needs to present a credible case or position; hence, you must provide supporting evidence and arguments (and clear acknowledgment of the sources of your ideas and data). Academic writing also needs to be analytical and critical; your role is to critique, not blindly accept data, opinion and research results, in order to present a reasoned case. See Chapter 4 for a discussion of the ethical aspects of academic writing.

Writing types and formats

As a professional in the health sciences, you will use a variety of types of professional writing, such as essays, journal articles, project reports, case notes and management plans. Each of these types of writing has a typical format or structure which may be particular to your profession, your workplace, or even your team or ward, in the case of client reports and records. Most universities produce a guide for written assignments that provides essential advice for students. If you are not sure of the format to use for a particular piece of writing, ask your lecturer or fieldwork educator for a good example of the type of writing required. Also, refer to other chapters of this book for advice on structuring essays, assignments, reports, clinical records, journal articles and theses.

Different types of writing serve different purposes. For example, essays typically argue, defend or critique a point of view. A thesis develops and provides evidence for a position. Clinical reports primarily inform clients or colleagues about a client's or group's needs or problems, and make recommendations for intervention. File notes inform relevant others about your treatment of a client to date. Community health proposals may include a needs assessment, program proposal, budget and plan for evaluation. Referrals for assessment or treatment by other professionals or colleagues are requests for an opinion or service. A case presentation informs colleagues, and can also serve to advocate for your client and persuade colleagues to adopt a particular view of the client's needs. Treatment plans, or self-management programs, explain to a client how to do something (such as self-care procedures at home). Technical reports describe a procedure and how to execute it. Public health reports may include the planning or evaluation of a community health education intervention program. Each of these kinds of writing belongs to a particular genre and has its own style.

TABLE 6.1 | WRITING PROBLEMS AND WAYS OF ADDRESSING THEM

WRITING PROBLEM	PROPOSED SOLUTION	EXAMPLES
1 Vague language	Make language clear and specific.	Avoid sentences starting 'This + (verb)', such as 'This had several consequences'. Always use a noun to explain what 'this' is referring to (e.g. 'This decision had several consequences').
2 Poor general vocabulary	Use correct vocabulary and expand your vocabulary.	Use a dictionary when you are unsure of the meaning of a word. If you have thought of a word and believe it might not be the most appropriate, use a thesaurus to find words with similar or related meanings. You can use the thesaurus on your computer.
3 Information not connected to the point being made	Ensure that information is relevant to the topic of the paragraph or heading.	Make sure a paragraph keeps to the topic announced or implied in its first sentence. Use a new heading to signal a complete change of topic.
4 Wordiness (too many words)	Be concise; use short, clear sentences.	An expression such as 'The problems which have been outlined in Section 3 …' can be condensed to 'The problems outlined in Section 3 …'. An expression such as 'They studied the effect that dehydration had on …' can be condensed to 'They studied dehydration effects on …'.
5 Important points not highlighted	Make sure important points are clear.	List or state your key point(s), particularly in an introductory sentence. Write more about the points that are most important in relation to your topic. Write about the most important points first and explain why they are important.

< cont. >

< cont. >

WRITING PROBLEM	PROPOSED SOLUTION	EXAMPLES
6 Illogical reasoning	Be sure that the reasoning is clearly explained.	When you have provided the necessary background information (such as information from other people's writings, information from observation of a patient, information from your research), you should draw conclusions that are supported by that information. Explain why you think the conclusions are justified.
7 Too much technical language	Use vocabulary that is generally understood; if you need to use technical language, define the terms you use.	Take into account which words your intended audience can understand. Remember that much health science terminology is unfamiliar to lay people. If you must use a technical word, explain what it means in simple words the first time you use it (e.g. 'Mr Smith has had a right cerebrovascular accident; that is, a stroke'). Abbreviations that are familiar to you (such as *CPR*) may not be familiar to your readers. Always explain an abbreviation the first time you use it (*cardio-pulmonary resuscitation*).
8 Poor overall organisation of writing	Organise writing to help the reader understand the sequence.	Make a plan of your writing (see Chapter 7). Use headings and subheadings as signposts to help your readers.
9 No clear overview	Include a clear overview.	At the beginning of your writing (e.g. essay, report or thesis), outline what is covered in that writing. This gives readers an idea of what to expect, and helps them have in mind an overview of the whole project.
10 Lack of continuity	Use strategies that help continuity of thought within and between paragraphs.	Use linkages between sentences and paragraphs, such as 'The problems described above have several consequences, which can be divided into individual and community consequences. Among the individual consequences …'.
11 Writing not adapted to diverse audiences	Adapt writing to suit the intended audience.	(See also Point 7 above.) When you come across new words in your lectures, practical work or reading, it can be difficult to know if they are new just to you, or if they would be unfamiliar words to most non-specialists. Similarly, when people with English as a second language learn a colloquial term, it can be difficult to know when that term can be used and for which audience. If this is a problem for you, ask lecturers and tutors for help. Ask your friends to explain the meaning of colloquial terms and their appropriate usage. In general, prefer simple, straightforward language.
12 Poor grammar	Ensure that grammar is correct.	Work to improve your use of grammar. Refer to style guides and books about style. If you receive feedback on your writing, make a list of the rules that have been highlighted in this way, so that you can refer to them in subsequent writing.

Building basic writing skills

All students learning to write in English encounter some common problems, whether English is their first, second or third language. The most significant of these problems, and ways of addressing them, are shown in order of importance in Table 6.1 (based on Huckin & Olsen, 1991). See also Bailey (2006).

Table 6.2 provides some general rules of grammar. A frequent difficulty in English expression, especially for those whose first language is not English, is the use of the English *article* (*a/an, the*, or no article at all). For others, use of the numerous verb forms and tenses is a mystery. If you can identify which aspects of English are especially difficult for you, staff at a learning support centre can suggest ways of finding help, or you can read a book on grammar and writing skills.

TABLE 6.2 | SOME BASIC RULES OF GRAMMAR

RULE	EXAMPLE
A singular noun subject takes a singular verb in the present tense. That verb commonly has –s added to it.	Wilson (2011) describes the behaviour of institutionalised children.
A plural noun subject takes a plural verb in the present tense. That verb does not have –s added to it.	Jones and Potter (2008) describe the functions of diet.
A singular, human noun is subsequently referred to using the words he, she, her, him, his or who.	Wilson (2010), who describes the behaviour of institutionalised children, gives her views on the causes …
A singular, non-human noun is subsequently referred to using the words it, its or which.	The diet, which is followed for four days, has as its main characteristic …
A plural noun is subsequently referred to using the words they, them or their. Further, the referent used is who for human and which for non-human nouns.	Jones and Potter (2009), who describe the functions of diet, outline their program for …
The (the definite article) refers to the specific or particular (noun). The indefinite article (a or an) refers to one or any (noun). (An is used if the noun starts with a vowel or a silent h.)	The poster presents an overview of my research. Mr Smith has an eye disease … The disease may require treatment using …
Past tense is used when actions, events or arguments occurred in the past. Present tense is used for current events, actions or arguments. As a general rule, keep the tense constant in a paragraph; use all past tense or present tense, as appropriate.	Smith (2007) discussed this technique as follows … In this essay I argue that … The patient reported that he had not eaten since last week. He said …

RESOURCES FOR PEOPLE WRITING IN ENGLISH AS A SECOND LANGUAGE

Various universities provide online writing labs that include resource pages, handouts and exercises among their materials for students with English as a second language. Check out Nordquist's (2011) top four online writing labs, at http://grammar.about.com/od/blogsandlinks/tp/wconline.htm

The effect of culture on writing

Culture affects writing in a variety of ways. Sentence structure and length, grammar and vocabulary selection may all show the influence of cultural preferences in relation to formality, directness and conceptual density of expression. As with face-to-face communication, levels of politeness used in writing vary from culture to culture. Western Anglo professionals would be embarrassed by a referral letter that began *Dear Esteemed Colleague* or *Honoured Doctor*; however, such formal titles are appropriate in some cultures. The level of directness in writing also varies with the 'politeness demands' of different cultures. Readers may be left to draw their own conclusions rather than be 'told' or directed. Westerners tend to make main points and recommendations early in a report, or even at the start in the executive summary. You need to learn how to write appropriately for your own situation (e.g. your university and country of enrolment).

The 10 Ps of academic writing

A common device in scholarly writing is to plan your writing around asking simple questions: 'Who ...?' 'What ...?' 'When ...?' 'Where ...?' 'Why ...?' 'How ...?' and 'So what ...?' These questions can be translated into various parameters (the 10 Ps) of academic writing: people, purpose, preparation, principles, process, progression, position, product, proofing, presentation (see Table 6.3).

TABLE 6.3 | THE 10 PS OF SCHOLARLY OR ACADEMIC WRITING © J. HIGGS 2004

	MEANING	GUIDELINES
People	Who is the author?	As author, consider your views and attitudes and how they might influence your writing.
	Who is the audience?	Identify your target audience and how you should write for these people—for example, formal compared with informal language, expected knowledge, level of language.

< cont. >

< cont. >

	MEANING	GUIDELINES
Purpose	Why am I writing? What is the goal of my paper or thesis?	Use different styles and approaches to explain, persuade and debate. Identify your goals and match your content and style to them.
Preparation	How can I investigate this topic? How do I sort and store the information, data and literature I collect? What are the findings of my research or topic investigation?	Consider what fields of literature you need to investigate—what information and data you need to collect. Spend time searching library databases to investigate your topic. Set a timeframe that will help you complete the task on time. Develop a system for sorting, collating and filing your data so that you can access it easily to write the various sections of the paper. Set up a reference-management system such as EndNote.
Principles	What are the rules of scholarly and academic writing and referencing? What styles or requirements are set by the school or the discipline?	Write with academic honesty. Reference appropriately; avoid plagiarism. Clearly indicate primary and secondary sources of ideas and quotes. Identify the writing style and product required by your school or discipline. Critique your work and that of other authors you are referencing.
Process	How can I turn my ideas and information into a paper?	Strategies include brainstorming, using a table of contents, flowcharts and concept maps to plan the content, and then writing sections in sequence or by preference.
Progression	How can I structure the argument throughout the paper?	Build the argument throughout the paper or thesis. Create a structure or framework for the paper. Build structure, flow and connections into the paper at micro (detailed) and macro (big picture) levels.
Position	What is the point I'm trying to make?	Identify the position or argument you wish to make and make sure that it is clearly expressed.
Product	What is the product of my writing—an essay, a paper, a journal article or a thesis? At the end of my work, how do I answer the 'so what?' question?	Consider the preferred or required mode of representing the argument or content. What place do stories, examples, graphs, tables, models and pictures have in illustrating the argument? What are the implications of your work for future research, education and practice (if these are applicable)?

< cont. >

< cont. >

	MEANING	GUIDELINES
Proofing	What fine-tuning or checking is needed to finalise the paper?	Before finishing your paper, essay or thesis, proofread it to check for clarity, sense, argument and technical correctness (accurate referencing, spelling, grammar).
		It helps to read your work aloud when proofing—this reveals problems such as incomplete sentences and lack of clarity.
Presentation	What are the presentation requirements and desired style of this work?	Identify the expectations of this work in terms of such presentation elements as word processing, length, writing style.
		Investigate what the typical thesis, essay or journal paper looks like for your field—look for such design elements as headings, language, layout and referencing style.

Dimensions of academic writing

Essentially, there are three parts to academic writing: the *big picture*, the *nitty gritty* and the *process*.

The big picture

The *big picture* refers to the fundamental argument or explanation you are presenting. For this task, you need to consider the *people*, *purpose*, *progression*, *position* and *product* items from Table 6.3. When crafting your argument, remember to structure your work. First, plan an overall structure. Your plan may take the form of a logical sequence of headings or questions, or a standard research report sequence, including: Introduction, Background Literature, Research Methods, Results and Conclusion. Second, within the argument, you need to think about creating the flow of the argument or building your case. This entails:

- creating signposts by, for example, starting with your endpoint ('In this essay I argue that …'), and then making your argument;
- using each paragraph to present a main idea and each section to make the next major point in your case;
- linking the ideas, through a logical sequence or through linking phrases, such as 'Having presented the background to this topic, my next task is to …' and 'On the basis of these results …'.

The nitty gritty

The *nitty gritty* refers to the technical aspects of writing; the details and the presentation of your work (see *principles*, *proofing* and *presentation* in Table 6.3). With all the tools available today (such as spell-checkers, online computer searches, style guides and reference manuals), there is no reason your work should not be well checked (with accurate referencing, spelling, grammar and punctuation) and well presented. These aspects of your work are largely invisible; if you do them well, they add a polish to your work. But if poorly done, they are glaringly obvious and detract from your argument. Even the strongest case or the most interesting research can be tarnished by poor presentation or spelling, and your grade or the impact of your work could suffer. You may need to learn these skills or improve your basic writing skills. Most universities have student learning centres where you can seek help. Learning these skills is an essential part of your tertiary education. Table 6.4 provides some valuable technical guidelines for academic writing.

handy hint 6.2

RESOURCES FOR GRAMMAR AND STYLE

Publication manual of the American Psychological Association (6th edn) (2010). Washington, DC: American Psychological Association. Although this manual is designed primarily for writers of journal articles and theses, it has useful sections on writing style, grammar and reducing bias in language. These sections deal with important matters that are subject to error in health sciences writing in general.

Ritter, R. M. (2003). *The Oxford style manual: The essential handbook for all writers, editors, and publishers*. Oxford: Oxford University Press.

Strunk, W. Jr. (2009). *The elements of style, with revisions, an introduction, and a chapter on writing by E. B. White*. New York: Pearson Longman.

Style manual for authors, editors and printers. (2002). (6th edn, rev. Snooks & Co.). Sydney: John Wiley & Sons.

Tyler, S., Kossen, C., & Ryan, C. (2002). *Communication: A foundation course* (2nd edn). Sydney: Prentice Hall Australia.

Zwier, L. J. (2002). *Building academic vocabulary*. Ann Arbor, MI: University of Michigan Press. Addressing academic writing in particular, this book provides many synonyms for words commonly used in essays, assignments and theses. Differences between similar terms are clearly explained, to help demonstrate the most appropriate usages.

The process

See Table 6.3 for the *preparation* and *process* items. Table 6.4 provides some strategies to help you write well. See also the other chapters in this book.

TABLE 6.4 | ATTENDING TO THE TECHNICAL ASPECTS OF WRITING

TASK/ITEM	GUIDELINES
Writing style, punctuation, grammar	Writing style is a combination of general expectations of academic writing (this is essential) and local instructions (such as university style requirements or specific essay instructions).
	Concentrate on clarity of expression and message; avoid long sentences or distracting layout and terminology.
	Grammar and punctuation should be accurate—this is required for academic writing, and it is an indication of the literacy and education of the writer.
Spelling	Use local (Australian) rather than American spelling (often set as the default in computers) of words like honour, practise (the verb), equalled, organise (except when writing for American journals). However, when quoting, retain the original spelling.
	Choose or follow local instructions about spelling options, but be consistent (except for spelling within quotes), for example: program or programme, aging or ageing, '-ise' or '-ize'.
Font	Use a font that is easy to read and not distracting, such as Times New Roman (TNR) or Arial. Avoid distracting the reader with fancy fonts. Use 12 point (= Arial 10), or 11 if there is a need to limit space.
	Use italic, not underlining, for emphasis. Use bold for headings only.
	Use quotation marks (inverted commas) or italics when you are citing new or jargon terms for the first time (add a footnote or endnote with definition, or explain the term in the text).
Layout and printing (general)	The aesthetics of your presentation or layout is a matter of taste. Make sure you follow any set requirements for your work (in particular, check your university's guide for presentation of assignments). Beyond that, make the text readable, the graphics clear and the overall appearance scholarly. Sometimes there is a place for more creative layout, as in posters with graphics.
	The layout of your writing, such as heading levels and paragraphs, has 'hidden meanings'—the reader will assume that each paragraph is a new point, or each same level heading is a section of equal importance and relevance. Recognise and use this factor.
	Avoid wasteful and distracting white space; avoid one-sentence or very small paragraphs (they also stop the flow of the argument).
	Justification refers to the left- and right-side alignment of your text. Left-sided justification is standard in text, and should be used in most tables. Double justification (both right and left) can be used for standard block text. In tables, right-justify or decimal-justify numbers, and include a consistent number of decimal places or use decimal tabs.

< cont. >

< *cont.* >

TASK/ITEM	GUIDELINES
Layout and printing (general)	*Portrait* page layout is most common and expected. Sometimes, as with a wide table, horizontal or *landscape* page layout is preferable.
	Check the requirements of your essay, paper or thesis. You may need to use double spacing or wide margins (especially for thesis binding).
	Different printers space text differently. A page of text from one printer might expand to a page and three lines on another. Check the layout on the monitor before your final print, especially if you are using manual page breaks.
Headings	You may use the heading system built into your software.
	Example of a system of headings:
	Chapter, title of essay: centred, capitals, bold, font size 16, two paragraph spaces after
	Major text headings: left-justified, bold, caps, two paragraph spaces before, one after
	Second-level text headings: left-justified, bold, sentence case, one paragraph space before, zero after
	Third-level text headings: left-justified, italics, not bold, sentence case, one paragraph space before, zero after
	Avoid complex section numbering such as *3.2.2.3*. It is hard to follow.
Headers, footers, page numbers, tabs	Headers and footers may be used if acceptable, but are generally used only in drafts, to keep track of the version or date of updating.
	Use page numbers.
	Use *tabs* rather than the *space bar* to ensure correct alignment of text.
Footnotes and endnotes	Footnotes (bottom of page) or endnotes (end of document) may be used for added information (such as definitions) that is not necessary in the text or slows down the flow of the argument.
	Check if such notes are acceptable, but do not use too many; they make the document hard to read.
	Many software programs allow you to insert these notes systematically, with sequenced numbers that adjust automatically if new notes are added.
Tables and figures	See Chapter 14.
Lists	In general, avoid using lists in essays, because they do not create a sense of flow or build up the argument, and often the message is obscure in the more cryptic and staccato style created by numbered or bulleted lists. Sometimes lists can usefully be placed in tables for reference, rather than as the main part of the text or argument.
	For an indented series of points, use numbers instead of bullets—e.g. *(1), (2) etc.*— if the sequence is important. If the sequence is not significant, use bullets. Use balance in the grammatical presentation of your points. For example, if the first point starts with a verb ending with *–ing*, all the other points in that series should start the same way.

< *cont.* >

< cont. >

TASK/ITEM	GUIDELINES
Lists	Delineation of a series of points within a sentence can be clarified for readers by the use of *(a), (b), (c) etc.* Use a comma between each point unless the points already have commas within them, in which case use semicolons.
Numerals written in words or in figures, dates	Write in words all numbers less than 10, and numbers starting a sentence. However, use figures for numbers relating to any unit of measurement, e.g. *6 months.* Use a consistent date format; e.g. *15 August 2008.* Decades are written without any added punctuation, i.e. *1980s* not 1980's.
Use of the first person, such as 'I', 'me', 'we'	This usage is becoming more accepted in academic writing, in appropriate instances such as when the writer needs to acknowledge the part that his or her involvement played in the study's outcome. At other times the convention is to use the *passive voice*, as in: 'Several factors were taken into consideration in designing the layout of the room'. Excessive usage of the passive voice can sound both detached and complex. Check if there are any local rules that apply to your institution for use of first person (I, me, my ...); e.g. 'You must write in the third person'.
Singular/plural	Singular subjects are accompanied by singular verbs; plural subjects take plural verbs. Avoid using single nouns such as 'the nurse' and then having to use 'his or her'. It's preferable to say 'nurses ... their ...'.
Tense	Use *past tense* to report what researchers or authors found, studied, reported, claimed, considered. When writing up your research methods, change the *future tense* (I will .../this research will investigate ...) of your research proposal to the past tense (I did .../this research investigated ...).
Inanimate/animate subjects	Some verbs do not suit inanimate subjects. Only *animate* subjects (researchers, authors, theorists) can discuss, contend, claim, assert, consider, argue or aim to. *Inanimate* subjects (studies, research, findings, chapters, theses) can demonstrate, present or provide.
Abbreviations and jargon	Use a full stop after abbreviations that do not end with the same letter as the full word, such as Prof., Fig. Don't use a full stop after abbreviations that end with the same letter as the word, such as Dr, Figs. Note the use of full stops in: 'etc.', 'i.e.', 'e.g.' and 'et al.'. Explain technical terms and abbreviations the first time they are used. This can be in the text or in a footnote (if acceptable). In longer works such as theses, a glossary of technical terms may be included.
Referencing and quotes	See Chapter 9 for details on referencing and quotes.

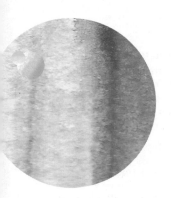

conclusion

After you have finished writing, it is time to reflect on the process of your writing and its product. Consider, for example, the following questions:

- Have you said what you wanted to say? Have you made your message clear?
- Did you complete your task (to critique, explain, debate, discuss or report)?
- What have you learned about your writing? What skills might you need to develop?
- What are the strengths and weaknesses of your writing?

references

Bailey, S. (2006). *Academic writing: A handbook for international students* (2nd edn). New York: Routledge.

Huckin, T.N., & Olsen, L.A. (1991). *Technical writing and professional communication for nonnative speakers of English* (international edn). New York: McGraw Hill.

further reading

Bazerman, C., & Wiener, H. S. (2003). *Writing skills handbook* (5th edn). Boston: Houghton Mifflin.

Creme, P., & Lea, M. R. (2003). *Writing at university: A guide for students* (2nd edn). Buckingham: Open University Press.

Fink, J. W., & Fink, C. P. (1990). *Writing for the allied health professional*. Englewood Cliffs, NJ: Prentice Hall.

Macquarie dictionary. Retrieved from http://www.macquarieonline.com.au/dictionary.html

Peat, J., Elliott, E., Baur, L., & Keenan, V. (2002). *Scientific writing: Easy when you know how*. Sydney: BMJ Books.

Soles, D. (2005). *The essentials of academic writing*. Boston, MA: Houghton Mifflin.

Villemaire, L., & Villemaire, D. (2001). *Grammar and writing skills for the health professional*. Albany, NY: Delmar.

CHAPTER

07

Learning to write essays and assignments

Lindy MCALLISTER | Fiona BOGOSSIAN | Iain HAY

key topics

This chapter covers the following topics:

- how to analyse an essay topic
- how to structure an essay
- how to support your case
- how to write well

key terms

STRUCTURE OF AN ESSAY

CONCEPT MAP

PROOFREADING

Introduction

Writing, one of the most powerful means of communicating, is also a thought-provoking, generative process, offering us the opportunity to present our work to others and seek feedback on our ideas. A good essay must clearly demonstrate your understanding and learning about the set topic, or justify a position or a course of action. This chapter will help you to achieve this end and provides advice on analysing your essay topic, structuring your essay, supporting your case and writing well.

Analysing the topic

A good essay *answers the assigned question* and deals in detail with the specific issues the topic raises. These matters are critical to essay-writing success. However, several steps can be taken to ensure that you are on the right track.

First, read the essay topic through carefully. Underline or highlight key words within it, as shown in this example:

Discuss the effects of the obesity epidemic on future health service delivery in Australia.

Second, dissect each of the key words and their relationships with others in the essay topic. Assignments commonly contain a *directional verb*; that is, a verb which tells you what to do—in this case, 'discuss'. When analysing an essay topic, it is important to understand the cognitive skill implied by the directional verb. See Table 7.1, which may be helpful as a guide.

It is not uncommon in health sciences to have an assignment task which has more than one directional verb and requires you to demonstrate more than one level of cognition; for example: 'Examine the effectiveness of high protein diets on weight management and propose the advice you would provide to an obese client on the basis of the evidence.' In this case, you are directed to examine and propose. A mistake students commonly make is to respond to the first direction and neglect the second.

Think about the word 'effects' in the essay topic. What kinds of effect? The topic makes clear that the paper should deal with effects on future health service delivery. But does this mean, for example, effects on the type and frequency of services available on public sector funding? In this assignment the specific area is unclear. You have at least two options in such a case:

- Ask your lecturer if there are any specific issues you should be focusing on. Be prepared to suggest some of the areas you would like to cover.
- Make it clear in your essay that, although a wide range of effects could be considered, you are choosing to focus on specific effects and justify why you are doing so.

Finally, it is evident from the topic that the paper must deal with health service delivery in Australia. Although you could use local examples, you must maintain a national focus.

The third step in preparing a good essay is to investigate your topic in depth. The recommended texts and reading lists for your subject are a starting point, but you will need to read more extensively. This requires judicious literature searching and careful reference-management. See Chapters 8 and 9, where these matters are dealt with fully.

TABLE 7.1 | COGNITIVE SKILLS, EXAMPLES AND DIRECTIONAL VERBS USED IN ESSAY TOPICS

COGNITIVE SKILL LEVEL	EXAMPLE	DIRECTIONAL VERBS
Knowledge: Recall information	List the actions in Basic Life Support as set out by the Australian Resuscitation Council.	Define, identify, list, name, recall, recognise, select, state
Comprehension: Understand the meaning	Explain Starling's Law.	Compare, describe, discuss, explain, express, identify, recognise, restate, paraphrase, translate
Application: Use concepts in a situation	Demonstrate the principles of thermoregulation in the care of pre-term infants.	Apply, complete, construct, categorise, demonstrate, employ, illustrate, interpret, modify, predict, solve, use
Analysis: Separate concepts into component parts to be understood	Examine the impact of primary health care in the care of individuals with chronic disease.	Analyse, appraise, contrast, debate, differentiate, distinguish, examine, question, test
Synthesis: Combine component parts together to form a whole and create new meaning or structure	Formulate an emergency department response plan to a catastrophic event.	Arrange, assemble, combine, construct, create, devise, formulate. generate, plan, propose, summarise
Evaluation: Make judgments about	Justify the use of long-term antibiotic therapy in the treatment of acne vulgaris in adolescence.	Argue, appraise, assess, conclude, critique, defend, evaluate, interpret, judge, justify, measure, rate, score, support

Structuring your essay

Consider the **structure of an essay**. At the global level, all good essays typically comprise three main parts: an introduction, body and conclusion. A good essay has a logical order of content that supports the argument or answers the question posed.

Introduction

Your introduction should include at least four characteristics. First, state your topic, purpose and 'case'. Let the reader know clearly what the essay is about. Do not simply restate the essay question as the statement of intent. Use something that rapidly engages the reader, such as an impressive statistic, an anecdote or, in

/ STRUCTURE OF AN ESSAY /

The structure of an essay has three main parts: the introduction, body and conclusion.

some cases, a controversial statement that focuses on key elements of your essay. Your paper might begin as follows: 'Over 60% of adult Australians are overweight or obese, and individual lifestyle choices are the root cause.' This highlights the second function of a good introduction: to capture the reader's attention. Third, the introduction explains the significance of the topic; something commonly described as the 'so what?' question. Why is this matter important? Who cares? Answers to these questions will give you a strong lead-in to identifying the significance of your work. Finally, a good introduction will usually provide a 'map' of the discussion to follow. Give your reader some idea of the intellectual journey you have planned, including the limitations or assumptions, and the analytical techniques to be used.

Essay body

The body of the essay is where you set out the reasons and evidence for the case or views you introduced earlier. You must substantiate each of your claims. If we return to the assertion made in our example essay, that individual lifestyle choices are the root cause of the prevalence of obesity, you must provide statistical evidence, quotations from experts or other evidence (figures and tables) to support this claim. Without good evidence, your assertions will never be anything more than your opinion.

Conclusion

The third and final part of an essay is the conclusion. Here, you should distil the essence of your answer to the question posed. The conclusion must be based on evidence set out within the body of the paper. It is not a place for new material. The conclusion needs also to be related logically to the introduction and should match the intent indicated in the introduction. To check this, read the introduction and conclusion together. Are they consistent and connected?

Developing your structure

A good essay has a coherent conceptual or thematic structure that breaks down the argument and contains evidence, examples and justifications. When a structure is not suggested, there are two particularly useful techniques for developing an essay's internal structure: the essay plan and the **concept map**.

/ CONCEPT MAP /
A concept map is a diagram of the relationships between each concept or element of an idea or theory.

Essay plan

To prepare an essay plan you need a clear idea of the general argument you wish to make before you start writing. With this in mind, list the major headings to describe material in different parts of the essay. Then look at their order, rearranging them if necessary so that the concepts flow in a logical fashion. Then, under each heading, add a series of subheadings and, under these, key points, data and reference materials to support your claims. Most word-processing packages include options (such as *Outline* view) that will help you develop and view your essay plan.

Concept map

If you have a less clear idea about the direction to take in your essay, or the essay deals with complex interrelationships between concepts, start by drawing a concept map (diagram of how each element relates to the others). Write on a sheet of paper all the concepts that relate to the essay topic. Eliminate any duplication. Arrange the concepts in a logical way. Draw connections between the elements and label the connections; for example 'relates to', 'reinforces', 'contrasts with'. Keep rearranging your diagram until you have generated an essay outline that reflects the flow of your arguments. Concept mapping is particularly useful for demonstrating higher-order thinking because, by its very nature, the process encourages synthesis.

Free writing

If neither of these strategies works, there is another, more challenging approach you can adopt: free writing. Simply start writing something related to the topic. The key idea is to get words onto the paper or screen. Once written, words can be edited, rearranged and otherwise massaged into the form of an essay. This approach should normally be your last resort.

Using headings for clarity and structure

Headings are useful organisational tools. For instance, once you have completed a draft of your paper, on a separate sheet of paper, write down all the headings you plan to use. Separated from the content of the essay, does the order of headings make sense and follow a logical sequence that contributes to a good essay answer? If not, think about rearranging the headings, or adding or deleting headings (and therefore sections in your essay). You may find that your summary of headings provides a helpful framework for your introduction.

Check the instructions for your essay topic to determine if the use of headings is permitted. For brief essays of 1500 to 2000 words, headings may not be appropriate. However, in their place, make sure that paragraph-linking sentences guide the reader through the flow of your argument. Generally, three levels of heading are sufficient.

Supporting your case thoroughly

Claims, contentions, arguments and allegations in an essay all require the support of high-quality evidence. Supporting evidence includes material such as data, quotations, examples and case studies that substantiate the case or position you are putting forward in your essay. Do not make assertions or generalisations (such as 'Women who have children young have a lower risk than older first-time mothers of getting breast cancer.') without including facts to back them up. Such evidence is a fundamental aspect of scholarly writing and compelling argument.

Reference material

A good essay will demonstrate that you have evaluated work written by others in relevant fields. Many beginning health sciences students express concern that they know little about a topic and feel largely condemned to quote the work of others. However, you can demonstrate your level of critical thinking by the judicious use and interpretation of reference material to support your argument. In some cases, this may mean that you need to be critical of or challenge the work of others. Scholarly critique is the foundation for the incremental development of knowledge or 'scientific progress'. If your learning style or previous educational experience has not prepared you to question the work of 'experts', this may be difficult at first.

Students commonly ask, 'How many references do I need?' There is no right answer to this question. Your examiner will expect to see references cited. In general, use fewer references for short essays. Examiners would prefer to see fewer references, but references that are high quality and well chosen, and which demonstrate that you have a grasp of the relevant literature, rather than a large number of references which are only vaguely related to the topic.

The evidence you employ should be *relevant, reputable, accurate, up-to-date* and *sufficient to support your case*. Such sources include scholarly books and refereed journals. A *refereed journal* is a journal in which the contents have been scrutinised carefully by peer reviewers who are experts in the field, before being accepted for publication. Using refereed journals as a source of evidence can generally provide some indication of the quality of a paper. However, in determining the quality of specific published research papers, you may need to be more rigorous in your evaluation. For example, if asked to review the evidence about the efficacy of high protein diets as a weight loss intervention, you should carefully screen the references you use. In this case, evidence equates to research, so ask yourself:

- 'Is it research?' as opposed to commentary or opinion;
- 'Is it primary research?' as opposed to secondary report;

- 'Is it credible?'—has it been subject to rigorous peer review or published in a highly regarded journal?;
- 'What is the level of evidence?' (e.g. NHMRC, 2000). Is it a personal account of experience or the gold standard of research—a randomised controlled trial; or
- 'Is the research high quality?'—you can determine this if you read critically and with a degree of scepticism!

Websites can also be useful, particularly those produced by professional bodies, or government or health agencies (such as the World Health Organization). However, when using web material to support your essay, remain sceptical of sources and critique them, using the following as a guide to determine the value of a website for your work (Curtin University, 2010):

- *Scope:* Does the site offer the information you really need? Does it relate directly to your essay topic or is it of marginal relevance?
- *Purpose and presentation:* What is the reason for the site's existence? Did you find the page through a sponsored link? Is the information likely to be biased? Is the site well organised and is the material presented clearly?
- *Authority:* Who are the authors, and what are their claims to credibility? Are the web pages written with specific—and possibly biased—intentions?
- *Currency and content:* When was the site produced? Are sources of information acknowledged?

When writing an essay, it is important to make reference to the thoughts and efforts of others upon whose material you have built your own essay. You can achieve this by citing fully and correctly the source details of quotations, evidence and ideas, using an accepted form of referencing or professional acknowledgment (see Chapter 9). To fail to do so can be interpreted as *plagiarism*, which is a form of intellectual theft. Universities increasingly use plagiarism detection software such as TurnItIn, something which students can also use prior to submission of assignments to check that they have not inadvertently incorporated unreferenced material in their writing. A good essay also includes a complete and correctly presented list of references.

Illustrative material

Plates, figures, tables and maps are often overlooked as useful illustrative or evidentiary devices in essays. Illustrations can be derived from other sources or you can create your own. You must ensure that every illustration is referred to in the text and that the reader's attention is guided to the key points of interest. See Chapter 14 for more information on tables and figures.

Writing well

Good written expression is critical to essay success. You can become a better writer by (a) practising writing, (b) following simple writing principles, and (c) listening to constructive criticism. Writing a good, well-expressed essay takes time. Do not be fooled into thinking that your first essay draft will be the final copy. It is vital to make the time to do ample research and rewrite drafts of your paper.

Short sentences

Have a look at essays you have written in the past. How long are the sentences? If you create sentences longer than about 25 words, you run the risk of creating grammatical minefields that may be difficult, confusing and frustrating to read. To avoid such problems, limit sentences in the first draft of your essay to between 10 and 20 words; break down longer sentences; and express ideas simply and succinctly. You will find not only that short sentences are easier to manage but also that they have greater impact.

Technical language

Expressing your ideas simply and succinctly does not mean resorting to the use of lay terms. It is important to use appropriate technical language to illustrate your argument. Indeed, in some cases, examiners look for the appropriate contextual use of technical terms to demonstrate your understanding of concepts. If you need to define a term, use an appropriate technical rather than a lay reference source.

Effective paragraphing

Another key to good essay writing is effective paragraphing. A paragraph is typically a self-contained expression of a single main idea, and generally consists of three parts. The first is a *topic sentence*. This introduces or states the main idea. For instance, 'Like many countries in the developed world, Australia has an aging population.' The second part is the *supporting sentence or sentences*. These provide evidence to support the topic sentence: 'In 1961, only 8.5 per cent of the population was over 65 years of age, whereas by 2031 it is anticipated that figure will have increased to 22 per cent.' The third and final part of a paragraph is known as the *clincher*. We might conclude our example paragraph with a statement like: 'Australia's changing demographic profile has important implications for health service planning and delivery.' While not all paragraphs contain these three components, you will find that an awareness of this structure is highly valuable as you develop your essay-writing abilities.

One difficulty many people face when writing is trying to link one paragraph to another. Without good links, an essay can read rather like a sequence of related ideas instead of a coherent, single work. Handy Hint 7.1 provides useful phrases to help bind one paragraph to another.

USEFUL LINKING EXPRESSIONS

Another matter to consider is ...   *Elsewhere ...*

On the other hand ...   *Other common ...*

A similar explanation ...   *A significant consequence is ...*

From a different perspective ...   *A number of issues can be identified ...*

Grammar and punctuation

Difficulties with grammar and punctuation often confound otherwise effective students. See Chapter 6 for more information on common grammatical errors. If you are confused about matters such as the correct location of an apostrophe or the right time to use a colon as opposed to a semi-colon, *do not guess*. Consult a good text on the topic, such as Peters' *Cambridge Guide to Australian English Usage* (2007) for advice.

Once you have completed your paper, put it aside for a few days. When you return to it, odd phrasing, flaws in your argument and typographical errors that simply were not evident before will become apparent! Another valuable idea is to read the paper aloud or ask someone else to read it. This will help identify many problems. You will quickly hear where problems exist with structure and clarity, logic, or the flow of the argument. It can sometimes be helpful to find a critical friend, someone whose skills as a writer in your field you value, to read through your essay and give you feedback. You may be able to reciprocate, critically evaluating and commenting on that person's work. However, a word of caution is necessary here: should you choose to share your work with another person, you must trust that your work will not be copied and submitted as their own.

Spelling

With the advent of powerful spell-checkers in word-processing programs, few excuses for spelling errors remain. However, you must always check the work of your computer! There will be occasions when you will have to outsmart the machinery and provide it with guidance regarding words such as *bow* and *bough*; *two, too* and *to*; and *affect* and *effect*. Remember to attach the appropriate national dictionary to your computer file, and set it as the default language on your computer for spell-checking. However, do not change the original spelling in quotes or references (e.g. from American to Australian English). If there is an actual spelling error in a quote, indicate this by '[sic]' after the misspelt word.

Presentation and word limits

Take care with the presentation of your essays. An essay that is nicely typed and formatted in accordance with your lecturer's requirements will make a better first impression than an essay that is sloppily handwritten, dog-eared and coffee-stained. Most essays have a word limit. Stick to it. Some markers monitor word limits closely, arguing that students who exceed the specified word limit may have an unfair advantage over those who keep to it. Also, in a large class, a hundred extra words on each essay quickly adds up to considerable extra reading, which can make for an unhappy marker! Make each word count. If you cannot meet the word limit, either stop writing, having said all you need to, or—and this is probably more advisable—do some more research.

Before submission

Plan your timeline for essay writing so you have sufficient time to undertake a final edit, quality check and proofread before the submission deadline. The first editorial process, called *substantive editing*, relates to the structure of your essay. To begin this process, reanalyse the essay topic: have you explicitly followed the directional verb/s? Have you responded to the specific issues in the question? Does your essay contain information that is inconsistent or irrelevant? Does your reference list represent the important sources of information in response to the topic? Review the sequence of headings or the topic sentences in each paragraph. Is there a logical flow of ideas? Do these lead to the logical conclusion you have drawn? Review your introduction and conclusion to check again that these reflect the topic of the essay.

/ PROOFREADING /
Proofreading is a process that involves a detailed review of the grammar, spelling, punctuation and mechanics of style of your submission.

Secondly, begin copyediting and **proofreading** your work. This process involves a detailed review of the grammar, spelling and punctuation, and mechanics of style of your submission. Attention to detail in proofreading and copyediting ensures that the examiner will not be distracted from the substance of your work by errors.

Next, consider the final presentation, ensuring that you have complied with any specific requirements. These may include formatting (e.g. font type and size, line spacing, margins, headers and footers, and page numbers); a cover sheet that includes the word count if requested; a statement attesting to the authenticity of your work or provision of a report form using anti-plagiarism software; the correct number of copies prepared as requested (e.g. printed on both sides of the page and stapled in the top left corner). Check that you have addressed all criteria in any marking guide provided to you.

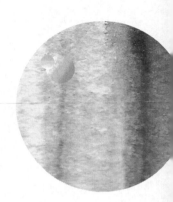

conclusion

Writing essays and assignments is a skill that can be learned and refined with practice. Writing good essays and assignments takes time: time to analyse what is required, plan out the writing task, structure it effectively and confirm that you have answered the question assigned. Time is also required to find references and other material to support your argument. Effective writing is about paying attention to the details of spelling, punctuation and grammar as well. Finally, you need to allow time for drafting (and redrafting) and for proofreading, so that your ideas and manner of expressing them can be fine-tuned. With good time management and regular practice you can learn to write essays and assignments that will be a pleasure to read and mark, and that demonstrate the depth and scope of your learning.

references

Curtin University School of Public Health. (2010). *Evaluation of health information on the World Wide Web Tutorial*. Retrieved from http://publichealth.curtin.edu.au/student/www/index.cfm

NHMRC. (2000). *How to review the evidence: Systematic identification and review of the scientific literature*. Canberra, ACT: National Health and Medical Research Council.

Peters, P. (2007). *The Cambridge guide to Australian English usage* (2nd edn). Melbourne: Cambridge University Press.

CHAPTER 08

Searching the literature and managing references and resources

Stephanie **SEDDON** | Claudio **DIONIGI**

key topics

This chapter covers the following topics:

- searching the literature and accessing information
- reviewing the literature
- managing references and resources

key terms

GREY LITERATURE

BIBLIOGRAPHIC DATABASE

LIBRARY CATALOGUE

SEARCH ENGINES

SYSTEMATIC REVIEW

Introduction

Whether you are writing an assignment, essay, review, report or thesis, a sound knowledge of the literature relating to your subject is fundamental to good research and communication. Literature comes in many formats, ranging from published books, journals and periodicals through to unpublished works such as government documents, technical reports and conference proceedings. Literature can be categorised into primary sources, original written work, or secondary sources, like a textbook that provides a critique or summary of one or more primary sources. You might also see a distinction between 'mainstream' published literature and what is referred to as **grey literature**. The latter can be difficult to find using regular search techniques, and might not have been peer-reviewed or through a formal editorial process. Examples include technical reports or 'white' papers. During your search for information, you may refer to several or all of these

/ GREY LITERATURE /
Grey literature is written work that is not published in easily accessible journals and may not be found in databases or through web searches.

forms of literature. A literature review can be a work in itself or it can be integrated into sections of a larger work, such as the introduction and discussion chapters of a thesis or research report—which is why developing skills in literature searching is so important.

Where to start?

Before you start searching and reviewing the literature, it is essential to have a clearly defined question or topic in mind. Sometimes this has already been decided for you, such as with an essay question for your course assessment; otherwise, you need to spend some time thinking about and framing your question or topic of enquiry. The way you word your topic or question will guide your literature search, as well as set the boundaries for the breadth and depth of information that you need to cover and incorporate into your written work. For example, you might want to ask a general open-ended question, such as: 'How has nursing practice changed since the introduction of graduate nursing degrees?' Or you might be interested in more specific information with clearer boundaries; for example: 'How has nursing practice changed in Australian children's hospitals since the introduction of postgraduate courses in paediatric nursing?' Although this second question gives more specific key terms to guide searching, it could narrow the field of literature too much if little has been written on this topic. Similarly, a study of 'The effects of diet on cholesterol levels' is a very broad topic, and the volume of information available is likely to be overwhelming. In that case, it would be helpful to limit the scope of the study to, for example, 'The effects of a diet high in saturated fat on the cholesterol levels of school-aged children'.

Now that you have defined your study question or topic, what type of information do you need? If you are writing an essay or report you might focus on secondary sources, but if you are writing a thesis or a paper for a journal you need to go to the primary literature for original data and interpretations, from which you can draw your own conclusions. If you are researching a topic in great depth, you can often find a wealth of information and detail in the grey literature. In any case, it is a good idea to start with a general textbook or a review to give you an overview and increase your understanding of the subject. Your lecturers or tutors usually provide a reading list or recommend texts that relate to your topic. They may also arrange for key books and other articles to be placed on 'closed reserve' in your library so that everyone in your course has an opportunity to read them. Specialist dictionaries and subject encyclopaedias are also useful for locating definitions around discipline-specific and specialised terminology.

FIGURE 8.1 | BOOLEAN SEARCH OPERATORS AND THEIR FUNCTION

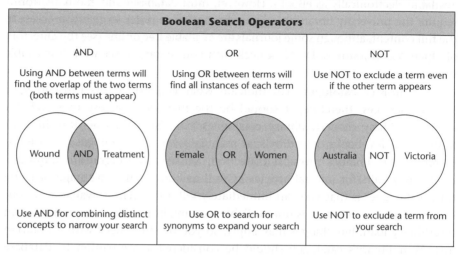

The main advantage of online databases is that they can be accessed at any time from your home or office or, indeed, anywhere in the world. Furthermore, you can refine your search in a database as you go—you can add terms to your search or remove terms that are not working, and you can access some articles well before they are available in print. With some software, you can add your own notes to articles that have been downloaded in PDF format (e.g. Adobe Acrobat Reader, Foxit Reader or Preview). Databases also offer many options for expanding or narrowing your search; for example, searching within a particular field, such as the title or the subject. Databases also allow you to limit your results to a specific date range. Instead of searching for articles in a database, you can browse through a list of journals and then view the table of contents for those publications.

/ SEARCH ENGINES /
Search eingines are computer programs that search documents based on given key words or phrases.

Search engines such as Google can help you locate many valuable online resources, as well as books and journal articles, including government documents and reports, statistical data, or the websites of key organisations for your discipline (e.g. Nursing and Midwifery Board of Australia). However, search engines often yield too many results and it is important to be able to filter them effectively, according to quality and relevance (Phelps et al., 2007). Other online resources, such as Wikipedia, can also give you a general overview of a topic when you first start reviewing the literature, but you need to be aware that these resources are not necessarily authoritative or adequately checked for accuracy. If you are unsure about the accuracy or reliability of a web-based resource, ask your librarian for help.

It is essential to constantly analyse the success of your searches and refine your search strategy if it is not working. There is no simple solution to searching for resources; searches take time and effort. The key is not to be discouraged when you do not get results. Remember to be organised and methodical in your searching.

Map out or list your search terms beforehand. Keep a search diary in which you can write down your searches and the databases you used. Most databases also allow you to save your search results into a permanent folder stored within the database itself. You can also export your search results to bibliographic management software such as EndNote or RefWorks.

Reference and citation tracking

Another way of finding relevant literature is to consult the reference list at the end of most books and journal articles. This is known as *reference tracking*. The disadvantage of reference lists is that the resources listed are older than the article that has cited them. This is where citation tracking can be very useful, because it allows you to work forward in time. Citation tracking uses the power of a specialised database called a *citation index* to allow you to find more recent articles that have cited the work you have discovered. Currently, there are three key citation indexes that are used for citation tracking: ISI Web of Science, Scopus and Google Scholar. The first two need to be accessed through your library, but Google Scholar is a free online resource.

You can conduct a topic search in a citation index, or you can look for a key article for which you already have the details. A citation index gives you a citation count for a particular article (i.e. how many papers have referred to that work in their reference list). In each of the three indexes listed above, you can then display the list of papers that have cited that work, essentially allowing you to find newer resources based on the original work you were looking at. If you have conducted a topic search in a citation index, you can identify the most influential works on the topic (based on how many times others have cited them). A citation index also allows you to track the development of a topic or field of research, or even an academic discussion based on published papers and critiques, and their rebuttals. Reference and citation tracking is particularly important if you are conducting a major research project, such as an honours, masters or doctoral thesis.

EFFECTIVE LITERATURE SEARCHING

- Make sure you understand and have clearly defined your study question or topic.
- Use the resources supplied by your study coordinator or lecturer as a starting point.
- Consult general texts and articles to increase your knowledge of the topic.
- Develop an outline that lists the headings and subheadings that you need to cover in your search.

- Brainstorm the key concepts and terms for your topic and identify any synonyms before you start searching.

- Conduct searches in all the databases that are relevant to your subject area.

- Use citation tracking to locate more recent articles.

- Use the references from any key articles that you find to expand your research.

- Document and keep track of the searches you conduct.

- If one search does not work, do not give up; change your search terms and strategy and try again.

- Analyse, interpret and critique the literature to ensure it is relevant to your topic, of high quality and authoritative.

- Be systematic in your storage of articles and use reference-management software to organise your research.

Reviewing the literature

Initially, you need to skim through the literature you have collected to decide whether the work is relevant—abstracts, executive summaries and conclusions are good for this. Then, read all the relevant literature carefully and critically. Keep an open mind, and consider that there might be alternative views and opinions expressed by different authors. Be aware of researcher bias, and ask yourself if the authors adequately explain their methodologies and if they provide evidence for the interpretations they make. Are their findings overgeneralised; that is, making conclusions beyond the scope of the study or work? Are there any conflicting views or contradictions? Identifying and communicating these issues in your writing will make your review all the more engaging and informative.

You also need to consider the quality of the literature. Has it been peer-reviewed? Whether you are dealing with primary, secondary or grey literature, all these sources of information can be of varying quality and rigour. It can be difficult to discern the reliability of any information, which is why the peer-review system is helpful. Brophy et al. (2008) discuss the 'hierarchy of evidence' in health research (Figure 8.2), a system which rates the level of the evidence provided based on the study design. That is not to say that you should avoid using anecdotal evidence and expert opinions in your writing; you just need to be clear about the reliability and source of the information. Evidence-based medicine is a relatively recent movement. It evolved as an attempt to move us away from a reliance on an individual's clinical expertise and a trial-and-error approach to new ideas, with some 'new ideas' having dire consequences for patients and the community. Sackett, Rosenberg, Gray, Haynes, and Richardson (1996) define *evidence-based medicine* as the 'conscientious, explicit, and judicious use of current best evidence

FIGURE 8.2 | HIERARCHY OF EVIDENCE (FROM BROPHY ET AL., 2008)

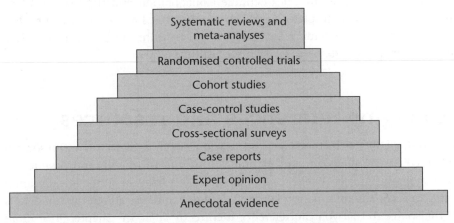

Anecdotal evidence – someone told you something works, or doesn't work.

Expert opinion – an editorial or a panel of experts draws up guidelines or gives a view of something based on many cases.

A case report – a systematic report using one example. It may be one hospital's experiences of a new system or one patient followed up after a new procedure.

Cross-sectional survey – a survey at one point in time.

Case control – people who have a disease as compared to people who do not have a disease in terms of things that might affect the disease. For example, people who have a stomach ulcer might take more anti-inflammatory tablets than people who do not have a stomach ulcer.

Cohort – Taking a group of people (the name comes from a cohort of Roman soldiers) and following them to see who develops the condition of interest. This is used for studies in work places where everyone in a certain job is followed but only some people may develop a disease. For example, those exposed to long-term noise may develop deafness. It could also be used to follow people with diabetes, some of whom attend a course and some who do not, and to see if control of the diabetes improves in those who attend a course. The important aspect of this study is that people should not have developed the condition or disease you are studying (e.g. deafness or improved control of diabetes) when the study starts.

Randomised controlled trial – assigning people to either receive a drug or attend a course (or any other intervention) in a random way (not dependent on, for example, the severity of their disease, the background of patients or the researcher's choice). This way those people who receive the drug and those who do not should be similar in everything except whether they are administrered the drug (that is, the same number of men and women, severe and mild disease, etc., in both groups).

A systematic review takes the results of completed studies – usually randomised controlled trials – and combines their results to give one overall answer.

A meta-analysis is the name for the statistical technique used to combine the findings of different studies on the same topic to give one overall, summary answer.

/ SYSTEMATIC REVIEW /
A systematic review
is a literature review
involving rigorous
critical assessment and
synthesis of all research
and evidence relating to
a particular question/
clinical issue.

in making decisions about the care of individual patients'. **Systematic reviews**, such as those produced by the Cochrane Collaboration and the Joanna Briggs Institute, are good examples of research studies that have been critically and rigorously assessed, providing best evidence to help inform practice. For more information about systematic reviews, see Griffiths (2009).

Managing references and resources

Developing effective methods for storing and retrieving references and resources will save an enormous amount of time during the writing-up and production phases of your project (Phelps et al., 2007). Make a habit of systematically filing hard copies of any information you find, and remember to attach the full details of the source so that you can reference it correctly later. See Chapter 9 for more detail on referencing strategies. If you are working on a smaller project, lists of references, related data and search words can be recorded in a spreadsheet (e.g. Excel) or a note-taking program (e.g. Microsoft OneNote). OneNote allows you to make notes about an article or book, create links between related notes, create links to documents and articles, and build relationships between all the literature that you have collected and your own notes and work.

For larger studies with many citations, reference-management software, such as EndNote, RefManager or RefWorks, is extremely useful. These tools allow you easily to create a database of citations (Phelps et al., 2007), as well as to export citation data for each article directly into a document created in a word-processing program such as Microsoft Word, using a selected referencing style, such as APA (American Psychological Association) style. These tools will insert in-text references and automatically generate a reference list at the end of your document. More recent reference-management programs allow you to attach a digital copy of journal articles to the references in your database. These can then be opened via your reference-management program. You can also add your own notes about a reference, or sort the references into groups according to topic, keywords, authors or various other criteria. Any notes can then be easily exported into an annotated reference list. A further advantage of using reference-management software is that all of your research and citations are stored and filed in one location.

Alternatively, if you prefer to do your referencing manually, and you like to keep hard copies or electronic copies of the references in your database or reference list, it is a good idea to develop a system to keep track of all of your research. For example, you can create an Excel spreadsheet that lists all of your research in groups or topics, or a OneNote file to keep notes about your research. Whichever tool or system you choose, it is important to maintain it consistently and accurately, and ensure that all your data is entered and stored there.

references

Brophy, S., Snooks, H., & Griffiths, L. (2008). *Small-scale evaluation in health: A practical guide*. London: Sage.

Griffiths, F. (2009). *Research methods for health care practice*. Los Angeles: Sage.

Machi, L. A., & McEvoy, B. T. (2009). *The literature review: Six steps to success*. Thousand Oaks, CA: Corwin Press.

Nieswiadomy, R. M. (2008). *Foundations of nursing research* (5th edn). Upper Saddle River, NJ: Pearson/Prentice Hall.

Phelps, R., Ellis, A., & Fisher, K. (2007). *Organizing and managing your research: A practical guide for postgraduates*. London: Sage.

Sackett, D. L., Rosenberg, W. M. C., Gray, J. A. M., Haynes, R. B., Richardson, W. S. (1996). Evidence-based medicine: What it is and what it isn't. *BMJ, 312*, 71–2.

useful web resources

For Google Scholar search engine, see
http://scholar.google.com.au/

For the Digital Object Identifier (DOI®) System, see
http://www.doi.org/

Bibliographic databases:

For the DAOJ (Directory of Open Access Journals), see
http://www.doaj.org/

For Ulrich's Periodicals Directory, Ulrichsweb, see
http://ulrichsweb.serialssolutions.com/

Systematic Reviews:

For The Joanna Briggs Institute, JBI COnNECT+, see
http://connect.jbiconnectplus.org/

For the Cochrane Collaboration, see
http://www.cochrane.org/

For the Nursing and Midwifery Board of Australia, see
http://www.nursingmidwiferyboard.gov.au/

For Occupational Therapy Critically Appraised Topics, OTCATS, see
http://www.otcats.com/

For Physiotherapy Evidence Database, PEDro, see
http://www.pedro.org.au/

Tutorials:

For PubMed tutorials, see
> http://www.nlm.nih.gov/bsd/disted/pubmed.html

For Virtual Training Suite: Developing Internet research skills, see
> http://www.vtstutorials.co.uk/

acknowledgments

We acknowledge Rola Ajjawi, Ann Sefton and Annette Street, who authored the chapter on this topic in the second edition of this book. Our chapter has revised and updated this earlier version.

CHAPTER
09 /

Reference systems and strategies

Joy **HIGGS** | Joan **ROSENTHAL** | Rola **AJJAWI**

key topics

This chapter covers the following topics:

- the place of referencing in scholarly writing

- referencing strategies

key terms

REFERENCES

PRIMARY SOURCE

SECONDARY SOURCE

Introduction

Referencing is about honesty, acknowledgment, legitimisation and accuracy. It is an essential component of authentic and high-quality scholarly writing. In most cases, written, verbal and electronic text is built on ideas and arguments that other people have already expressed. It is honest and responsible to acknowledge the original authors of these ideas by referencing their publications or communications in your work.

Referencing and sources

/ REFERENCES /
References acknowledge
the sources of the ideas,
information, data and
arguments you present
in your work.

/ PRIMARY SOURCE /
A primary source
is a work that gives
you direct or primary
knowledge of an event,
period, original thought
or research findings.

/ SECONDARY SOURCE /
A secondary source
provides commentary
written about a primary
source.

References acknowledge the sources of the ideas, information, data and arguments you present in your work. There are two main types of source (Spatt, 2003). A **primary source** is a work that gives you direct or primary knowledge of an event, period, original thought or research findings. A **secondary source** provides commentary about a primary source. Secondary sources are valuable when they summarise, critique or comment upon a range of primary sources. They can save you a great deal of time finding and reading all the original works, particularly if those works are difficult to obtain (such as unpublished manuscripts and old publications). However, your work, particularly research work and thesis, needs to demonstrate *your* original ideas and insights, your critiques and your interpretations of primary sources; so do not rely heavily on secondary sources. You have two broad ways of indicating that you are the source of an idea or argument:

- Implicitly: if no source is mentioned, then you as the author are assumed to be the source. All the arguments you present will be attributed to you.
- Explicitly, using the first person (such as 'In my opinion …') or using the third person (such as 'It can be argued that …'). Note that use of the first person in academic writing is not acceptable in some schools and disciplines.

The importance of referencing style and conventions

The style of referencing used in scholarly writing and referencing conventions is influenced by the writing situation—the referencing system used by your institution, school or teacher; the expectations of your field; the journal or publisher; and your own preferences. For assignments, you may be required to format the references according to a particular institutional style. Copy the required style exactly. If you have any questions, ask your lecturer before you start formatting. If there are no specific requirements, choose a well-known referencing style and use it consistently.

Bibliographies and reference lists

All the references you have used in your work must be included in your *reference list* at the end of your document. Alternatively, if your arguments have been indirectly influenced by a range of readings that you want to acknowledge, even if you have not mentioned them directly, you can include them in a second list called a *bibliography*.

Major referencing systems

Two common methods for referencing in the health professions are the APA (American Psychological Association) and Vancouver systems. The APA system uses the *author, year* format in the text. The Vancouver, or *numerical*, referencing system uses superscripted numbers to designate references in the text (such as 'Three major studies[1–3] involved …') and lists the references in numerical sequence in the reference list. See the resources list below for instructions for using these referencing systems.

Examples of references using the APA system

In-text references

References in the text are written as follows:

- *One reference, one or two authors:* 'It has been argued (French, 2009) that …' or 'Henry and Smith (2010) demonstrated that …' References come before the full stop if they occur at the end of the sentence.
- *One reference, more than two authors:* '(Jackson, et al., 2000)'. However, if this abbreviated format does not differentiate multi-authored references that were published in the same year, include as many authors as are needed to identify the reference; for example, '(Jackson, Black, et al., 2000)' contrasts with '(Jackson, Morton, et al., 2000)'.
- *Multiple references:* list in alphabetical order (unless directed otherwise, perhaps by a journal's style guide, which may require the references to be in chronological order).
- *Quotations:* include page numbers. The page number may be stated as part of the reference, as in '(Wentworth, 2011, p. 96)', or at the end of a block quote.
- *Personal communications:* '(Arrilla, June 2009, personal communication)'. Use this if you have had a conversation with someone. It does not need to be included in the reference list.

References in the reference list or bibliography

Journal articles

Finset, A. (2007). Nonverbal communication: An important key to in-depth understanding of provider–patient interaction. *Patient Education and Counselling, 66*, 127–8.

Edited books

Boud, D., & Lee, A. (Eds.) (2009). *Changing practices of doctoral education*. London: Routledge.

Authored books

Gannon, S. (2008). *Flesh and the text: Poststructural theory and writing research.* Saarbrücken: VDM Verlag.

Book chapters

Grant, M., & McMeeken, J. (2009). The physiotherapy workforce. In J. Higgs, M. Smith, G. Webb, M. Skinner & A. Croker (Eds.), *Contexts of physiotherapy practice* (pp. 44–57). Melbourne: Elsevier Australia.

Web publications

Innes, A., Macpherson, S. & McCabe, L. (2006). *Promoting person-centred care at the front line*. York: Joseph Rowntree Foundation. Retrieved from www.jrf.org.uk/bookshop/eBooks/9781859354520.pdf

VERIFYING WEBSITES

Websites change over time. They may even disappear. Check that the website is live and accessible at the time of publication.

Lectures and lecture notes

You may want to quote or refer to information provided in a lecture you attended. If this information was not published, provide the name of the course and the year:

> Communication Studies 301. (2000). Lecture notes.

Newspaper and magazine articles

If the author is named in a byline in a newspaper or magazine article, write the reference in the same way as for a journal article, stating the date of publication instead of the volume number. If no author's name is provided, use the name of the newspaper or magazine:

> *Australian*. (2003, June 15). Where are they now? p. 25.

Quotations

Quotations are verbatim extracts from published material. You must attribute this material to the original author or source. This is done by referencing the source and including the page number (if published), transcript reference (if research data) or date (if verbal information) pertaining to the quote. The following are some guidelines for formatting and reporting quotes:

- Use *inverted commas* or *quote marks* for quotes; for example, 'The incidence of influenza in this population rose to 13% in the subsequent two years' (Francis, 2007, p. 42). (Note that the reference is within the sentence, before the full stop.)

- Use *double inverted commas* for quotes within quotes, that is, when the original author was using quotation marks already. For example, 'Review of the various reports led to the conclusion that there had been "a significant misrepresentation" of the findings in several cases' (Kennedy, 2010, p. 339).

- For large quotes (more than five lines), use a left-indented paragraph, without inverted commas; for example:

  > Although clinicians may have knowledge of 'best practice', according to professional standards or the literature for a particular condition, they recognise that such generic best practice might not be the most appropriate for a particular patient's context, or best according to that patient's own perspective and priorities (Trede & Higgs, 2003, p. 67).

- Omit words from a quotation if you think they are unnecessary to your discussion and their omission will not change the original author's meaning. Use an ellipsis (…) to indicate that words have been deleted.

- Add words if necessary to make sense of the quotation (in order to explain words like 'it' and 'they') or to maintain the flow of the text where you have inserted the quotation. Put square brackets around the added words to show that this is *your* comment, not that of the person quoted; for example, 'For many patients this [increased waiting time] was a major problem.'

- If the text you are quoting contains inaccurate or undesirable spelling, words, or grammar, you may insert '[sic]' in the quote to show that you note the inaccuracy but you are quoting correctly from the original. For example, 'Practitioners who are in a sole practice needs [sic] to develop networking skills …'

- If desired, you may add emphasis within a quotation by *italicising* a word or words. Then write [emphasis added] after the quote.

Specific referencing strategies and tools

The following points explain some of the finer details of referencing:

- *Referencing in drafts*: use the author and year (and page number if required) method when writing so that you can reference accurately, even if you later have to change to another method, such as superscript numbers.

- *a and b references:* you may be referencing two papers by Smith and Hauser, both published in 2001. In this case, you need first to ensure that when you are making notes from those papers and when you are writing about them, you keep note of which paper you are referring to at each point. Second, list the references in the reference list as '(a)' and '(b)', using the authors and title alphabetically. In your paper, refer to the sources as 'Smith & Hauser (2001a)' and 'Smith & Hauser (2001b)' consistently throughout the text; for example:

  > Smith, R. E., & Hauser, L. S. (2001a). *Researching lived experiences.* Cambridge: Smithson.

  > *Smith, R. E., & Hauser, L. S. (2001b). Textual analysis.* Chicago: Perrington Books.

- *et al. ('and others'):* the use of 'et al.' saves the reader having to read many authors' names and possibly lose the flow of the text. If you have used 'et al.' in the text, be sure that the reader can determine exactly which reference you are referring to in the list.
- *Paraphrasing:* you paraphrase when you are using an idea or data from a source but are not quoting it directly, such as when the section is extensive and you want to abbreviate it, or to avoid excessive quotations. Paraphrases should be referenced the same as any idea derived from another source. Page numbers are not essential.
- *Describing your own work:* there are times when you are describing your research activities and you need to reference some aspect, such as the method used. Remember that the author of the work you are referencing did not write about your work. It is incorrect to write:

  > I used a reflective practitioner approach to the focus groups (Schön, 1983).

Instead, write:

  > I used Schön's (1983) notion of 'the reflective practitioner' to frame the focus-group discussion.

- *Citations:* sometimes you are using a secondary source and the author refers directly to a work by another person. The format for reporting this is:

  > Example 1: (Johns, 2000, p. 225, citing Graveney, 1982).

Here, Johns mentioned Graveney but did not provide the reference details. In your references, list Johns only.

Example 2: (Graveney, 1982, p. 84, cited in Blakehurst, 2001, p. 21).

Here, Blakehurst quoted from Graveney and provided the full reference details. In your references, list Graveney and give details of both the Graveney and Blakehurst publications within that reference.

Developing and storing your own reference lists

When developing a system for storing your references, record enough information to report the reference (and relevant content) accurately later and, if needed, to track it down again. Comprehensive bibliographical data can also help to retrieve references when you have only a limited recall of important components. For a writing task, you might have a long list of sources but only use some of them. Do not spend more time making your database than you do writing your essay! Keeping an electronic reference database is ideal, but remember to back it up regularly. Keep at least one copy away from the main computer, on disk, CD or server.

Electronic reference-management systems

The best bibliographic reference-management systems are electronic, because of their convenience in storing data and relative ease of searching through data (e.g. Endnote, ProCite and Reference Manager). Your university library will probably have online tutorials and site licences for these programs. You can also use standard software, such as word-processing and spreadsheet programs. The reference database(s) you develop will be invaluable in your future professional life and will support publication of your work. Once the information is entered accurately, it need never be retyped; the program can reformat the reference to the requirements of different referencing systems. Electronic references inserted into your paper, essay or thesis ensure that citations in the text will match the list of references at the end. References can also be downloaded automatically (without retyping) to your reference manager from literature search databases such as MEDLINE, CINAHL and ProQuest (see Chapter 8), or the information can be cut and pasted into your reference database.

Principles of storing references

Enough information should be stored to allow you to access and cite a specific work without ambiguity. Be thorough in recording information at the beginning; it will save time in the long run. References are stored electronically in *fields* that can be searched independently. The number and types of field you need to include in your references vary; check the journals in your area of study and your university's referencing guide. Record the locations (e.g. 'library') and reference numbers of hard copies in libraries.

Using keywords can help you retrieve references easily from your reference database. Be systematic in developing your own keyword systems. Software like EndNote allows you to create 'groups' and 'group sets' which are readily accessible without conducting a search. These may be linked to your keywords; for example:

- *for science:* topic, issue or discipline; experimental strategy; body system, organ and/or region; original paper or review; issues specific to your interests; location of source;
- *for clinical studies:* topic, discipline and/or diagnosis; nature or type of study; issue of concern; original paper or review; issues specific to your interests; location of source.

Developing a set of references as you write an assignment, thesis or paper

When writing, open both the word-processing file and the master reference database (often called a *library* in reference programs). To insert a citation into your text, toggle to the database, select one or more references that you want to insert in the text, copy them, return to the word-processing file and paste. Or, you may be using a program such as EndNote, which has a toolbar link to Word. Check the instructions for transferring references between the library and text. Citations appear, each with a unique identifier, in the text. When ready for formatting, the in-text citations are replaced by a number, or by a citation with the name(s) and date. Each in-text reference will be matched precisely with an item in the bibliography.

Leave yourself enough time for this formatting component of your task. Be sure to proofread and spell-check the reference list at the end of the process, and go back to correct any errors in your database. If you are citing from British, American and Australian books and journals, you might find differences in spelling within the references (e.g. in the titles of book, articles and journals); these should always be left as published.

conclusion

Referencing has two main purposes: it demonstrates the academic honesty of your writing and it informs readers of the sources of your ideas and information. If your readers want to follow up any of the sources you mention to find any published background material, they should be able to obtain all the details they need from your writing. Take care to acknowledge and record accurately any sources that have contributed to what you write.

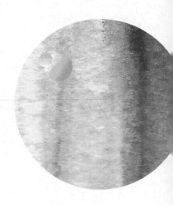

references

Note: Some references in this chapter have been included for illustrative purposes only. They are not included in this reference list.

Spatt, B. (2003). *Writing from sources* (6th edn). Boston, MA: Bedford/St Martin's Press.

resources for referencing

Murdoch University. (2011). *Referencing.* http://library.murdoch.edu.au/Getting-help/Referencing/

This has information for APA, Vancouver, Chicago, and a number of other commonly used reference systems.

APA referencing system

American Psychological Association. (2010). *Publication manual of the American Psychological Association* (6th edn). Washington, DC: American Psychological Association. This book contains detailed instructions for APA referencing of all types of material.

American Psychological Association. (2011). *APA style.* Retrieved from http:/www.apastyle.org/. This website contains links to APA blog, Twitter, Facebook, FAQs, and more.

Style manual for authors, editors and printers. (2002). (6th edn., rev. Snooks & Co.). Milton: John Wiley & Sons Australia.

Formatting and text styles

Charles **HIGGS** | Joy **HIGGS** | Ros **ALLUM**

key topics

This chapter covers the following topics

- using styles in Word documents

- using preset and customised styles

- managing large documents

key term

STYLE

Introduction

Presentation and layout are important in reports, papers, assignments and theses. It is valuable to learn strategies and functions that help with these tasks, such as the use of inbuilt and optional styles in software programs to streamline word processing. Functions such as styles, automated tables of contents and templates make creating your documents easier, and help achieve greater consistency of layout and format.

A note about versions before you begin: the instructions in this chapter relate to Microsoft Word 2010 (Word). There are differences between the various versions of Word and other software programs.

What are styles and how can they save me time?

When we make a word bold, we change only one characteristic of the word's *format*. When we apply a **style** to a word or sentence in Word we can change an entire set of characteristics at once, and by changing the style again later you can update a whole document at the same time.

Styles enable you to format different types of text consistently and in line with your preferences, right throughout your document. Styles give structure to your document. For example, when a style has been applied, Word will know whether the words you have typed are meant to be a heading, subheading, body text etc.

Managing long documents in Word

Many people ignore the time-saving functions in word-processing packages like Word 2010. Manually formatting short documents is fine, but when it comes to more complex documents like theses, reports or books, it is worth spending a little time to learn some of the more advanced features of the software. Heading styles can save you a considerable amount of time. They make it easy for you to find your place in a long document such as a thesis and can assist you in building a table of contents.

Activating Styles panel and applying styles

When you are creating the structure of a document, it is helpful to display the *Styles* panel. This can be activated by clicking on the small arrow in the bottom right corner of the *Styles* box, located under the *Home* tab. The *Styles* panel shows all the styles available for that particular document.

It is easy to find out which style is currently applied; simply place your cursor on a particular piece of text, scroll through the styles in the *Styles* panel, where a blue box indicates the style for that text. To apply a particular style, place your cursor on the text you want to change, then click on the selected style name in the *Styles* panel.

Predefined styles

Microsoft Word comes with a large number of built-in or predefined styles. Word automatically attaches a style to each paragraph—the default style is called *Normal*. The default font for *Normal* style in Word 2010 is Times Roman 12 point, with no paragraph spacing. If you want to change the style of your paragraph, you need to change the characteristics of the *Normal* style.

/ **STYLE** /

When we apply a style to a word or sentence in Word we can change an entire set of characteristics at once. Styles enable you to format different types of text consistently. Styles give structure to your document.

Planning the structure of your document and customising your styles

It is worth spending a few minutes selecting and then customising a significant new document with the styles you prefer, especially when creating lengthy documents. You might also set up a personal style in a blank document (see the section on Templates, below) and use this for all your assignments and other documents. A very small number of styles can cover the vast majority of your work. For example, most documents would not require more than body text, three heading levels and a bullet list.

To select your preferred font, size, and paragraph spacing, right-click on the *Normal* style in the *Styles* panel and select *Modify*. Select a font and size and then click on the *Format* button. Choose *Paragraph* from the drop-down menu. Next, select the amount of spacing you would like to use before or after your paragraphs, or whether you would like your paragraphs indented (it is better to use spacing or indenting but not both). For example, you could choose to insert a 6-point space after each paragraph to break up text blocks and give some visual space.

Now, turn your attention to the default headings offered in Word. The *Heading* styles define the hierarchical structure of your document and enable you to use other Word features like creation of tables of contents and *Outline* view (see below). Start by choosing the default headings or modifying three heading levels in line with your preferences. Right-click on *Heading 1*, choose *Modify*, then make your selections. Similarly, follow this procedure with *Heading 2* and *Heading 3*. Finally, scroll through the *Styles* panel and select *List Bullet 1*. Right-click on it and select *Modify* then click on *Format* in the bottom-left corner. From the drop-down menu, select *Numbering*, click on the *Bullet* tab and choose your preferred bullet. Click on *OK*.

Changing styles

If you decide to change the look of your document, you can modify the selected style. Word will instantly update all instances of that style throughout the document, no matter how large the document. For instance, if you consider that your document needs a more spacious look, you can change the *Body Text* style to increase the space between lines or after each paragraph.

Templates

The styles you apply to a document will stay with that document, even when opened by someone else who uses different styles. You can also save your preferred style as a *template* (i.e. a blank document with preserved format for repeated use) for use in other documents. To do this, select *Save As (a template file)*, and navigate to the *Templates* folder. The document can then be accessed via *My Templates* under the *Available Templates* dialog box. Note that templates are stored in the computer on which you are working. If you want to move a template from one computer to another, you must copy the template to the second computer. Each time you open the template you should save the file as a document file with a relevant name.

Table of contents

Once a document is complete, styles make the creation of a table of contents very simple. Under the *References* tab, select *Table of Contents*, then *Insert Table of Contents*, from the drop-down menu. Decide how many levels of heading you would like to show in the contents and then select *OK*. If you edit the document further, the table of contents can be quickly updated by selecting the table and either pressing the **F9** key or selecting the *Update Table* option within the *Table of Contents* tab.

FORMAT PAINTER

Have you ever found yourself continually formatting different aspects in a document? Perhaps changing font size, colour or bolding?

By using the *Format Painter* button 🖌, you can copy *just the formatting* from a highlighted section of text to another item. Highlight the text you want to copy, click the *Format Painter* button, then highlight the text to which you want the formatting applied— the formatting is instantly applied.

If you have more than one item to format, double-click the *Format Painter* button. This will turn on the *Format Painter* for as long as you need. When you have finished, simply press the **Esc** key. ●

Serif and sans serif fonts

Readability is central to good typography. There are two main kinds of typeface: *serif* and *sans serif*. The small decorative finish at the end or bottom of a letter is called a serif. Observe the differences in these fonts:

$$gp \quad gp$$

Sans serif typeface   *Serif typeface*

The characters on the left do not have the decorations, so are in a sans-serif font (*sans* is the French word for 'without'). The characters on the right have serifs, and are called *serif fonts*.

Serif typefaces are clearer and more familiar in design, as well as easier to read in large blocks. Newspapers, books and magazines generally use this kind of typeface. Some commonly used *serif* typefaces include Garamond, Times New Roman and Georgia. *Sans serif* typefaces can place more strain on the eyes, but are commonly used in headlines, as they can have greater impact. Some commonly used *sans serif* typefaces include Arial, Verdana and Tahoma.

WHY DOES MY DOCUMENT LOOK DIFFERENT WHEN VIEWED ON ANOTHER COMPUTER?

Ever noticed that a document you have been working on looks different on your work and home computers?

1. The most common reason that the layout of your work changes when viewed on different computers relates to the printer. When your document is viewed in *Print Layout* view, the properties of the selected printer can affect the layout. Consequently, aspects such as the default paper size and margins can result in a document looking noticeably different when viewed on other computers. Changes to the document can also be seen if your computer is connected to more than one printer. To view the changes, go to *Print*, selecting a different printer each time. Depending on the characteristics of the individual printer, the changes could be either significant or subtle.

2. Another possible reason for different layouts is the use of fonts that are not available on both systems. If a document is created using a unique font that is installed on only one of the computers, Word will attempt to substitute a similar font. This can affect the layout and readability of your document. It is advisable, therefore, if you are working on a document that will be viewed on different computers or in PowerPoint presentations, to select a commonly used font such as Times New Roman or Arial, unless you plan to embed the fonts (look this up in *Help*) in your document. ●

Outline view and the *Navigation Pane*

Once a document becomes larger than a few pages, the ability to move between sections and to reorganise or restructure your document is important and can save you a considerable amount of time. To take advantage of the time-saving features offered by *Outline* view or the *Navigation Pane*, it is important that your document is created using Word's styles. The drag-and-drop function in *Outline view* allows you to move an entire section (including subheadings) very easily.

Outline view

We typically view a page in either *Draft* or *Print Layout* view. In *Outline* view, you can view an entire document or only specific headings in the document, and you can move sections or change formatting using *Outline*. You can also see all your headings minimised to any level of heading you select. In *Outline* view you can navigate rapidly around a very large document before switching back to an alternative view. As well, subheadings can be promoted to higher level headings or main headings can be demoted to subheadings, simply by clicking on the right- or left-arrow keys.

The Navigation Pane

The *Navigation Pane* offers the same functions. To view the *Navigation Pane*, click on the *View* tab and ensure that the *Navigation Pane* section is ticked. By clicking on any heading in the *Navigation Pane*, you can readily move to different sections in your document.

TIPS FOR PREPARING DOCUMENTS

1. Ensure you add page numbers to your document.

2. Do not use too many different fonts in the one document, as this makes a document look disorganised. Avoid using bold and underlining together as this is considered bad practice.

3. Avoid *hard page breaks* (breaks that force the document to stop and restart on the next page)—if your document is printed using a printer with a slightly different print area, hard page breaks may result in a small amount of text flowing onto a separate page.

4. Don't overcrowd your pages with too much content.

5. Make use of Word's built-in *Document themes* which ensure fonts, colours and graphic effects have a coordinated look. These can be accessed via the *Themes* gallery in the *Page Layout* tab.

6. Apply *styles* to your document to provide a consistent look.

7. Add visual interest to your document by illustrating key points. A large variety of professional quality graphics can be created using *SmartArt* in Word. Many different layouts can be selected, including lists, diagrams, organisational charts, timelines, process or cycle diagrams. The *SmartArt* icon can be found on the *Insert* tab under *Illustrations*.

8. Make use of Word's *Cross-reference* feature, to refer to a footnote, endnote, figure or table elsewhere in your document. These update automatically if content moves. The *Cross-reference* feature can be found under the *References* tab, in the *Captions* section.

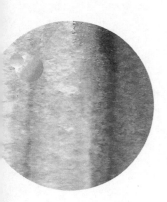

conclusion

Presentation and layout are important in undergraduate reports, theses and journal articles. The features in your word-processing software can help you to improve the layout and aesthetic presentation of your work. The features can also increase the ease and efficiency of creating and managing large documents.

useful web resources

For useful tips and step-by-step instructions to help make the most of Word's features, see http://www.shaunakelly.com/word

For *answers* to readers' questions, simple computer tips and general online technical support, see Leo Notenboom's website http://ask-leo.com/.

Communicating in problem-based learning classes

Stephen **LOFTUS** | Rola **AJJAWI** | Sarah **HYDE**

key topics

This chapter covers the following topics:

- problem-based learning (PBL) as an active, self-directed learning process

- the roles of students and tutors in PBL

- optimising participation in PBL tutorials

key terms

PROBLEM-BASED LEARNING

SELF-DIRECTED LEARNING

FACILITATE

Introduction

Problem-based learning (PBL) is increasingly being implemented in health sciences curricula. The focus in this chapter is on PBL programs where clinical problem-solving is a part of professional practice. The general strategies described in this chapter are also applicable to PBL tutorials in other professional education courses. Students are active participants in these programs, determining their own learning topics and constructing their understanding together. To be effective, the process requires styles of participation, interaction and learning that are different from those of traditional university classrooms. Mutual trust and support between group members, and also between the group and the tutor, is essential. In this chapter you will learn what characterises PBL and how you can make the most of the method.

What is PBL?

/ PROBLEM-BASED
LEARNING (PBL) /
Problem-based learning
(PBL) is one particular
method of case-based,
active learning which
has been growing in
popularity in higher
education for many
years.

/ SELF-DIRECTED
LEARNING /
Students are
encouraged to assume
responsibility for their
self-directed learning by
identifying knowledge
gaps, then finding and
appraising information
to close those gaps,
and following up
any learning issues
pertinent to the case
(Taylor & Miflin, 2008).
Identifying knowledge
gaps is an important
part of PBL.

/ FACILITATE /
To facilitate, the tutor
uses questions to
explore and stimulate
student thinking, and
helps the group set
standards for depth and
breadth of knowledge,
develop reasoning
ability and enhance
communication skills.

Problem-based learning (PBL) is one particular method of case-based, active learning which has been growing in popularity in higher education for many years. This is because the process both models realistic clinical problem-solving and encourages the understanding of underlying mechanisms in health and disease. Students work cooperatively as a team, now a common practice reality for many health professionals. There are many variations on the original version. Common to most variations is that learning starts with a patient encounter, often a paper or virtual case, requiring some action or management. Through this experience students can integrate their knowledge of anatomy, physiology and other discipline areas within the scope of the patient case. Students are encouraged to assume responsibility for their **self-directed learning** by identifying knowledge gaps, then finding and appraising information to close those gaps, and following up any learning issues pertinent to the case (Taylor & Miflin, 2008). Identifying knowledge gaps is an important part of PBL.

Problem-based learning requires students to work in small groups to explore and resolve clinical problems devised by curriculum staff. Each problem typically extends for a week, sometimes longer. Tutors do not teach content knowledge per se, but act to **facilitate** the learning and group process.

Problem-based learning has been shown to be effective in supporting students' self-directed learning and in enhancing other skills: effective communication, the confident use of clinical and scientific language, integrating knowledge, practising critical reasoning and identifying gaps in personal understanding (Boud & Feletti, 1997; Schmidt, Vermeulen, & van der Molen, 2006). Other studies have shown that medical students from PBL curricula demonstrate deeper learning approaches (Van der Veken, Valcke, Muijtjens, De Maeseneer, & Derese, 2008) and greater propensity for self-regulation of learning (White, 2007). Students are able to solve realistic cases safely through PBL. If the group gets it wrong nobody is hurt. Problem-based learning can be particularly effective when it is integrated across disciplines, and it lends itself to inter-professional learning programs. Occasionally, variants of PBL are used within a single subject, perhaps relating to complex issues and research questions. For example, a group might work through a case of cancer, complicated by advanced diabetes, where there are numerous problems to be sorted out, many of which are the subject of active research programs at the institution.

The role of a PBL tutor

It is important to appreciate the tutor's responsibilities in PBL. Tutors facilitate the learning process and encourage all students to participate. A good tutor will be a 'guide on the side' and not a 'sage on the stage' (King, 1993). This means that tutors will rarely, if ever, formally 'teach' in a conventional sense. Neither will tutors be quick to indicate that ideas are 'right' or 'wrong', although they will subtly encourage the group to challenge and review unclear or dubious statements. When groups are working smoothly, tutors might intervene only rarely. Problem-based learning offers the potential for extensive communication among the members of the group. Tutors ensure smooth interactions and encourage a single shared conversation. They encourage and empower quieter group members, and may make suggestions when the conversation stalls. Sometimes they help the group to manage an over-enthusiastic, dominant or even disruptive personality. In the review of each problem, tutors provide feedback and make suggestions about the group's process. They may invite the students to make comments on the group's progress. It is important for discussion to be honest, but also for everyone to be sensitive to the feelings of others.

Your tutor might meet with all group members individually, to discuss each student's contribution, develop knowledge and address concerns. A perceptive tutor will offer insightful comments about your progress, highlighting your strengths and weaknesses in the PBL process so as to enhance your skills in group settings.

The PBL process

The PBL cycle begins when the student group is introduced to the problem. In health sciences, the problem, usually developed around a patient, might emphasise diagnosis, management or social issues, depending on the focus of the profession. Groups typically meet two or three times for discussion. The tutor may reveal information progressively in tutorials, or further data may be presented on paper or via the web. In some programs an online forum is used to facilitate the learning process, particularly if people are out in the field and want to link into the support network. Virtual patients are increasingly being used in the PBL process to promote clinical thinking.

A *trigger* is presented on paper, video or computer. Triggers can be short (such as that in Case Study 11.1), stimulating immediate interaction and responses. Alternatively, substantial and detailed information might be provided in an initial handout of a few pages.

CASE STUDY II.I
EXAMPLE OF A SHORT TRIGGER

Antonio Rinaldo, aged eight, presents in distress at the local dentist's surgery with his mother after falling off his skateboard in the park an hour ago. His mouth is bleeding and his mother has one of his teeth in a handkerchief.

During brainstorming, a typical group would raise the following issues: How do we deal with his distress? What are the first things we should say to him and his mother? Where is the bleeding coming from? Is it a 'baby tooth'? What should we do with the tooth? Is it possible to reimplant it? What about germs? He has a Mediterranean name: why might that be significant? What do we need to know about his family? And so on. These issues are prioritised before the group goes on to develop a set of questions to ask Antonio and his mother.

Although in PBL the discussion is often free-flowing and lively, there is an underlying structure. One common structure is the so-called Maastricht '7 jump' approach (named after the medical school where it originated) (Schmidt, 1983):

1. clarifying terms and concepts
2. defining the problem
3. analysing the problem/brainstorming
4. categorising (critiquing possible explanations)
5. formulating learning issues/objectives
6. self-study
7. discussion of newly acquired knowledge (and sharing with the rest of the group).

After the trigger, a brainstorming session ensures that issues are identified and noted, usually on a whiteboard. It is important at first to think broadly and record the ideas, exploring everyone's prior knowledge of relevance in the process. The hypotheses listed are subsequently organised and scrutinised critically in a general discussion. The group rejects obviously incorrect or unlikely possibilities. Hypotheses are then generated to try to explain the key data presented in the trigger. During these processes, the group identifies and records learning issues that members will need to understand to advance towards resolution of the problem. As a group member, you may note additional items for your individual follow-up after the class meetings.

When the group breaks up, students study the issues identified, using the textbooks or resources provided (either online or in libraries) to advance their understanding. Informal learning or study groups can be effective supports. Practical classes, online resources, lectures, seminars, skills sessions or clinical encounters may be provided to help students understand the issues raised by the problem and develop skills needed to deal with it in real life.

In subsequent meetings, the group reassembles for members to share their new understanding in discussion, and to identify and organise further information needed from the 'patient'. In response to appropriate questions, the tutor may provide information or offer a handout or online access to data. The group agrees on a tentative diagnosis or list of problems (if that is the focus), and constructs a mechanism to explain the patient's problems or symptoms, taking into account basic and clinical sciences, and geographic and social factors. In discussion, the group usually identifies additional learning issues for individual study. A final resolution and management plan is agreed jointly.

Students' roles in a PBL group

The degree of interdependence between the tutor and the group, and between individual students within the group, is one of the unique characteristics of PBL. This interdependence can affect the way PBL groups function and may also influence the extent to which the tutor regulates the group, and the ability of students to regulate and transfer their learning.

As a group member, you have a responsibility to contribute actively but sensitively to the problem-solving process. When a new group forms, it is a good idea to agree on some simple expectations (also known as *ground rules*) with your tutor. Although it is important to challenge ideas, the PBL process depends on mutual trust and respect for others. Each person must have a chance to express his or her ideas. In groups, the collective knowledge may be enough to resolve the problem, but that understanding must be constructed in collaboration with all the individuals in the group.

Most groups elect a secretary to ensure that information is passed between the tutor or faculty and students. The group should ensure that the secretary has everyone's email and phone contact details. At each tutorial, a scribe records the discussion (e.g. on a whiteboard or computer) by summarising and organising the points raised, so that important ideas are not lost. It is customary to rotate this task around the group, as it helps develop valuable skills such as critical listening, comprehension and summarising.

When the problem trigger is introduced, everyone contributes to the brainstorming, discussion and refining of ideas. If you have particular knowledge of the subject it can sometimes be frustrating not to take over, but all need to participate and develop their own understanding, as well as the understanding of the group as a whole. You will probably eventually get the chance to share your knowledge, but should avoid simply delivering information to the others.

Some institutions use senior students as facilitators, and developing these skills will be useful for you in the long term.

After each tutorial, you will usually identify key issues to study. At the next tutorial, presenting and discussing the information is important to ensure that all members are informed on the key issues. You should feel comfortable questioning ideas that seem unclear or incorrect, and expanding on others when you have specific knowledge. Be sure that everyone's conceptual understanding is clear, but remember to confine any criticisms you have to the content, not the individual presenting it. You have an obligation to participate in feedback or problem review sessions (commonly held at the end of each problem or case). You are usually expected to complete evaluation forms, and it is important to give honest opinions. Try, however, to suggest improvements rather than simply offer criticism.

WORKING IN PBL GROUPS

- Your first priority is to be an active participant and to always be willing to offer suggestions, be critical of information, encourage others to participate, provide feedback and come prepared to contribute to the discussion.

- Maintain ground rules and know your role within the group for each particular session.

- Treat the other members of your learning group with respect and honesty, and expect the same from them.

- Be prepared both to listen and to take your turn in discussion. While you must avoid putting your colleagues down, it is important to critique faulty logic and to challenge information you think is wrong.

- You have an obligation to work on the group's agreed study topics, not only for yourself but also to contribute to later discussions. Work out early which textbooks are most appropriate and use them. Consult any web-based resources provided, and check the validity and reliability of information you find.

- You may find it particularly helpful to work with a few other students in an informal cooperative learning group outside tutorials.

- Be prepared to reflect on the group's progress and on your own performance. Contribute to evaluation sessions each week.

- Suggest ways to improve the group's work, but be sensitive to the feelings of others. Positive suggestions are usually better received than negative remarks.

- Think carefully about any criticism of your contributions—do not just assume that it is ill-informed or wrong. Reflect on any personal feedback you receive, and seek further advice from the tutor or your colleagues if you need it.
- Be prepared (tactfully) to raise issues of concern about the group's functioning, the tutor's style or the process itself. Complete evaluation forms if asked. ⬤

Being a good group member

Active participation and collaboration are essential to the PBL process. Offer to share the different roles; you will find it a rewarding experience. Be careful not to dominate, even when you have special knowledge or experience. On the other hand, avoid being passive. You will learn most by actively suggesting and exploring ideas, even if they turn out to be wrong. Although some of your group may not be particular friends of yours, everyone brings something to the group. In professional life you will usually not be able to choose the members of working teams. See Chapters 26 to 29 for discussions of group dynamics and the roles of group members.

It is particularly important to manage your time. It is easy to become absorbed in certain fascinating issues, but you must ensure that you understand and learn the core elements of the problem. Study plans are also important (see Chapter 5). If you find interesting information, be sure to record it accurately so that you can find it again, and remember to share it with the group.

Issues in PBL

Students in PBL programs are sometimes uncertain about what to learn and how much depth is required, especially in the early days. If goals seem unclear, discuss them within your group and ask staff for clarification. Take advantage of any guidelines on skills, competencies or the depth and breadth of knowledge. Use formative assessments (trial examinations, past papers or questions on the web) to identify your strengths and weaknesses without penalty; you will gain confidence by doing them.

The presence of a disruptive group member or interpersonal differences between members can create difficulties. Raise concerns frankly but sensitively, and encourage the group and the tutor to explore solutions. The group may also need to consider approaching (tactfully) a tutor who intervenes too much or too little. At worst, remember that group members (and tutors) often rotate each term or semester!

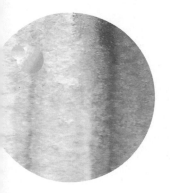

conclusion

In many courses, student participation in PBL is seen as an important part of the curriculum. Proponents of this method describe it as both effective and enjoyable, with major advantages over more traditional models of education (see Schmidt et al., 2006). Problem-based learning can provide realistic learning, and gaps in student knowledge are not only accepted but are seen as providing the motivation to learn. However, successful PBL needs all group members to participate actively. We hope you make the most of your PBL experiences.

references

Boud, D. J., & Feletti, G. (Eds.) (1997). *The challenge of problem-based learning* (2nd edn). London: Kogan Page.

King, A. (1993). From sage on the stage to guide on the side. *College Teaching, 41*(1), 30–5.

Schmidt, H. G. (1983). Problem-based learning: Rationale and description. *Medical Education, 17*, 11–16.

Schmidt, H. G., Vermeulen, L., & van der Molen, H. T. (2006). Longterm effects of problem-based learning: A comparison of competencies acquired by graduates of a problem-based and a conventional medical school. *Medical Education, 40*(6), 562–7.

Taylor, D., & Miflin, B. (2008). Problem-based learning: Where are we now? *Medical Teacher, 30*(8), 742–63.

Van der Veken, J., Valcke, M., Muijtjens, A., De Maeseneer, J., & Derese, A. (2008). The potential of the inventory of learning styles to study students' learning patterns in three types of medical curricula. *Medical Teacher, 30*(9–10), 863–9.

White, C. (2007). Smoothing out transitions: How pedagogy influences medical students' achievement of self-regulated learning goals. *Advances in Health Sciences Education, 12*(3), 279–97.

acknowledgments

We would like to acknowledge the contribution of Professor Ann Sefton, a pioneer of PBL, who was an author of this chapter in earlier editions of this book.

CHAPTER 12

Giving effective presentations in class

Narelle **PATTON** | Maree **SIMPSON**

key topics

This chapter covers the following topics:

- importance of effective presentation skills

- delivering an effective presentation

- assessing your own performance through reflection

- listening, viewing and responding to presentations

key terms

PRESENTATION SKILLS

CASE STUDY PRESENTATIONS

ROLE-PLAY

Introduction

As a health professional, you will be required to give presentations in a variety of contexts, including case presentations, health promotion programs and client group education sessions. Thus, the ability to develop and deliver effective presentations is critical to successful health professional practice. As a student, you will be required to deliver a range of presentations in class to assist development of the appropriate communication skills required for professional practice. These class presentations may include formal presentations, **case study presentations** and role-plays.

In this chapter we discuss the importance of **presentation skills** to health professional practice, and we describe many contexts in which health professionals may be required to give and respond to presentations. We also provide tips for development and delivery of effective presentations, including reflective processes that facilitate the improvement of future presentations, and we consider how you can fulfil your responsibility as an audience member.

/ CASE STUDY PRESENTATIONS / Case study presentations involve you being able to briefly describe your client's progress to date, treatment interventions, response to treatment, anticipated timeframes and future recommendations.

Importance of effective presentation skills

/ **PRESENTATION SKILLS** /
Effective presentation skills form a significant component of the raft of communication skills integral to successful health professional practice.

The importance of oral presentation skills to professional practice is generally recognised, with many university lecturers and tutors requiring students to make oral presentations (De Grez, Valcke & Roozen, 2009). As a student, you will likely be required to give a presentation to your peers in a class situation at some stage. Like many other people, you may initially react to public speaking with fear and trepidation, and a tight knot developing in the pit of your stomach. You may ask yourself some of the following questions: Why is this being asked of me? Is this because the lecturer/tutor does not have time to research evidence-based information on all of these topics? In fact, you will be asked to undertake a presentation because your lecturers and tutors recognise that giving a presentation in class is good preparation for workplace learning and, ultimately, professional practice. Clinically, high-quality oral presentations have the potential to enhance client care (Davenport, Honigman & Druck, 2008) and facilitate sharing of important client-related information between healthcare professionals (Green, DeCherrie, Fagan, Sharpe & Hershman, 2011).

Through engagement in class presentations, students become active participants in the learning process and improve their understanding of a topic by being required to research, organise content and articulate their understanding to an audience. Students also learn to present their ideas clearly and concisely, a skill that is integral to successful healthcare practice, for example when presenting case summaries at team meetings. Student class presentations provide a perfect opportunity for students to gain feedback from three perspectives: the tutor, peers and self, thus further broadening the learning experience (Sterling, 2008). At the conclusion of a presentation, when students respond to their audience they are required to acknowledge the viewpoints of their peers and, in so doing, are able to check their understanding of a topic with that of their peers, and potentially extend their own understanding.

Different styles of presentation

You may be asked to undertake many different styles of presentation while at university, during workplace learning and throughout your professional career. Presentations are context-dependent and vary in level of formality, length and desired outcomes.

Class presentations

Class presentations are often formal, with students electing to use multimedia; PowerPoint is a popular choice to assist delivery of the message. See Chapter 13 for advice on creating effective PowerPoint presentations. The presentation may be assessable, and may be undertaken individually or as part of a group. Group presentations provide a unique set of challenges, including managing conflict if certain members are not pulling their weight. It is important to remember during class presentations that, as presenter, you are responsible for facilitating the learning of the group.

Discussion groups

Discussion group presentations are often less formal, perhaps requiring you to report back to your class on key points generated by your group during a discussion. These reports are usually brief, and you should clearly, comprehensively and concisely summarise the group discussion. It is important in this report that the views of all group members are represented, not only those that agree with your own.

Role-plays

Role-play in a classroom environment usually involves acting out a clinical scenario in front of fellow students. Participation in role-play helps students to translate theoretical knowledge to clinical practice, encourages social interaction, and can reflect a wealth of humour, creativity, sensitivity to cultural issues and analytic thinking (Higgens-Opitz & Tufts, 2010). Active engagement in role-play opportunities provides a rich learning opportunity for all students.

/ **ROLE-PLAY** /
Role-play involves students acting out a clinical scenario in front of fellow students.

Case study presentations

As a health professional, and even as a student while undertaking work placement, you may be required to speak at a team meeting or case conference. This will usually involve briefly describing your client's progress to date, treatment interventions, response to treatment, anticipated timeframes and future recommendations. When you present case studies to your peers in the classroom, following this structure will provide excellent practice for delivering case presentations during workplace learning. See Chapter 23 for information regarding presenting at case conferences.

Presenting research to professionals at a team meeting

You may be required to present findings of research or an ongoing quality assurance project to your colleagues at a team meeting. Students often find presenting to professional colleagues a nerve-racking experience. Do not be afraid to generate discussion in these situations as, in this way, everyone learns from the shared wisdom generated by the group.

Developing and giving an effective presentation

Effective presentations are clear, concise and follow a logical sequence. Effective presenters are excellent communicators who connect with an audience by making eye contact and smiling. Presenting is a skill like any other, and can be developed with time and effort. Think back to a presentation you enjoyed and which made a lasting impression. Try to identify the positive aspects of this presentation; for example, was it logical and clearly articulated? Did it use images that appealed to you? You can use your experience of other people's presentations, as well as the helpful tips provided below, to develop your own presentation skills.

Preparation

The first step in presentation development is to identify the aims of your presentation and, most importantly, your core message. Reynolds (2008) advises that presentation development is a creative act, best undertaken away from the computer, to enable you to see more clearly the bigger picture without the distraction offered by multimedia software such as PowerPoint. Once you have identified your key messages, you need solid content and logical structure for your presentation. At this stage, you may need to undertake research to develop the content for your presentation. Your finished presentation should include appropriate content arranged in an efficient, logical and aesthetically pleasing manner.

Having recorded your key points and assembled an outline or structure, you can now use multimedia software to develop your presentation. Inclusion of appropriate images is an effective way to assist an audience to understand your point and provide a more visceral and emotional connection to your ideas. Images in slide presentations should be chosen carefully to ensure that they support and emphasise the messages you want to convey to the audience. Appropriate images can more than double audience comprehension and retention, but use of inappropriate images can be worse than using none at all (Wing, 2009).

Oral rehearsal of your presentation is crucial to effective delivery. Practise your presentation aloud, with timing, to ensure that you will be able to complete your presentation comfortably in the allotted time.

Delivery

Good presentations are about conversing, sharing and connecting at an intellectual and emotional level, in an honest and sincere way with an audience (Reynolds, 2008). One of the most important things to remember when delivering a presentation is to be fully present at that moment in time. A good presenter is fully committed to the moment, committed to being there with the audience (Reynolds, 2008). Before you start your presentation, take a deep breath, establish eye contact with the audience and smile, in order to establish a connection with your audience.

It is also important to remember that your mannerisms during a presentation form a critical part of the communication process. Presenters who appear trustworthy, confident and enthusiastic will make a favourable impression with their audience. Specific delivery traits most often associated with successful presentations include eye contact with the audience and vocal variety, incorporating clear diction and appropriate volume, and avoiding unnatural pauses and pronunciation problems (Leeds, Raven & Brawley, 2007). Less reliance on reading from presenter notes will help you to develop a good rapport with your audience. Credibility and confidence can be negatively affected by performance anxiety. Fear of speaking can lead to behaviours such as speaking too softly and quickly, shifting body weight repeatedly and avoiding eye contact. Nervous mannerisms distract audiences and can be interpreted to mean the presenter is unsure of the content, and detracts from overall presentation quality (Wing, 2009).

The opening words of your presentation are important because they establish your topic and create rapport with the audience. Effective beginnings command audience attention, highlight your main messages and set out the framework of the presentation. If you are feeling nervous it is useful to memorise the opening words of your presentation, as a good start will build your confidence.

Finally, your points will be more persuasive and easily understood if you illustrate them with an anecdote, story or use of metaphor throughout your presentation. At the conclusion of your presentation, summarise the key points and emphasise the main message to enhance audience understanding.

Fielding questions

After a presentation you will often be required to answer audience questions. Many presenters feel nervous about this. Experienced presenters anticipate likely audience questions and prepare responses in advance. Fielding questions after a presentation requires a certain level of tact, as you need to listen carefully and sensitively acknowledge views sometimes different to your own. When a question is asked, avoid rushing to answer; repeat the question so that all can hear, and give yourself time to consider your answer. If you are unsure of the meaning of a question, repeat or paraphrase it in your own words. If you do not know the answer to a question, say so—you may consider asking members of the audience and thereby gain knowledge from the shared wisdom of the audience.

Speaking to an audience you know well

Many presenters find speaking to an audience they know well at best difficult and at worst intimidating. When giving a presentation to your class you are likely to know your audience well, which may have the adverse effect of increasing your nervousness. It is therefore important when presenting to your peers to start strongly, and gain their respect and attention from the beginning of your presentation. To maintain audience attention, consider what your audience knows already and focus on information that will be new and interesting. This will encourage them to take you seriously, and respect your information and analysis.

PRESENTATIONS ARE ABOUT MAKING A CONTRIBUTION

Remember that presentations are about making a contribution to audience knowledge; you are the expert on the topic you have researched. Do not get bogged down in a sea of measurement, comparing yourself to others and worrying about whether you are good enough or know enough to be making the presentation, or whether somebody else could be doing it better. Instead, realise that at this moment in time—right here, right now—you are the gift, and your message is the contribution.

Source: based on Reynolds (2008)

Reflecting on your performance

Reflective practice capabilities are crucial for lifelong learning, and are skills that students should take seriously and strive to develop to facilitate improvement of future performance (Sterling, 2008). When reflecting on your presentation, identify aspects of your performance that went well, in addition to those that did not go so well. To improve the accuracy of your review, underpin your reflections with a clear understanding of your presentation goals, as well as any assessment criteria, because students' self-assessment is often lower than both tutor and peer assessments. You should also seek and consider feedback from trusted peers regarding specific aspects of your performance. For example, you might ask for feedback on the appropriateness of your material or the effectiveness of images you employed. Once you have identified areas for further development, consider strategies you could implement to achieve an improved performance for your next presentation. As an example, if you have identified excessive reliance on your notes as an area for improvement, consider increased rehearsal time or inclusion of key points only in speaker notes, to avoid the temptation to read your presentation.

PROMPTS TO GUIDE REFLECTION ON YOUR PERFORMANCE

- How did I feel at the end of the presentation?
- How did the audience react throughout and at the end of the presentation?
- Was I able to maintain eye contact with members of the audience?
- How reliant was I on my notes?
- Was I able to complete my presentation in the time allowed?
- How does peer and tutor feedback compare to my self-assessment?

Listening, viewing and responding

It is essential that, as a healthcare professional, you develop the ability to acknowledge another's point of view, and to respond sensitively and critically to ideas presented by colleagues. As a student, and throughout your professional career, you will often be required to respond to other people's presentations. When responding to a colleague's presentation you should provide constructive feedback in a supportive manner that identifies areas to both 'grow' and 'glow' (Sterling, 2008). Feedback should encompass presentation style, information presented, clarity of visual information and interest of examples.

Responding to other people's presentations assists your ability to accurately assess your own work through an increased awareness of the many factors that influence the quality of presentations. Focused observation of presenters encourages you to emulate good presenters and avoid poor behaviours exhibited by ineffective presenters. Put simply, when viewing presentations, you should embrace the opportunity to learn from the experience of others—you cannot live long enough to learn everything from your own successes and mistakes (Roush, 2008).

conclusion

Delivering presentations provides students with valuable opportunities to develop communication skills integral to their future healthcare practice. Effective presentations have a logical flow, engage the audience and, importantly, have the potential to increase the quality of client care in healthcare practice. While delivering presentations can be anxiety-provoking it can also be immensely rewarding as you develop communication skills required for successful health professional practice.

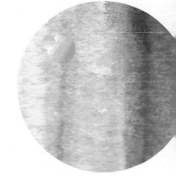

references

Davenport, C., Honigman, B., & Druck, J. (2008). The 3-minute emergency medicine medical student presentation: A variation on a theme. *Academic Emergency Medicine, 15*(7), 683–7.

De Grez, L., Valcke, M., & Roozen, I. (2009). The impact of goal orientation, self-reflection and personal characteristics on the acquisition of oral presentation skills. *European Journal of Psychology of Education, 24*(3), 293–306.

Green, E. H., DeCherrie, L., Fagan, M. J., Sharpe, B. A., & Hershman, W. (2011). The oral case presentation: What internal medicine clinician teachers expect from clinical clerks. *Teaching and Learning in Medicine, 23*(1), 58–61.

Higgens-Opitz, S. B., & Tufts, M. (2010). Student perceptions of the use of presentations as a method of learning endocrine and gastrointestinal pathophysiology. *Advances in Physiology Education, 34,* 75–85.

Leeds, E. M., Raven, A., & Brawley, D. (2007). Primary traits of oral business presentation: Translatable use for assessment in a virtual learning environment. *College Teaching Methods & Styles Journal, 3*(4), 21–33.

Reynolds, G. (2008). *Presentation Zen: Simple ideas on presentation design and delivery.* Berkeley: New Riders.

Roush, R. E. (2008). Being 'on stage': Improving platform presentation skills with microteaching exercises and feedback. *Gerontology and Geriatrics Education, 29*(3), 248–56.

Sterling, D. (2008). Assessing student presentations from 3 perspectives. *Science Scope, 31*(5), 34–7.

Wing, K. (2009). Simple secrets of power presenters. *Strategic Finance,* June, 21–22.

further reading

Reynolds, G. (2008). *Presentation Zen: Simple ideas on presentation design and delivery.* Berkeley: New Riders. In this book you will find valuable hints to improve presentation delivery and slide design.

useful web resources

For free high-quality photographs for use in your presentations, see www.morguefile.com.

acknowledgments

We acknowledge Annette Street, Ann Sefton and Stephen Loftus, who authored the chapter on this topic in the second edition of this book. Our chapter has revised and updated this earlier version.

I3 / Projected presentations

Peter **MILLS** | Tony **MCKENZIE**

key topics

This chapter covers the following topics:

- planning and preparation
- constructing the presentation
- delivering the presentation

key terms

MULTIMEDIA PRESENTATION

STORYBOARD

TEMPLATE

Introduction

Imagine this scene: your group has to present a report to your class on your group project. Or this: you have completed a major assignment and now you must present your results to the class. Either way, you know that your performance will be judged by how informative and well prepared your talk is, and how well you bring the topic alive for your audience. Everyone will be expecting the presenter to employ some kind of visual media and do a good job. In this chapter we demonstrate how you can exploit the powerful features of presentation software to create your message, highlight content and maintain audience attention.

Many of our readers will be giving presentations to classmates, so this chapter is intended for those situations; however, we have chosen principles that apply to all presentations.

Planning and preparation

Where will the presentation be given?

The spatial relationship between you and the members of your audience will be a key factor in your presentation planning. Consider the following questions:

- Will you be in the same physical space as your audience?
- Are you giving a live presentation to an audience located at another venue through the use of technology?
- Will this be an online presentation to a distributed (scattered) audience?

What kind of experience do you want your audience to have?

There are many possible answers to this question. You may want your audience to understand the material presented, remember the material, or engage with you and your material.

And what is 'the material'? Written texts can be classified into several genres or text types—descriptive, discursive, persuasive and narrative texts. The same genres occur in presentations that use visual or audiovisual aids:

- A *descriptive* presentation predominantly offers a glimpse or a representation of your subject.
- A *discursive* presentation is a presentation whose main purpose is to analyse or evaluate a situation, phenomenon, framework or point of view.
- A *persuasive* presentation is a vehicle a presenter uses to draw an audience towards a particular viewpoint.
- A *narrative* presentation has parallels to storytelling.

Presentations, like texts, can combine more than one of the above genres. Be aware of your intentions.

PREPARATION

Do your homework on the purpose of your presentation and your audience: their demographics, background, experience, expectations, culture and special interests. Adapt your presentation accordingly. ●

Choosing a visual presentation medium

Choosing your visual presentation medium is one of the early decisions in your presentation planning. You need to end up with a plan that suits: (a) the spatial arrangements for the presentation; (b) the audience; and (c) the purpose or goal of the presentation—the kind of experience you want your audience to have. The decision about what presentation technology to use for your visual aids should rest upon three factors: (a) what technology options you have available; (b) your ability to use them; and (c) how well they will support your oral presentation. You and your projected presentation will be a double act. You want your double act to have maximum impact on as many audience members as possible.

This chapter focuses on projected presentations. A projected presentation is supported by technology. But the success of a presentation does not depend only on the projected material and medium; it is also a function of the audience's interest in the topic and, most importantly, the personality and style of the presenter.

The initial plan

In planning, focus on: the specific objectives of your presentation; the audience dynamics you want to promote; the message to be delivered or the topic to be explored; the discussion strategies you wish to employ; and the structure and timing of the presentation (see De Wet, 2006; Harden, 2008). Your plan might commence as a digital **storyboard**—a logical superstructure of ideas (see Farkas, 2005). You will engage your audience better if you can link your approach to the audience's experiences or expectations. If the topic is unfamiliar to the audience, plan how the use of visuals and language can help you draw the audience to engage in the presentation.

/ STORYBOARD /
A storyboard is a sequence of images and text used to plan a presentation.

Like stories or structured arguments, presentations have a beginning, a middle and an end. Spend approximately 10 per cent of your time on the beginning and end, and the rest on the middle.

The beginning should provide an overall description of the situation—the big picture view; draw attention to the topic using something dramatic (like a story, anecdote, picture, some groundbreaking finding) or do something that will dramatically engage the audience's interest. You also need to explain the benefits of the topic (why this topic is important to the audience—what will they get out of it?). Establish the credibility of the presenter or the topic, then provide the objectives for the session and outline the presentation—what is going to be covered and what is not.

The middle provides details and examples. When using projected presentations, it is best to break up the middle into several distinct themes or sections. At the beginning of each section, use 'identification slides' (as advised by Farkas, 2005) to alert the audience to topic changes and provide an overview of the coming topic. These slides provide pauses that allow the audience a moment to absorb previous content or anticipate new content, or give the presenter some time to gather thoughts (Farkas, 2005).

The end of the presentation allows for a summary of the main points; questions—from the audience and/or the presenter; reflection on what they have learned; and an opportunity for discussing 'what's next' (after Sandars, Murray, & Pellow, 2008).

Do I use the templates provided or make my own?

Audiences prefer presentations not to be plain, but to be delivered with some design flair and variation (after Clark, 2008). This maintains audience attention and interest.

Some presenters prefer one consistent design throughout a slide show; others prefer to use several styles. Software programs typically provide templates to achieve consistency of design. You might stick to one **template** or design throughout, or change your template at a topic change or to highlight particular content.

/ TEMPLATE /

A template is a pre-formatted page layout in presentation software that assists in the creation of slides that all have a similar design.

TEMPLATES

Use available templates or create your own if those provided are inappropriate for the audience, topic or theme. See Murley (2006) for a quick guide on how to create your own templates.

What genre shall I use?

The next step is to determine what genre or combination of genres to use. If you want to engage the audience by making the presentation interactive, then break it up into shorter segments to allow for interaction with the audience: ask questions; allow questions from the audience; do an exercise or other activity. For advice and examples see De Wet (2006) and Clark (2008).

An important aspect to consider is your live presentation style. This affects the construction of the slides. In some cases, for example, a presenter might use a free-form arrangement of items on a slide, which may seem disjointed until the verbal explanation makes sense of it (after Farkas, 2006). Make sure that your oral presentation or discussion helps the audience make sense of your slides. In other instances, you might use various levels of bullet points that help you to proceed deliberately and logically through a topic (Farkas, 2006).

Slide show construction

Follow the suggestions below to create successful slides and avoid technological pitfalls that can sabotage the presentation.

How many slides? How much information on a slide?

In Clark's (2008, p. 42) words, 'slides must not be useless in their brevity, nor burdensome in their detail'. The amount of information or text and visuals on a slide will depend on the slide category (e.g. title, outline, example or summary) and the genre of the presentation. Often, presenters cram too much information on one slide, to have fewer slides. It is better to have more slides, each with only a little content.

The general opinion is to cover one idea, topic or theme on each slide. However, in a two-hour presentation, 'one idea' or 'one theme' might utilise multiple slides (Farkas, 2005). It is important to avoid excessive content on any one slide.

Audiences prefer slide text to contain key phrases rather than sentences; the slide text should be expanded by the presenter's commentary, through use of examples and elaboration (Apperson, Laws, & Scepansky, 2008). With text slides, the optimum is to have a heading and three points per slide, with an image. Do not use more than five or six lines per slide, and use a maximum of six words per line (Holzl, 1997; Burke, James, & Ahmadi, 2009). Leave 'white spaces' to separate text, to enhance reading and distribute the slide features (De Wet, 2006). For definitions and terms, however, sentences or paragraphs are appropriate for a slide (Farkas, 2006). For large tables or data-intensive slides, most software packages have the facility to link presentations (e.g. PowerPoint) to spreadsheets or other files so that more complex information can be presented (Farkas, 2006).

handy hint 13.3

VERBAL COMMENTARY FOR THE PRESENTATION
When developing your commentary for the slides, use analogies, metaphors, stories and examples, to enhance the presentation.

Typeface

There are two main groups of typeface: *serif*, which have 'little tails' (properly called serifs) at the ends of the letter strokes, and usually have variable line thicknesses (e.g. Times New Roman); *sans serif* typefaces do not have the tails, have simple shaping of letters and their line thickness is even ('*sans*' = 'without' in French). See also Chapter 10.

On slides, use sans serif typefaces (e.g. Verdana or Arial), which have simple shape and uniform line thickness and are easiest to read (Holzl, 1997). Unless you want to emphasise or make a point of difference, avoid fancy typefaces (e.g. Brush Script) as they are difficult to read in electronic presentations, especially from a distance.

Use sufficiently large letters or font sizes. Text should be readable by all members of the audience, including those at the back of the venue, whether you are in a small classroom or large lecture theatre. Holzl (1997) recommended that the size of headings should be 32 point and text 24 point in small classrooms (fewer than 50 seats); or 36 point for headings and 28 point for text for large lecture theatres. Check whether the font is the right size by testing the slide show in the venue.

Using two different fonts on each slide can be helpful: one for headings and another for text (Holzl, 1997). You can also draw attention to particular text, for example, by placing a text box on a slide with a font and colour different from the rest of the slide.

Words in all capital (upper case) letters, can be difficult to read. However, capitals may be used for headings or for particular emphasis (Holzl, 1997). For bullet points, use lower-case letters or start with a capital letter and then use lower case.

What about visuals?

/ MULTIMEDIA
PRESENTATION /
A multimedia
presentation is a
combination of multiple
forms of media,
including more than
one of the following:
text, graphics, pictures,
audio, animation, video
and others.

In projected presentations, words are for listening to; they are not visual aids. It is desirable therefore to incorporate **multimedia material**: pictures, graphs, charts, diagrams or short movie clips into the presentation (Sandars et al., 2008). Audiences prefer this and can gain more from presentations. Visuals must be relevant to the message and not be superfluous. Use your own pictures, or borrow from the software's clip art library or the internet, but check copyright. Acknowledge the source of graphics—include author and year at the bottom of the slide. Limit the number of visuals on each slide: they should be appropriately sized according to their detail or emphasis; and they should not duplicate or be covered by text (see Holzl, 1997).

Use different colours, typefaces, outlines, shadows or word logos to create focal points; or use arrows, labels, borders, underlining; but limit these attention grabbers to 10 per cent of the slide (De Wet, 2006), otherwise it becomes too busy and distracting.

Should I use motion and sound?

In general, special effects are sometimes interesting, entertaining or even spectacular, but often they are distracting and annoying to an audience (after Mullen, 2003; Murley, 2006), especially if they do not work or take up too much time. There are situations when motion and sounds may be used, but these instances should be appropriate to your objective (Holzl, 1997). If you need to emphasise or distinguish points, use only simple effects (Mullen, 2003). The same comments apply to slide transitions—keep them simple (Holzl, 1997).

SPECIAL EFFECTS

Make sure that the 'media does not mask the message'.

And colours?

Audiences prefer colour, so use three or four compatible colours. These colours may appear in the background, the heading and text. If there are already visuals and text on a slide, adding too much colour can make the slide appear 'busy'. Use common sense here. Avoid black text on white or other bright backgrounds (Apperson et al., 2008), as this tends to strain the eyes. Audiences prefer any colour background to white, but text and graphics should be distinguishable from the background. Use dark typeface on light backgrounds or light typefaces on dark backgrounds. Avoid combining red and green, as some people are red–green colour blind (Burke et al., 2009).

With colours, be consistent throughout the presentation, and then change colours when you want the audience to pick up cues (Apperson et al., 2008). Avoid shades of the same colour, especially in graphics such as pie and bar charts, as your audience may find it hard to see the difference; rather, use bright contrasting colours to distinguish between the different components.

Delivering the presentation

If at all possible, practise and test the presentation in the same (or a similar) venue, to ensure a satisfactory and smooth delivery, test the hardware and software for compatibility and functioning, and test the projection. This practice also helps to optimise the duration of your presentation, improve diction, find and correct mistakes, and make improvements in the flow of the presentation (after Giardiello, 2006; De Wet, 2006).

BEING PREPARED FOR DELIVERY

Arrive at the venue well before the start to set up; review your checklist; have a back-up option; be in good shape, physically and mentally. Take a copy of your presentation to refer to—rather than reading it verbatim.

Do not regurgitate full sentences directly from the slides, without explanation or discussion (De Wet, 2006; Apperson et al., 2008; Clark, 2008), as this reduces retention (Harden, 2008), shows lack of confidence in the material and can annoy audience members. Aim to use your slides as support material for the presentation, not as a replacement for good discourse.

When there are several points on a slide, it is good practice to reveal them one by one, rather than showing the full slide all at once. This allows the audience to focus on each particular point rather than being distracted by the points to come (Murley, 2006). Farkas (2005) suggests a technique called 'synch and launch'. The presenter focuses on the bullet point or visual aspect of a slide and then provides commentary, elaborating beyond the slide (Apperson et al., 2008). Do not bypass bullet points: audiences find this disconcerting.

Judge the timing for the presentation: not too fast or too slow (Clark, 2008). This requires practice. According to De Wet (2006), people read on-screen text 28 per cent more slowly than printed text. Therefore, when presenting text, visual or graphic material, it is important not to rush. Allow the audience to record and process the information (Apperson et al., 2008). You might also want to think about the venue's lighting: students prefer lights to be dimmed rather than fully off or on (Apperson et al., 2008); otherwise, they prefer them to be fully off, rather than fully on.

Some useful tips on presenting include: speak slowly and with clear diction; do not digress from the planned presentation—you can run over time very easily; beware of joking and injecting humour unless appropriate and relevant to the slide or topic; be enthusiastic and animated; do not turn your back on the audience (Giardiello, 2006). Use a pointer with skill, without distracting the audience—point, then talk; do not wave the pointer around; put it down when not in use (after Mullen, 2003; Farkas, 2006). Ensure that you are appropriately dressed; remember that you and your image are part of the presentation.

In lectures or student presentations, it is critical that the projected presentation is not so closed or powerful that it shuts down argument, conversation and debate (Turkle, 2003). The slides should provide information, and they should also be vehicles to promote interaction with your audience.

HAVE A BACK-UP PLAN

Be prepared with a back-up plan should the software or hardware fail (Holzl, 1997; De Wet, 2006). This might be as simple as a thumb drive or perhaps another computer or projector; or it might be an alternative such as a flipchart version of the presentation. Other alternatives are printed handouts, overhead projector slides, white- or blackboard, cards or pinboard materials. ●

Useful technical features of presentation software

A number of features within presentation software can provide useful flexibility in lectures. For example, use of a remote-control device to change slides allows the presenter to move around and interact more readily with the audience.

Make use of the **B** and **W** keys on the keyboard, which turn the screen blank—either black or white—to serve as a break in the lecture for some other activity; this avoids any on-screen distractions (Murley, 2006). Use highlighting or felt-tip pen mouse options to emphasise something on the slide during the presentation (Murley, 2006). An alternative and more sophisticated technology is the use of the package in combination with a Sympodium (Clark, 2008). The Sympodium pen can be used to draw and write over projected slides, to annotate diagrams or graphs or to emphasise features of a slide. You can also combine blank white or black screens with the Sympodium. The blank screen can serve as a white- or blackboard for drawing demonstrations or recording audience contributions.

To provide slides as handouts or not?

Depending on the genre of the presentation, the presenter may consider the use of handouts. If the presentation is a lecture, the provision of handouts before a lecture has been proven by research to: help track the presenter's place in the presentation; reduce the burden of taking notes; allow the audience more time to read slide content and listen to the presenter, and better process the information; make more complex visual materials easier to follow; and support interaction between presenter and audience. Students learn more and retain more when: (a) handouts are made interactive, such as requiring students to label diagrams, annotate visuals or fill in missing points; (b) slides are formulated as questions rather than statements; (c) open-ended brainstorming slides are included; (d) quizzes are included on slides; and (e) students are assigned to co-lead classes (after Farkas, 2005, 2006; Apperson, Laws, & Scepansky, 2006; De Wet, 2006; Clark, 2008).

If the presentation is intended to stand alone, then perhaps the slides need to be more comprehensive; or they can be printed, with notes below them representing the presenter's narrative.

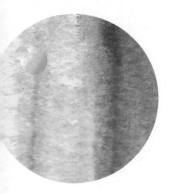

conclusion

Projected presentations are now ubiquitous in universities and, in most cases, are here to stay. They should be a support to the delivery of presentations, not a substitute for a good talk. With careful planning, using appropriate construction techniques, and then delivering the presentation in an improved manner, projected presentations can contribute to an effective and interesting presentation, engage the audience, highlight content and deliver the required messages effectively. It is important that the presenter remains audience-focused and not presenter-focused, using auditory and visual stimuli to encourage engagement and participation.

references

Apperson, J. M., Laws, E. L., & Scepansky, J. A. (2006). The impact of presentation graphics on students' experience in the classroom. *Computers & Education, 47*(1), 116–26.

Apperson, J. M., Laws, E. L., & Scepansky, J. A. (2008). An assessment of student preferences for PowerPoint presentation structure in undergraduate courses. *Computers & Education, 50*, 148–53.

Burke, L. A., James, K., & Ahmadi, M. (2009). Effectiveness of PowerPoint-based lectures across different business disciplines: An investigation and implications. *Journal of Education for Business, March/April*, 246–51.

Clark, J. (2008). PowerPoint and pedagogy: Maintaining student interest in university lectures. *College Teaching, 56*(1), 39–45.

De Wet, C. F. (2006). Beyond presentations: Using PowerPoint as an effective instructional tool. *Gifted Child Today, 29*(4), 29–39.

Farkas, D. K. (2005). Understanding and using PowerPoint. *Proceedings of the Society for Technical Communication Annual Conference*, 313–20.

Farkas, D. K. (2006). Toward a better understanding of PowerPoint deck design. *Information Design Journal & Document Design, 14*(2), 162–71.

Giardiello, F. M. (2006). Powerful PowerPoint presentations. *Gastrointestinal Endoscopy, 64*(3), 393–4.

Harden, R. M. (2008). Death by PowerPoint – the need for a 'fidget index'. *Medical Teacher, 30*(9–10), 833–5.

Holzl, J. (1997). Twelve tips for effective PowerPoint presentations for the technologically challenged. *Medical Teacher, 19*(3), 175–9.

Mullen, D. (2003). *Train the trainer*. Dar-es-Salaam, Tanzania: FAO.

Murley, D. (2006). Making presentations visual. *Law Library Journal, 99*(2), 451–9.

Sandars, J., Murray, C., & Pellow, A. (2008). Twelve tips for using digital storytelling to promote reflective learning by medical students. *Medical Teacher, 30*, 774–7.

Turkle, S. (2003). From powerful ideas to PowerPoint. *Convergence: The International Journal of Research into New Media Technologies, 9*(2), 19–25.

further reading

Lambert, J., & Cox, J. (2011). *MOS 2010 Study Guide for Microsoft® Word, Excel®, PowerPoint®, and Outlook®.* Redmond, WA: Microsoft Press. This book is useful for improving your expertise in using PowerPoint. It has clear instructions and visuals to help practise and prepare presentations.

useful web resources

For ideas, suggestions and examples of how to prepare and deliver great presentations, see http://www.m62.net/

acknowledgments

We acknowledge Charles Higgs and Joy Higgs, who authored the chapter on this topic in the second edition of this book. Our chapter has revised and updated this earlier version.

Designing tables and graphics

Alison **GATES** | Joy **HIGGS** | Charles **HIGGS**

key topics

This chapter covers the following topics:

- commonly used graphics and tables: their forms and purpose

- guidelines for the presentation of graphics and tables

key terms

TABLES

FIGURES

/ **TABLES AND FIGURES** /

Tables are characterised by horizontal rows and related vertical columns. All other forms of graphics, including diagrams, charts, photographs, pictures, maps, icons, graphic organisers and drawings are called figures.

Introduction

Graphics are important communication devices and can often be used effectively to represent information in less space and with greater clarity than written prose (Durbin, 2004). There are many instances where images are more powerful, entertaining and stimulating communicators than words; they fire the imagination, prompt pattern recognition (of illnesses, for example), and communicate relationships (such as locations, levels and rates). In academic writing, everything outside the main text body is either a **figure** or a **table**. A table is characterised by horizontal rows and related vertical columns, each with its own heading. Tables are used to communicate both qualitative and quantitative data. All other forms of graphics, including diagrams, charts, photographs, pictures, maps, icons, graphic organisers and drawings are called **figures**.

TYPES OF GRAPHICS

In academic writing, a table has related columns and rows, and every other kind of graphic is called a *figure*. ●

Effective figures and tables

To be effective, figures and tables (Hay, Bochner, & Dungey, 2002) need to be relevant, concise, comprehensible, meaningful as 'stand-alone' items without the text, and referenced (i.e. any sources—other than yourself—for the data or the graphic must be acknowledged). Tables and figures need clear and comprehensive titles, legends, labels and footnotes. The format of tables and figures is a matter of convention and preference. In this chapter we make some recommendations for simple, clear and consistent data presentation. It is important to recognise the conventions of the audience you are writing for. You should check the common practice in relation to assignments or theses in your school, follow your university's guide to presentation of essays and assignments, or use the style of the journal for which you are submitting a paper.

Types of figures and tables

There are many kinds of figures and tables. Generally speaking, graphs are best for showing trends and patterns, or highlighting differences between data sets. Tables are better when the data *values* are more important than the *trends* (Annesley, 2010). Let us take a minute to look at the various types of figures and tables that you can consider incorporating into your writing.

Graphs

There are many types of graphs, including scattergrams, line graphs, bar charts, histograms, population pyramids, pie charts and logarithmic graphs. Hay et al. (2002) give instructions for constructing all these graphs. It is important to plan the construction of your graph carefully in order to demonstrate that you have handled the data with integrity. Much has been written about common student pitfalls of dealing with data.

Durbin (2004) gives the following helpful recommendations for dealing with data in tables and figures:

- Do not include the same information in both a figure and a table.
- Do not reiterate in the text what is already conveyed in the figure or table.
- Avoid unsubstantiated extrapolation between or beyond data points.

- Avoid truncating, compressing or enlarging the axes in such a way that could mislead your reader.
- Discrete points should not be connected with a line.
- Use a single typeface and font in a table as much as possible.

Figure 14.1 shows a bar chart that was created using Microsoft Excel. The raw data for the graph is given within the figure so that you can use it to create your own graph. Excel readily allows you to include the raw data annexed to the table in your figure; however, it is not usual in student writing to include this information. With a reasonable amount of practice you should be able to create and modify charts in Excel from a variety of data sets. Note also that Figure 14.1 contains both a graph and a table, and is correctly labelled as a figure.

FIGURE 14.1 | EXAMPLE OF A BAR CHART: PRE-TEST AND POST-TEST SCORES FOR GROUPS A–D

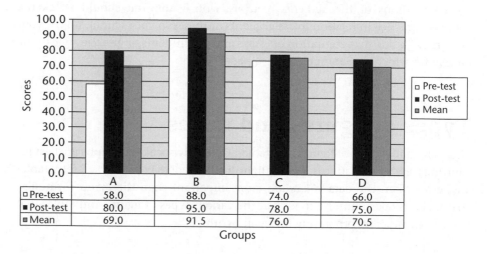

	A	B	C	D
Pre-test	58.0	88.0	74.0	66.0
Post-test	80.0	95.0	78.0	75.0
Mean	69.0	91.5	76.0	70.5

Groups

YOUR TURN...

Using the guidelines listed above, produce a figure from the data in the table at the bottom of Figure 14.1.

Tables with word data

Table 14.1 is an example of a table that contains word data. This is an excellent way of summarising literature and reducing the word count of your text.

TABLE 14.1 | EXAMPLE OF A TABLE WITH WORD DATA: THEORIES OF BENCHMARKING

THEORY	KEY CONTENT	REFERENCE
Best current national practice	3 key indicators measured Top national scoring hospital identified	Frederickson 1999
Best international model	10 key indicators measured Top scoring unit for each indicator identified	Schmidt & Abrendt 2001
Achievable growth target	Own unit as benchmark Achievable growth on indicators set	Wu & Fenwick 2000
Ideal position model	Use of research data and theoretical models Ideal position for 6 key parameters set	Trendle 2000

PUTTING WORDS INTO TABLES OR FIGURES

Work smarter: information in figures and tables does not usually count toward the maximum word count of student work and of some academic publications. If you are struggling to edit your work to within the prescribed word limit, ask yourself: 'Can I say this with a figure or a table?'

Tables with numerical data

A number of texts provide detailed instructions for the construction of tables (e.g. see Thomas, 2000; Anderson & Poole, 2001; Baker, Barrett, & Roberts, 2002; Annesley, 2010). Table 14.2 provides an example of a table containing numerical data; it has been created using Excel spreadsheet software. Note that the decimal points are aligned vertically and the variables are clearly labelled.

TABLE 14.2 | EXAMPLE OF A TABLE WITH NUMERICAL DATA: SCORES ON THREE TESTS OF MEN'S AND WOMEN'S ATTITUDE TOWARDS CHILD-REARING

	TEST 1: ACMT (MAX. 60)*			TEST 2: PPS (MAX. 110)*			TEST 3: ATPS (MAX. 100)*		
	MEAN	SD**	%	MEAN	SD**	SA	MEAN	SD**	%
Men	44.3	8.2	73.8	78.3	7.2	71.2	25.4	8.2	25.4
Women	27.5	25.5	45.8	81.4	4.2	74.0	79.9	25.5	79.9
Average	35.9	16.9	59.8	79.9	5.7	72.6	52.7	16.9	52.7

*max. = maximum possible score on test
**SD = standard deviation

Pictures

At times your text, poster or talk can be enhanced by the inclusion of a picture such as a cartoon, photograph or drawing. Sometimes you can find the image you are looking for in another publication, and sometimes you need to create it yourself.

In unpublished student work, including assignments and theses, when you are using pictures or graphics that are not your own creation, it is usually sufficient to acknowledge the source of the original figure. In books, chapters or journal publications, it is usually necessary to obtain copyright permission from the publisher if you want to include a diagram that is not yours in your work. This can be time-consuming and it is important not to leave this task until the last minute.

Graphic organisers

Graphic organisers include flow charts, timelines (e.g. treatment protocols), concept maps, fishbone diagrams, Venn diagrams and many other schemas for representing data and ideas. Graphic organisers are used to represent complex relationships and ideas in an easily accessible manner. Some journals require particular graphic organisers to accompany manuscripts, such as patient flow charts in clinical trials (as shown in Figure 14.2).

FIGURE 14.2 | A FLOW CHART DESCRIBING A CLINICAL TRIAL

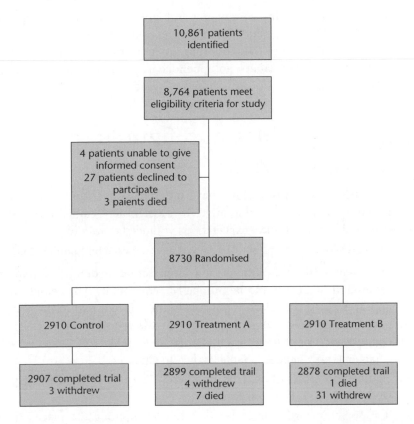

There are many templates for graphic organisers, SmartArt, in the Microsoft Office suite of programs (see also Chapter 10). These are easy to modify to accommodate your data or the concept you are trying to represent. Perusing the SmartArt library is a good way of finding inspiration for your next figure. If you cannot find what you are looking for in the SmartArt library, consider searching Google Images for the particular graphic organiser you wish to use, such as 'fishbone diagram template'.

INCLUDING SMARTART

It is easier now than ever before to produce professional graphics and tables in your documents. Microsoft Word, Excel and PowerPoint all contain wizards and templates for the production of charts and so-called SmartArt (graphic organisers).

Perusing the available templates in the SmartArt menus can be a helpful way of deciding which form of graphic best suits the idea or data that you are trying to represent.

Designing figures and tables

Time spent carefully planning your figures and tables will improve the quality of your work. Take a blank page and sketch a representation of the data or idea that you need to present. Choose the most appropriate format, bearing in mind that you can always place raw data in an appendix. Pay careful attention to labels, titles and references.

Integrating tables and figures into your written work

Different professions and disciplines have different conventions for using and labelling graphics. Check with your university's assignment guidelines or ask your lecturers to find out which local expectations you need to follow.

In the absence of any prescribed format, we suggest a few general guidelines:

- Placement of tables and graphics in your presentation or report is important. Tables and figures should be numbered sequentially, labelled clearly and appear in the text as close as possible to the relevant part of the text. They may be numbered sequentially through the whole work (e.g. Figure 1, Figure 2 etc.) or through each chapter (e.g. Table 1.1, Table 1.2 etc. in Chapter 1, and Table 2.1, Table 2.2 etc. in Chapter 2).
- Figures and tables should be numbered separately: Figure 1, Figure 2, Figure 3, Table 1, Figure 4, Table 2 etc.
- It is sometimes recommended that the label should be placed below a figure and above a table (Cargill & O'Connor, 2009).

It is most important, however, to be consistent and follow any publication, university rules or style guides.

Generally speaking, raw data is rarely included in the main body of an academic report or presentation; if it is, it is generally presented as a figure or table. It is important that any figure or table is referred to in the text *before* it appears on the page, to avoid confusing the reader. Each figure and table needs a concise label explaining what it is about. A longer description or discussion of the illustration should occur in the text, but it is not necessary to reiterate in the text the data conveyed in a figure or table (Durbin, 2004). All illustrations and tables must be referred to in the text, to indicate how they relate to your argument.

Referencing tables and figures

It is important to correctly reference any information in figures or tables that is not your own work. If a graphic contains no citation, you are communicating to your reader that it is your own work (see Chapter 17, 'Avoiding plagiarism'). The citation is usually placed under the heading of the graphic.

If the entire graphic is reproduced from another work, reference your source below the heading of the figure or table; for example '(Source: Smith, 2000, p. 7)'. This is the case even if you have only slightly modified the format of the graphic (e.g. changed colours, reorganised shapes). If you have modified the diagram to include new information or findings, or if you have merged work from several authors, you should cite this in the following way: '(After Jones, 2000; Smith, 2004)'. You can also include references to different sources within different sections of the graphic. For example, each column of a table might have a particular source, or each balloon in a flow chart or concept map could have a different source. Your referencing style should be consistent throughout your document; thus, if you use footnotes in the text, you should also use footnotes in the tables and figures. Citations in figures and tables require matching references in the main reference list at the end of your work.

CHECKLISTS FOR TABLES AND FIGURES

These checklists for figures and tables will help you to ensure that your work meets the required standard for presentation. You can add extra bullet (dot) points to each checklist to accommodate any particular requirements of your discipline or school.

Checklist for figures:

- Does the figure have an appropriate label/title? ✓
- Is the source of the figure properly acknowledged? ✓
- If the figure is a chart does it have all axes labelled (including units/ scale)? ✓
- Is the figure in the right place (main body or appendix)? ✓
- Has the figure been referred to in the text? ✓
- Does the figure appear after it has been referred to in the text? ✓
- Are the figures numbered sequentially and in the order they appear in the work? ✓

Checklist for tables:

- Does the table have an appropriate label/title? ✓
- Does each row/column have an appropriate heading with units specified? ✓

- Is the source of the table properly acknowledged? ✓
- Is the table in the right place (main body or appendix)? ✓
- Is the table referred to in the text before it appears in the work? ✓
- Are the tables numbered sequentially and in the order they appear in the work? ✓ ●

conclusion

Tables and figures are an important part of your academic writing, and they need careful consideration and planning. It is important to be consistent when labelling, referencing and producing tables and graphics, and to follow the conventions of your institution with respect to style and formatting.

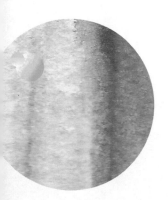

references

Anderson, J., & Poole, M. (2001). *Assignment and thesis writing* (4th edn). Milton, Qld: John Wiley & Sons.

Annesley, T. M. (2010). Bring your best to the table. *Clinical Chemistry, 56*(10), 1528–34.

Baker, E., Barrett, M., & Roberts, L. (2002). *Working communication*. Milton, Qld: John Wiley & Sons.

Cargill, M., & O'Connor, P. (2009). *Writing scientific research articles: Strategies and steps*. Oxford: John Wiley and Sons.

Durbin, C. (2004). Effective use of tables and figures in abstracts, presentations and papers. *Respiratory Care, 49*(10), 1233–8.

Hay, I., Bochner, D., & Dungey, C. (2002). *Making the grade: A guide to successful communication and study* (3rd edn). Melbourne: Oxford University Press.

Thomas, S. A. (2000). *How to write health sciences papers, dissertations and theses*. London: Churchill Livingstone.

further reading

Jelen, W. (2010). *Charts and graphs: Microsoft Excel 2010*. (MrExcel Library) USA: Que Publishing.

Lindsay, D. (2011). *Scientific writing = Thinking in words*. Sydney: CSIRO Publishing.

Giving and receiving feedback

Lindy M^cALLISTER | Jennifer SCHAFER

key topics

This chapter covers the following key topics:

- what is feedback?

- why do we give feedback?

- when to give feedback

- how to give feedback

- principles for giving and receiving feedback

- having difficult conversations

key terms

FEEDBACK

DIFFICULT CONVERSATIONS

Introduction

Whether we realise it or not, we are constantly sending and receiving feedback, as we interact with those around us, which influences our behaviour. Learning how to use this feedback to enhance relationships, teach and learn new skills, and improve performance is an invaluable communication skill.

As students, you will learn to give feedback to clients and their families, peers, your educators and healthcare team members, and to receive feedback from them as well. Giving and receiving feedback is complex and potentially problematic. Giving feedback that preserves dignity, and receiving feedback in an open and non-defensive way that facilitates ongoing communication between the communication partners, but that also leads to behavioural change, is a challenge. It requires self-awareness, awareness of others, and understanding of the principles and strategies for giving and receiving feedback.

What is feedback?

/ FEEDBACK /

Feedback includes 'information about a person's performance of a task which is used as a basis for improvement'. It is based on observation and is formative.

According to the *Oxford Dictionary* (2009), the definition of **feedback** includes 'information about a person's performance of a task which is used as a basis for improvement'. Feedback is not the same as praise or criticism—these are judgments—although they may be delivered at the time as feedback. Feedback provides very specific information, is based on observation and is formative. This is in contrast to evaluation, which reflects the judgment of the observer (Ende, 1983).

Why give feedback?

Table 15.1 highlights some reasons for giving feedback. There are a range of outcomes we aim for in giving feedback. Effective feedback can enhance social and professional relationships, improve educational outcomes, foster positive change in an organisation, build therapeutic alliances, reinforce desired behaviour, improve compliance with healthcare advice, motivate change, promote trust and candid dialogue, and provide valuable self-awareness and self-knowledge. You will be given feedback regularly during your health profession program, but you may also be required to give feedback to your peers as part of your education program. Research evidence suggests that giving feedback is likely to be more beneficial to learning than receiving it because it promotes higher-order thinking (Nicol, 2010).

TABLE 15.1 | EXAMPLES OF REASONS FOR GIVING FEEDBACK

PURPOSE	EXAMPLE
To provide feedback to someone learning a new skill	A physiotherapy student teaching a patient a new exercise: 'Your position is just right and your feet are in line with your shoulders—perfect. Now, remember to tighten your core muscles before you lift the weights.'
To reinforce skills	A nurse to a student nurse learning how to use a sphygmomanometer: 'Well done. You chose the right-sized cuff for this patient and applied the cuff over the middle third of the arm.'
To provide feedback on behaviour	One student to another: 'You mightn't realise it, but when you spoke to that patient's relatives this morning, everyone in the ward could hear. There's a quiet room just down the corridor that we can use for interviews. Let me show you where it is.'
To encourage	An oral hygiene student consulting with a patient with gum disease: 'I can see that you have been working on regularly brushing and flossing. Your gums are much healthier. Excellent work!'
To affirm	A team leader talking to a colleague: 'Thanks for your work on this. Your willingness to take on an extra project means that we can meet the deadline.'

< cont. >

< *cont.* >

PURPOSE	EXAMPLE
To confront	A manager to a member of staff [or a clinical teacher to a student] who is repeatedly late in submitting reports, despite receiving previous feedback on this matter: 'When you don't complete your reports on time, I feel angry and anxious: angry because, as your manager [or fieldwork educator], I'm the one responsible for problems arising from the absence of treatment guidelines for our patients which are provided in your reports, and anxious because without your reports the team can't coordinate the management plans and patients can't receive quality care. If you want to continue to work here after your probationary period expires [or pass this fieldwork placement], you need to have your reports in on time or notify me if there is a reasonable delay. I have noted your tardiness in your file and will review your progress towards meeting the report timelines at our next review meeting. If you need help with report writing, please make an appointment to see me or another colleague. I am happy to review draft reports at any time and provide feedback on them. Is there anything further you would like to say about this matter? Would you like me to explain anything further?'

When to give feedback

Timing of feedback

Effective feedback is delivered as close to the relevant event as possible. It is difficult for people to recall their behaviour if it took place some time ago. This is particularly the case when people are learning something new or complex, or if they are anxious about their learning or performance. As well, the timing of feedback needs to take into account a person's emotional state. If either the giver or the receiver of feedback is upset, angry, fatigued or overtly resistant, it would be wise to find another time. Receivers of feedback should feel empowered to say if the timing is not right for them. However, postponement of confrontation needs careful thought, as the timing may never feel right for either party, but it may nonetheless need to be done. Avoid the trap of too little feedback delivered too late for change to occur; it is not fair for the recipient of the feedback and can compromise patient care and student learning outcomes. As a student, you should actively seek feedback from your educators, peers and client, be able to receive it with grace and respond appropriately.

Frequency of feedback

Feedback works best if it is frequent enough to help people make immediate changes to their behaviour. It should be frequent enough to build incrementally towards long-term behavioural change and to be supportive for the receiver. Frequent feedback is important for behaviours that affect the welfare or safety of others. For example, if you are running a balance program for people in aged care, you will need to instruct, assist, observe and provide feedback several times before learners can do the tasks safely.

Providing informal feedback regularly and frequently also normalises the feedback process, provides opportunities to reward and reinforce desired behaviour, modify other behaviours and resolve misunderstandings quickly before they escalate. However, this can often be perceived as normal conversational banter. Students sometimes feel that they 'never get feedback' (Branch & Paranjape, 2002), so check with your educators if what they are saying is feedback they expect you to act on. Similarly, preface your comments to peers or clients by saying, 'I would like to give you some feedback about…'.

Where to give feedback

Consider the need for privacy in delivering and receiving feedback, particularly in busy clinical settings. Positive feedback shared publicly can be an accolade that rewards and encourages the recipient. Corrective feedback may be more appropriately and respectfully delivered privately. This may not always be practical, however, in the clinical environment, particularly if the feedback is in the context of providing patient care. In such environments, words need to be chosen carefully, especially if the patient is listening to the interaction. Be careful not to say anything that will undermine a client's confidence in the healthcare they are receiving.

How to give feedback

The methods for exchanging feedback include combinations of oral, written and online communication, review of video and audio recordings, as well as self-evaluation. Face-to-face feedback is very powerful. Although it takes more time, there are significant advantages to written feedback. Aim to achieve a balance of affirming and corrective feedback. The receiver is less likely to hear and recall 'only the negatives' or 'only the positives', and can refer back to written feedback for detail that might have been missed in the emotion of the moment of hearing oral feedback. Written feedback is particularly helpful in supporting learning and you should feel comfortable in requesting this from your educators.

Principles to consider when giving and receiving feedback

Effective feedback is based on a number of principles, including:

- The foundation for effective feedback is good interpersonal communication skills, which we practise daily in our personal and professional environments. Effective clinical communicators are attentive, non-judgmental, empathic, enquiring and informative (Groves & Fitzgerald, 2010).

- Many people dislike or feel anxious about giving and receiving feedback, perhaps because they confuse feedback with criticism. Remember that feedback is an opportunity for positive change. It can be easier to approach both giving and receiving feedback if you frame it as a journey to improvement. For any particular skill, each of us is on a continuum from novice to expert. The purpose of feedback is to move the recipient in a positive direction on that continuum. Even experts aspire to improvement.

- Feedback is two-way. It can be invaluable to invite your educators, peers, colleagues or patients to share their views on what they expect from you, your performance, and how you can best assist them to achieve the goals that you have negotiated.

- Feedback should be used as an opportunity to self-assess performance against that of an external source. There is a tendency to deflect feedback when there is a mismatch between the learner's and teacher's perceptions (Molloy, 2009). Learners may re-interpret the feedback to conform with their own hope, intention or interpretation of their performance (Carless, Salter, Yang, & Lam, 2011).

TECHNIQUES FOR GIVING AND RECEIVING FEEDBACK

Focus on the needs of the person receiving the feedback. It can be useful to clarify, specifically:

- What is their goal?

- Where do they think they are on the spectrum of performance?

- How do they think they are progressing?

- What is going well?

- What are the challenges and barriers?

- Is there any extra information that you should know? (e.g. special needs or difficult circumstances)

- What do they see as the next steps or solutions to problems?

- Is there some aspect of their performance about which they would appreciate feedback?

When giving feedback:

- Communication should be authentic, sincere, respectful, and considerate of the other person's best interests.

- Identify the topic or issue that the feedback is about.

- Gather data to support your feedback.

- Encourage self-assessment and then build on that information. A commonly used technique is to invite the recipient of feedback to begin by identifying his/her strengths, followed by the mentor reinforcing and adding further information. The recipient is then asked to identify areas for improvement, which is (again) reinforced and added to by the mentor.

- Provide your perspective on the stage that they have achieved on their journey to improvement.

- Honesty and lack of ambiguity are essential. Be direct—beating around the bush creates confusion and mixed messages.

- Be specific about the behaviour observed, the impact or outcome of the behaviour, and how to improve.

- It is easier to focus on your observations rather than your judgment by starting with: 'I have noticed', 'I have seen', 'I have observed'.

- Acknowledge if feedback is 'secondhand'; for example, by saying, 'It has been reported to me that...'

Choose your language:

- Consider starting with a positive statement about the level of performance that the recipient has achieved to date.

- In most situations, choose words that are affirming, encouraging and promote change, while still clearly and accurately identifying areas for improvement or serious errors.

- Avoid words such as 'but', 'however' and 'although'—they negate whatever comes before. For example: 'Your patient notes are very comprehensive, but your handwriting is terrible.' End the first thought before starting with the next. For example: 'Your patient notes are very comprehensive. I note that your handwriting is difficult to read—that creates confusion for the other staff and is a patient safety risk.'

- If the feedback is affirming, you can add comments that reflect your appreciation of the good work.

- If the feedback is corrective, a tone of 'concern' can convey the importance required. Expressing anger, frustration, disappointment and sarcasm can turn feedback into criticism. The desired outcome is positive change, rather than humiliation.

- Avoid negative strategies such as public humiliation, judgments about personality, talking at rather than with the person, showing no personal interest, making comments that are general or non-specific (e.g. 'that was awful').

- Help your patient/student/colleague to identify the next step towards improvement.
- Be specific about how they can improve. Providing examples can be helpful—and check for understanding.
- Allow opportunities for practice, followed by further feedback.
- Follow up (including support when needed) should be arranged to assess progress.

When receiving feedback:

- Be open to the feedback being given; remember it is intended to help you learn.
- Try to avoid 'deflecting' feedback when it does not match your self-perception.
- Engage in constructive dialogue with your feedback provider rather than adopting a passive or defensive position.
- Ask for specific examples of behaviours that need to change.
- Be aware of your responses to feedback, both emotional and cognitive.

Difficult conversations

Not all feedback that we give and receive is positive, supportive or encouraging. Although most of the behavioural change we want to foster in our peers, and clients and their families can be achieved using positive feedback, there are times when that is not enough. When direct instruction and coaching have been tried and have failed, we have a duty to confront our colleagues, clients and family members if their behaviour is impeding learning, quality care or professional relationships. For students, the supervisor should lead such **difficult conversations** with clients and families. Handy Hint 15.2 provides some tips for preparing for and having difficult conversations.

TIPS FOR HAVING DIFFICULT CONVERSATIONS

- Prepare yourself by thinking about the principles for giving feedback.
- Choose an appropriate time and location—it is better to avoid feeling rushed or on display.
- Stay calm, and keep your voice slow and steady.
- Start with the positives before moving to the negatives.

/ **DIFFICULT CONVERSATIONS** /
We have a duty to confront our colleagues, clients and family members if their behaviour is impeding learning, quality care or professional relationships. Difficult conversations often require assertive communication to ensure feedback is provided with clarity and respect.

- Focus on the observed or reported behaviour, followed by its impact or outcome, while avoiding inferences about personality, feelings, intentions or motives.
- Ask the recipient of the feedback for his/her perspective.
- Use active listening skills that include reflection and summarising; empathise appropriately, seek clarification of areas of confusion, acknowledge concerns and issues, identify the problem and work together to create a 'management plan'.
- Choose language that maintains respect and dignity while avoiding emotionally charged wording or personalising the problem.
- Aim to be fair and unbiased.
- Keep the conversation constructive and improvement-focused, not destructive.
- Be prepared for the 'fight or flight' reaction and don't take it personally.
- Challenging the recipient's defence mechanisms is unlikely to be successful.
- Trying to understand and empathise with the reaction may help to build rapport and trust.
- If the situation becomes emotionally charged, be prepared to provide time out or to re-convene at another time.
- Consider following up with a written summary.

The final example in Table 15.1, of confronting feedback from a manager to a junior health professional, illustrates the use of principles of assertive communication:

- 'I' statements ('I feel anxious …')
- Clear references to problematic behaviours ('when you don't complete your reports on time …')
- Clear statements about the impact of the behaviour ('…because without your reports the team can't coordinate the management plans and patients don't receive quality care')
- Clear statements of what alternative behaviour is expected ('You need to have your reports in on time or notify me if there is a reasonable delay.')

As well, the manager or supervisor has:

- Offered support to achieve the desired behaviour ('If you need help with report writing, please make an appointment to see me or another colleague. I am happy to review draft reports at any time and provide feedback on them.')

- Outlined the consequences ('If you want to continue to work here after your probationary period expires, you will need to …')
- Invited feedback and continued communication about the matter ('Is there anything further you would like to say about this matter? Would you like me to explain anything?').

conclusion

This chapter considers many of the factors that can help improve the effectiveness of giving and receiving feedback, important skills for health professional practitioners.

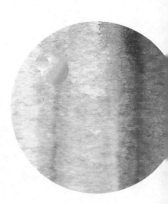

references

Branch Jr, W. T., & Paranjape, A. (2002). Feedback and reflection: Teaching methods for clinical settings. *Academic Medicine, 77*(12, Part 1), 1185–8.

Carless, D., Salter, D., Yang, M., & Lam, J. (2011). Developing sustainable feedback practices. *Studies in Higher Education, 36*(4), 395–407.

Ende, J. (1983). Feedback in clinical medical education. *JAMA: The Journal of the American Medical Association, 250*(6), 777–81.

Feedback. (2009). In *Oxford English dictionary online*. http://dictionary.oed.com/

Groves, M., & Fitzgerald, J. (2010). *Communication skills in medicine: Promoting patient-centred care*. East Hawthorne, VIC: IP Communications.

Molloy, E. (2009). Time to pause: Giving and receiving feedback in clinical education. In C. Delany & E. Molloy (Eds.), *Clinical Education in the Health Professions* (pp. 128–46). Sydney, Elsevier.

Nicol, D. (2010). From monologue to dialogue: Improving written feedback processes in mass higher education. *Assessment & Evaluation in Higher Education, 35*(5), 501–17.

Digital communication in a networked world

Helen **WOZNIAK** | Philip **UYS** | Mary Jane **MAHONY**

key topics

This chapter covers the following topics:

- overview of a range of digital communication technologies
- digital identity and the associated pitfalls and risks
- choosing the best tools for your communication needs
- managing your networked world for learning

key terms

ELECTRONIC COMMUNICATION DEVICES

DIGITAL COMMUNICATION

MOBILE LEARNING

PERSONAL LEARNING ENVIRONMENT (PLE)

ASYNCHRONOUS COMMUNICATION

SYNCHRONOUS COMMUNICATION

EPORTFOLIO

Introduction

Studying in the health sciences will involve you in new methods of communication because of:

- opportunities for interacting with professional practitioners and other industry experts located off-campus
- professional practice placements being undertaken as part of your studies away from campus

- the demands of managing your studies along with other responsibilities (e.g. work, family, community, sport)
- expectations that as a graduate you will be prepared for involvement in e-health activities.

You are likely to be already using a range of informal **electronic communication devices** in your everyday life, which can be described as a 'networked world'. Many of these same devices will be used in your academic and professional life, leading to a blurring of the boundaries between your home life and study life. You will now need to use these devices and many more to communicate with other students and your lecturers from home, your workplace, a library or computer access centre, or another location. You are also likely to be separated by distance and/or time.

A range of terms can be associated with your communication patterns with variations in the mode, time or place; for example: 'blended', 'distance', 'electronic', 'multimode', 'distributed', 'online', 'off-campus' or 'off-site'. Whatever the label, at least some of the time, you will be using a range of communication methods which will mirror your likely communication experiences as a professional.

In this chapter we emphasise the importance of taking control and being responsible for your part in using **digital communication** technologies to enhance your learning, including how to manage your digital identity and the associated risks. We ask you to consider how these forms of communication differ from your prior experiences and what they may now require of you. We would like to encourage you to explore digital communication alternatives and select those that work best for you, and thus build your **personal learning environment (PLE)**. We also include some tips on how to use the various digital communication alternatives efficiently and effectively.

/ ELECTRONIC COMMUNICATION DEVICES /
Electronic communication devices are tools such as telephones that are used for multiple forms of verbal and written communication. They create a 'networked world'.

/ DIGITAL COMMUNICATION AND PERSONAL LEARNING ENVIRONMENT (PLE) /
Explore digital communication alternatives and select those that work best for you and thus build your personal learning environment (PLE).

Digital identity and communication style

You will already be aware of the risks associated with revealing your identity in a digital world, maintaining your personal privacy and avoiding cyber bullying, but how do such risks affect you in developing identity as a health professional? It is helpful to map out the many dimensions of privacy in your academic and professional world. Figure 16.1 represents the various levels of privacy that you should consider when deciding which aspects of your identity you will reveal to others.

FIGURE 16.1 | SPACES IN A NETWORKED WORLD OF LEARNING
(ADAPTED FROM LOWENTHAL & THOMAS, 2010)

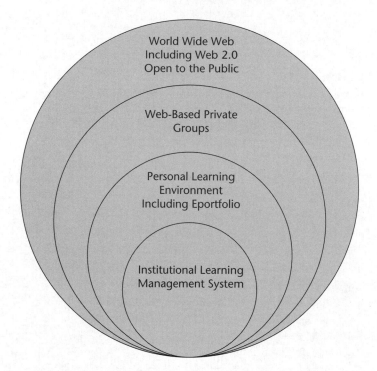

When you commence formal academic study at the tertiary level, you are provided with an academic identity in the form of a student ID and email address. This ID links to all your personal information, and universities are required to protect your personal identity through a range of complex security measures and institutional firewalls. This identity is used in formal online activities most often connected to the learning management system (LMS) where you engage in your study-based online assignments and discussions. Make sure you review your institution's information technology (IT) policy documents about this, and make yourself aware of the support that universities provide if you experience any mistreatment as part of your interactions during your study. This closed system is represented in Figure 16.1 as the innermost circle.

Depending on how your lecturers have set up the digital environment for your study, you may engage in a range of collaborative activities with other students enrolled in your units of study, where your name or ID is displayed. Occasionally, outside experts will be given access to this 'protected' digital environment to participate in your activities. Your lecturer should always inform you if this is to occur. During your study you will further develop your personal learning environment to include other digital communication tools. Here, you will have greater control over who you invite to participate and who can see your work (next circle in Figure 16.1). This situation occurs in the case of an **electronic portfolio or eportfolio**. Usually, it is the institution that provides the system for you to create your own portfolio, where you can create evidence to support your learning and invite others to view your work. Increasingly in the health professions, eportfolios are being used to demonstrate continuing competency for your profession.

Alternative spaces may be utilised for your learning, which 'live' or are hosted outside of the institutional boundaries in computing 'clouds'. These spaces can provide a rich learning environment, and allow you to access a broader range of opinions and facilitate a wider community engagement with your work. Be careful when you sign up to these systems; ensure that you understand what control you have over your identity and the work that you display on these sites. You should always use an alias (not your university ID) when asked to join these networks, and make sure you are familiar with the privacy levels of these spaces. You are responsible for the content that you post. You also need to respect copyright: provide URL links to content developed by others, rather than cutting and pasting content that you have not created yourself (see Chapter 17, 'Avoiding plagiarism'). Finally, information such as your grades should never be accessible in any public spaces. The outermost circles of Figure 16.1 represent these externally available spaces, which have the option of providing a more private group space or a space open to everyone.

The use of digital media for professional communication can create problems in meeting expectations about politeness. Emails allow brief and informal communication. When time pressure exaggerates this trend to brevity, the result can be disconcerting. When emailing someone from another country or culture, take care to write in an appropriate style, in terms of the degree of politeness and formality (such as the use or non-use of given names). It can be helpful to consult a guide on 'netiquette' for the rules of good cyberspace communication.

/ ELECTRONIC PORTFOLIO (EPORTFOLIO) /
Using an electronic portfolio (eportfolio) you can create evidence to support your learning and invite others to view your work.

A plethora of possibilities

As you progress from your study life and enter your professional life, you will rely on digital communications to develop a broad network of colleagues. This initially encompasses your lecturers, clinical supervisors, other health professionals and your fellow students (peers). Over time, these relationships will develop into your professional colleagues; relationships that you will maintain throughout your career. It is important to be mindful of this change over time as you begin your interactions with your lecturers and peers.

Interaction with your lecturers now goes beyond the scheduled face-to-face lectures or tutorials. With the introduction of online LMSs, your lecturers are more accessible than ever and can potentially respond to your queries outside the scheduled class or meeting times. Make sure you are aware of any university policies or guidelines associated with student-to-lecturer interactions, and clarify this with your lecturer at the commencement of your study. Lecturers have a range of responsibilities beyond their teaching role, so you need to show respect and ensure you manage your interactions with them efficiently. For example, lecturers may set up an online forum for students to post their study queries. This enables all students to benefit from the questions posed by all students. Check this area before sending unnecessary email messages to your lecturers.

Another important type of interaction is that conducted with your peers. Student-to-student interaction is increasingly occurring across the years of study and between different health professional groups. Your fellow students are a valuable source of support, as well as being able to assist you in your learning. Although you will benefit from reading the contributions of your fellow students, you will gain a deeper understanding about the subject content if you actively participate in discussions with your peers. Handy Hints 16.1 and 16.2 provide some practical tips for sending and replying to digital messages.

WRITING AND SENDING DIGITAL MESSAGES

- Compose the *Subject* to give the essence of your message. This helps retrieval and helps your peers manage information overload. An ideal subject line provides keywords that best characterise the contents of the message.

- To continue the conversation use the *Reply* function, so that messages related to the subject appear in one thread. Otherwise, the discussion appears as one long list of unrelated single messages.

- If you are shifting the topic or direction of the discussion, use a new subject title.

- Keep your message short, with paragraphs between 3 to 5 sentences in length. Paragraphs should be separated by white space to make your messages easy to read on–screen.

- Aim to build on the contributions of others by asking questions, offering reasons for your ideas and support for your claims, and offering sources linked to further information (such as web pages or references).

- Make visible how you feel, as well as what you think. Brief statements such as 'I laughed out loud when …' or 'I felt uncomfortable when …', or common emoticons such as the smiley face :-) or the sad face :-(can also help in informal communication. This more casual language should not be used when you are communicating with your lecturers (when submitting assignments or asking questions about your studies or enrolment).

- Do not use abbreviations commonly used in online and text-messaging social interactions (such as '4U'). You are communicating in an academic or professional environment.
- Do not use all capital letters. That is considered impolite, the equivalent of shouting.
- Avoid losing your work if your online connection times out or drops out. Compose your more thoughtful, complex or substantial messages in a word-processing document, then copy and paste them into your online message.
- If you include an attachment, give it an informative name.
- Do not wait too long before joining the discussion.
- Make sure you allow enough time for others to respond to your messages.
- Before you hit *Send*, be sure your message is going only to the person or persons you want to read it. Re-read it to make sure your message is clear.
- Remember, you are communicating with people. Offer your online colleagues courtesy and respect. Treat others as you would wish to be treated. Inappropriate comments can damage your reputation.

RECEIVING DIGITAL MESSAGES OR FILES

- Acknowledge emails received. A brief 'thanks' assures the sender that you received the message.
- Avoid replying in haste or in heat; think over your contribution before sending it. Composing your message offline helps.
- Develop time-management strategies so you do not feel overwhelmed; for example, designate specific times to check and respond to email.
- When sharing documents, make sure you label each version, consider using 'track changes' or comments, and clearly identify who is reviewing and making each change.
- When working in groups, establish a timeframe for replies and responses, and share your schedules so you can determine the best way to work together.

< cont. >

EXAMPLES	ADVANTAGES	DISADVANTAGES
Teleconferencing Video conferencing Skype Web conferencing or a virtual classroom with an electronic whiteboard, shared document, chat, audio and video all possible	You may have a record of the event. Use of audio, or audio with video, can enhance your social experience with fellow students and your lecturers. Can have a lively conversational tone that moves quickly.	You may require additional hardware, headset with a microphone or webcam. In chat and instant messaging, you can feel frustrated or left behind if your keyboard skills are slow or if others take over the discussion. In chat, the message is short and limited in length so may lack depth and detail, moving quickly from one topic to another, making it more difficult to follow. In audio- or videoconferencing (especially desktop), you may find the standard of picture or sound unsatisfactory for the intended communication.

Social media for learning

Social media practices are increasingly being used for learning and teaching purposes. These types of interaction can occur when students use an external program like Facebook for their learning or within a LMS that is provided by the educational institution.

Social media emphasise the social aspects of learning; that is, that learning is often collaborative and goes beyond the mere exchange of ideas. In learning, you can get to know the other students and the lecturers, so that learning occurs in this network of peers and can include lecturers as well.

There are many ways to communicate when social media are used for learning purposes. You can share information through textual, pictorial or moving images. Others can express their 'liking' of information, comment on the information through textual, pictorial or moving images. Microblogging (e.g. Twitter) allows only very short comments.

The social network provides opportunities to 'follow' those that you particularly would like to learn more from. One can set up sub-groups or channels to work on specific projects or assignments.

You should feel free not to accept requests to join groups that do not relate to your studies and to contribute only what you feel comfortable in exposing about yourself; for example, if you would rather not display a photograph feel free to say so.

Mobile learning

It is becoming common to use mobile devices such as *smart* (internet-enabled) phones and tablet devices for communication and accessing information for learning purposes (Uys, 2011). Some of the biggest challenges for educational institutions are to provide ubiquitous network access on campuses and to deliver learning materials to a plethora of mobile devices.

An interesting aspect of **mobile learning** is that it often occurs in the student's environment, off-campus and also away from work and home. In some geographical regions in Australia (and often in developing contexts) mobile networks are far more robust than internet access.

There should be clear information as to which websites of your educational institution and which aspects of its LMS are mobile-enabled, and which applications (apps) can be downloaded for mobile learning.

Mobile learning can occur in many ways:

- using mobile phones to respond to polls in class;
- using a tablet to access your LMS modules and communicating with other students in the class using the chat tool;
- using mobile devices to access online forums to see how your peers are going and to share your experiences;
- making new friends with your peers from a number of different subjects through a Facebook group that can be set up for a generic group of students, such as all first-year students;
- receiving notifications from your lecturer (using SMS) regarding the availability of new internet resources as they are posted, so students know when they need to get online;
- being able to aggregate and share content on your tablet from a variety of sites and applications in one central location.

There are further possibilities that are described elsewhere (Charles Sturt University, 2010).

Some particular issues need to be addressed when mobile learning occurs. Contact your lecturer if you cannot access mobile-enabled materials and there are no alternatives. Manage your time in a way that allows for a reasonable cognitive load ('head space') and do not get sucked into thinking that you need to be continually engaged. Spaces are not neutral, and the various localities in which mobile learning can take place could influence your interactions. This can be particularly critical in assessment and evaluation settings. Handy Hint 16.3 provides some suggestions about how to use a range of different media to enhance your learning with digital communication tools.

/ **MOBILE LEARNING** /
Mobile learning uses mobile devices such as smart phones and tablet devices for communication and accessing information for learning purposes.

LEARNING TO COMMUNICATE WITH DIFFERENT DIGITAL MEDIA

General

- For synchronous meetings, be there ahead of the scheduled time. If you are located in a different time zone, be sure you know the local time you are due to commence.

- Read all instructions provided in advance, to increase your confidence and minimise surprises. This includes completing pre-reading or preparation for tutorial discussion.

- Practise informally with others to increase your familiarity with the technology.

Voicemail

- State your name, the time and date of the call, specific details as to the topic of your message, and your contact details.

- Spell out your name if it is difficult, and repeat any phone numbers and other contact details.

Chat rooms

- If you are making a presentation, prepare it in advance, then copy and paste it into a message.

- Use short messages with a sign indicating that receivers should continue the discussion (usually +), to minimise waiting time for other participants.

Telephone and video conferencing

- Distribute any illustrations you want to use, ahead of time.

- Ensure you have a quiet background for the period of the call.

- Arrange to sit where you can write, and (for video) adjust the camera settings to place yourself in the centre of the screen with the appropriate zoom.

- Always introduce yourself when you make your first comment and speak distinctly during the conference.

- Remember to turn your microphone on and, for video, turn your microphone off when you are not participating, otherwise all the sites will hear your background noises such as paper shuffling and other unwanted sounds.

- Always introduce yourself when taking a turn: 'It's Helen speaking.' Do not be afraid to ask who is speaking. It helps you situate the content and tone of interaction.

- Make a conscious effort to put colour into your voice; let your voice indicate when you are smiling.

- For telephone and if in a group, help with communicating the group's responses; for example, 'Everyone here nodded in agreement with your views.' From time to time, ask for an indication of non-verbal information; for example, 'I wish I could see you, you sound like you are happy/puzzled. Are you?'

- For video conferencing, be careful with the lighting, close blinds behind you so you don't appear as a dark shadow on the screen.

Web conferencing

- Practise ahead of time to ensure that you are comfortable with the basic procedures and their implications (e.g. ensure you are familiar with the process for displaying files on your computer to other participants during the conference). Will people understand your presentation? Would a diagram help?

- Ensure that you have checked your microphone and speaker settings. Using a headset with both is best.

- Ensure that your documents are not overloaded with graphics, which can prevent other participants from viewing them easily.

- If you are presenting through a webinar, it can be helpful to have a collaborator assist you by monitoring the synchronous chat and troubleshooting computer issues or alerting you to questions from the audience.

Building your personal communications environment

In this chapter, you have been introduced to a number of digital communication and learning tools. You can now create and expand your own PLE of digital communication tools of your preference by exploring these different tools for learning purposes. Your PLE can include tools provided by your educational institution and tools that you have selected externally. Your networked world of learning will enable you to interact with a wide variety of people, many that you would not otherwise have the opportunity of meeting, but it requires you to be mindful of maintaining the respect of others and developing a digital identity that will remain with you throughout your career.

references

Charles Sturt University. (2010). *CSU mobile learning investigation*. Retrieved from http://www.csu.edu.au/division/landt/resources/mobilelearning/index.htm

Lowenthal, P. R., & Thomas, D. (2010). Death to the digital dropbox: Rethinking student privacy and public performance. *EDUCAUSE Quarterly*, *33*(3). Retrieved from http://www.educause.edu/EDUCAUSE+Quarterly/ EDUCAUSEQuarterlyMagazineVolum/DeathtotheDigitalDropboxRethin/ 213672

Uys, P. M. (2011). *mLearning collection*. Retrieved from http://www.globe-online. com/mobilelearning

useful web resources

For an overview of the role of new technologies in learning, see www.educause. edu/ELI7Things

For seven things you should know about privacy in Web 2.0 learning environments, see http://net.educause.edu/ir/library/pdf/ELI7064.pdf

For Megan Poore's blog: Essential information for students using Web 2.0 services, see meganpoore.com/2009/09/22/lifeline-essential-information-for-students-using-web-2-0-services/

To check your understanding about netiquette, complete the quiz at www.albion. com/netiquette/

For resources with tips for electronic communication, see the PennState University site tlt.its.psu.edu/suggestions/etips/stuguide.html

For Salmon G.5 stage model of online learning and teaching, see http://www. atimod.com/e-moderating/5stage.shtml (a useful model for tracking your development as a user of online communication tools.)

For a catchy Youtube video which examines privacy and public issues for using social media in the workplace, see the Victorian Department of Justice site http://www.youtube.com/watch?v=8iQLkt5CG8I

CHAPTER

17 /

Avoiding
plagiarism

Susie **SCHOFIELD** | Rola **AJJAWI**

key topics

This chapter covers the following topics:

- what plagiarism is

- why it should be avoided

- how it can be avoided

key terms

PLAGIARISM

REFERENCE MANAGEMENT SOFTWARE

PLAGIARISM DETECTION SOFTWARE

Introduction

In February 2011 the German Defence Minister Karl-Theodor zu Guttenberg admitted that substantial parts of his thesis were copied from other sources (BBC, 2011). He claimed it had been an unintentional mistake, blaming the error on his busy schedule. His crime was **plagiarism** and his penalty was to be stripped of his PhD. Dubbed 'Baron cut-and-paste' and 'zu Googleberg' by the German media, his suitability for the role of Defence Minister was questioned. How could someone guilty of academic dishonesty stand in front of troops and talk of matters of honesty? In March 2011, he resigned from his ministerial role, the Bundestag (German parliament) and his role in local politics.

What is plagiarism?

As you can see from this example, universities take plagiarism very seriously. Honesty in academic writing is also seen as part of the professional behaviour of health professionals. In the United Kingdom, doctors have been severely reprimanded for plagiarism (Dyer, 2011). It is important, therefore, for students and future health professionals to understand what plagiarism is and how to avoid it.

The word **plagiarism** comes from *plagiarius*, the Latin for 'kidnapper'. The *Merriam Webster Online Dictionary* (www.merriam-webster.com) defines it as 'to steal and pass off (the ideas or words of another) as one's own: use (another's production) without crediting the source; to commit literary theft: present as new and original an idea or product derived from an existing source'. From this we can see that there are two parts to plagiarism: theft (of a thought or words) and fraud (presenting them as our own).

/ **PLAGIARISM** /

Plagiarism contains two parts: theft (of a thought or words) and fraud (presenting them as our own).

Types of plagiarism

Walker (1998) identified seven types of plagiarism. If you look at the description of each one, you'll recognise the first two examples as coming from the first paragraph of this chapter. Becoming aware of the different types of plagiarism and thinking about your attitude towards each will help you to avoid it (see Handy Hint 17.1).

Sham paraphrasing

The material is copied word-for-word and acknowledged with a citation but lacks quotes:

> In February 2011 the German defence minister Karl-Theodor zu Guttenberg admitted that substantial parts of his thesis were copied from other sources (BBC, 2011). He claimed it had been an unintentional mistake, blaming the error on his busy schedule. His crime was plagiarism and his penalty was to be stripped of his PhD. In March 2011 he resigned from his ministerial role, the Bundestag (German parliament), and his role in local politics. (Schofield & Ajjawi, 2012)

To avoid this we should make sure we include quote marks around anything written verbatim. Note that, as a general rule for good academic writing, you should avoid lengthy quotes, as you are not demonstrating your understanding of the text.

Illicit paraphrasing

The material is paraphrased without citing the source.

> Being too busy to cite your references is no defence against plagiarism, as the then German defence minister Karl-Theodor zu Guttenberg found out in 2011. He was stripped of his PhD and lost his ministerial job.

Although the author has used her own words she has not included a citation, so the reader cannot follow up the writing to check the facts and learn more about the case.

Other plagiarism

The material is copied from another student's assignment with the knowledge of the other student. In this case, both students could be deemed to have been dishonest if the tutor thought the authoring student knew of the intention of the plagiarist.

Verbatim copying

The material is copied word for word without citation:

> In February 2011 the German defence minister Karl-Theodor zu Guttenberg admitted that substantial parts of his thesis were copied from other sources.

Recycling (also known as duplication)

The same assignment (or part of it) is submitted more than once for different courses. Universities should not give credit twice for the same piece of work, yet there may be times when, for example, you want to use a particular experience twice. If in doubt, always check with your tutor, who might suggest you add it as an appendix, explaining that it has been previously submitted.

Ghost writing assignment (also known as commissioning)

This is where a third party writes the assignment and the student presents it as his or her own work. There is a growing market in online writing services where students pay for an essay, often of unknown quality. The companies claim there is no plagiarism in the assignment. This may be true, but as soon as you present it as your own work you are plagiarising. The point of assignments is to develop your skills, to alert yourself and your tutor to your learning needs, to reinforce what you are doing well. How can feedback from your tutor on a ghost-written assignment do any of those things? By using such a service, not only do you have to pay someone else to do your work, you are also depriving yourself of an educational experience.

Purloining assignment

A student copies from another student's work without the other person's knowledge. Clearly, here the original author is not to blame.

ATTITUDES TO PLAGIARISM

- How well do you understand each of the types of plagiarism listed?

- Which do you still need to learn more about?

- Consider each type and rate how serious you think it is, from 1 'not at all serious' to 3 'very serious'. Compare your answers to those of your friends. Did any differences come as a surprise?

Reasons students plagiarise and ways of avoiding it

There are many reasons students might plagiarise, either intentionally or unintentionally. Understanding these reasons will also help us to be on our guard and learn how to avoid them.

Not understanding the rules

It is important to understand the rules of your own institution and profession relating to academic writing and plagiarism. If you are at all unclear, find someone who can explain the rules to you, such as your subject librarian. If you are unsure about your work, there may be a writing support service offered by your university or your tutor might be happy to answer particular concerns.

Poor referencing skills

Make sure you know how to reference. Guidance should be available from your institution. Again, your subject librarian would be a good source, and may offer training and/or online guidance. Different disciplines use different formats.

This book uses a format whereby the citation (the part in the text) contains the author(s) surname(s) and year of publication (or just the year if coming straight after the author's name), and the full references are listed in alphabetical order by surname at the end of the chapter. In health science literature you will also come across the Vancouver style, where the citation appears as a superscript number and the full references are in the order in which they appear in the text. You might find that some of your lecturers have a preference for one referencing style, some for the other, so it is always worth checking. Your institution may provide **reference management software** such as Endnote or ProCite to help you to manage bibliographies and references. Make sure you access training in the use of such software, keep backups and always use your most up-to-date copy.

/ **REFERENCE MANAGEMENT SOFTWARE** /
Reference management software helps you to manage bibliographies and references.

Not keeping citation close to relevant text

Consider these two examples:

> Levels of pollution have long been known to affect health, an effect confounded by deprivation levels as more affluent families move out of high deprivation areas (Lee & Ferguson, 2009; Stafford & Marmot, 2003).

> Levels of pollution have long been known to affect health (Lee & Ferguson, 2009), an effect confounded by deprivation levels as more affluent families move out of high deprivation areas (Stafford & Marmot, 2003).

> They contain the same information but in the second it is much clearer which reference informed each part of the sentence.

Using secondary sources

You may find a paper referenced in the literature you are reading. Wherever possible, seek out the original (primary source), as the second author could have misquoted or misrepresented the first author's work. If that is not possible, you must make clear in your referencing that it is a secondary source; for example, by writing (…, cited by Bloggs, 2012).

Poor time-management skills

Make sure you leave enough time for your assignment. Searching the literature, selecting relevant sources and creating a well-structured, correctly referenced assignment takes time. When you have finished your assignment, ask someone else to read it, or leave it for a couple of days then re-read it yourself. Are there places where it is not clear where the ideas or facts came from?

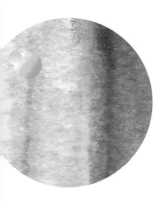

conclusion

As discussed in this chapter, there are various reasons students might plagiarise, either intentionally or unintentionally. Universities take plagiarism seriously and, with care, it can be avoided.

references

BBC. (2011). *German Defence Minister Guttenberg resigns over thesis.* Available from http://www.bbc.co.uk/news/world-europe-12608083

Dyer, C. (2011). GMC suspends surgeon for plagiarism. *BMJ*, 342, d3457.

SafeAssign® by Blackboard. Available from http://safeassign.com/

Turnitin®. Available from https://turnitin.com/static/index.php

Walker, J. (1998). Student plagiarism in universities: What are we doing about it? *Higher Education Research and Development, 17*(1), 89–106.

Communicating

in the workplace

Talking with colleagues, patients, clients and carers

Diane **TASKER** | Anne **CROKER** | Lindy **M^cALLISTER** | Annette **STREET**

key topics

This chapter covers the following topics:

- the nature of talking with others in healthcare

- dealing with challenging communication situations

- developing capability for meaningful talk for healthcare

key terms

RAPPORT

ACTIVE LISTENING

AUGMENTATIVE COMMUNICATION

Introduction

Talking within professional and therapeutic contexts is a complex, though often taken-for-granted phenomenon. Effective and meaningful talk is not necessarily easy or straightforward to achieve. In this chapter we explore the nature of talking with others in healthcare. We explore some challenging communication situations, and make suggestions to assist you to develop your ability to talk meaningfully as a healthcare professional. Talk is one aspect of communication, which also includes listening, writing and use of body language. See Chapter 1 for more information regarding communication.

The nature of talking with others in healthcare

A key aspect of talking with others in healthcare is that it involves people; talking is by people, with people, for people and about people. Talking involves communicating by speaking, and is supported by the use of facial expression, gestures and body language. People's roles, experiences, situations and needs, together with their communication styles and preferences, all influence how they talk with one another. Talking is dynamic rather than formulaic; it needs to respond to the people involved and their situation, needs and styles of communicating.

Being responsive to the purpose of talking

There are many reasons we might need or want to talk with people as we practise healthcare. We need to adapt our talk for different purposes; for example, connecting with people, providing information, understanding issues, discussing situations, negotiating solutions and providing support. The purpose of the talking influences how issues are framed and dealt with. We need to understand this in order to approach and respond to situations appropriately. In Case Study 18.1, a practitioner demonstrates the ability to move seamlessly between informal interpersonal communication and more formal transfers of clinical information.

CASE STUDY 18.1

PULLING THE WORKDAY TOGETHER WITH TALK

This case study, set in a paediatric ward, shows how talk can be used for different purposes, ranging from careful but practical exchanging of information to sensitively supporting people. A practitioner briefly touches base with a patient, then seeks relevant information before continuing the interaction; spends time obtaining and clarifying clinical information from other staff; communicates understanding of a sensitive issue; and indicates an awareness of maintaining (appropriately timed) social bonds between colleagues.

John makes his way down the long corridor to the children's ward. Walking into the ward, John sees Jenny looking out the window towards the car park, from her bed. He guesses that her mother has just left to go to work. He remembers that Jenny hates to have her daily blood test without her mother there. He smiles at Jenny, saying, 'Back in a few minutes' and she tentatively waves back at him. Reaching the ward office, he checks the in-tray for Jenny's test results while asking the other staff how things were in the ward overnight. There have been new admissions. Through questions asked and answered, John builds a picture of the tasks he needs to deal with and how to prioritise his day. He then returns to the laboratory results, but when an experienced staff member mentions her concern about possible child abuse for a newly admitted child, John stops flicking through results and looks up. His attention and his murmured 'Mmm, thanks for that' indicates that this concern has been heard and will be taken it into consideration when he assesses that child's condition. Locating Jenny's blood results he notes that the last results look very good and goes to tell her that she will not need another blood test today. 'It's all good, Jenny. You don't need to have another blood test today.' Jenny bounces up in her bed and returns the 'thumbs up' sign that John gives her. Although it was only a small event, John smiles as he walks back down the corridor to see his next patient, commenting to another staff member on the way, 'I'll catch up about your weekend game at morning tea'.

Although it all seems straightforward and easy, there is a lot happening at any one time for this practitioner.

Establishing rapport

/ **RAPPORT** /

Rapport is a close and harmonious relationship in which there is common understanding (*Concise Oxford Dictionary*, 2008).

Rapport is an important part of the development of a working alliance between healthcare professionals and their clients, and most often involves particular verbal behaviours on the part of the healthcare professional. In some situations rapport builds up over years (e.g. between colleagues working in a team or practitioners working with long-term clients), whereas other situations require that rapport is established quickly (such as on first interaction with a client). Establishing rapport encompasses the notion of having the time and inclination to engage with others using respect, empathy and genuineness.

Introductions offer a valuable opportunity for establishing rapport. It is important to introduce yourself and explain your status. For example, if you are a student, make this clear. Ask patients how they want to be addressed; if they want you to use their title (such as Mr, Mrs, Miss, Ms, Reverend, Professor or Dr). If the person says 'Call me Sam', then do so. If you are discussing clients with other practitioners or presenting their cases, refer to them by their formal title. As a general rule, address older people and people from cultures other than your own by their formal title, unless asked to do otherwise.

When establishing and maintaining rapport, good communicators do not talk or relate the same way to all people, but adapt their communication to the needs, assumptions, expectations and abilities of the other person or audience. This allows them to better learn and understand about a client's personal and healthcare situation. The practitioner's existing skills and knowledge, and the client's contribution may then interplay in a collaborative form of reasoning to create a new form of knowledge (Edwards, Jones, Higgs, Trede, & Jensen, 2004). Edwards et al. (p. 80) argue that this altered view of the practitioner–client exchange may emancipate either or both the participants 'from previous limited or distorted perspectives concerning their situation(s)'.

Balancing listening with talking

A good conversation requires a balance between talking and listening. Practitioners may be able to balance this process if they 'wait to hear' in the silences that occur naturally within conversation. Relaxing and waiting can give the other person more opportunity to talk, and also helps them to relax. By combining silence with **active listening**, the practitioner can encourage the other person to confide important information that might not otherwise be volunteered. Active listening involves combining communication strategies to help you to listen and respond to another person in order to better understand them. It includes sensitivity on the part of the healthcare practitioner to any differences between themselves and the other person that may interfere with the telling of those confidences. Active listening also involves behaviours such as maintaining eye contact, nodding, mirroring the other person's key vocabulary, modulating pitch and phrasing, gesturing appropriately, adopting an appropriate posture, giving verbal encouragement (such as 'mmm' and 'uh huh'), summarising to show you have understood the essence of what the person is saying, and requesting clarification when necessary.

/ **ACTIVE LISTENING** /
Active listening involves combined communication strategies that help you to listen and respond to another person to better understand them.

Using grammar, vocabulary and body language effectively

The grammar and vocabulary we choose to express an idea, together with the pitch, volume, rhythm and stress patterns we use to deliver it, all affect how our message is received and understood. Our speech is also imbued with layers of meaning or *nuance*. A statement as simple as 'I got your report' could mean anything from 'Thank you for your report' or 'About time I got your report—why are you always late?' to 'I really disagree with your diagnosis and proposed treatment'.

Body language is also important. When 'I got your report' is said by a speaker with hands on hips, it might convey irritation that the report is late or a desire to argue about the contents. If said with a quizzical look, it might convey a lack of understanding of what is in the report or disagreement about the contents. Interpretation depends not only on the sentence construction and delivery, but also on who you are, who the speaker is, whether you share a common culture or language, your previous history of interaction, the background and context, and your expectations as well as those of your client about the communication.

Maintaining confidentiality

An important and well-recognised element of communication in healthcare relates to confidentiality.

> Confidentiality is the right of an individual to have personal, identifiable medical information kept private; such information should be available only to the physician of record and other health care and insurance personnel as necessary (*Encyclopaedia of Nursing and Allied Health*, 2011).

Talking in healthcare often involves information that is confidential. Talk with clients, patients and carers needs to be conducted carefully, with attention to where it is conducted and who might be able to hear. This can be particularly difficult in ward situations where people have to give confidential information in the presence of others, particularly where only a curtain separates the patient from other people in the ward or at clinic desks. Maintaining good peripheral awareness of possible leaks will help you to respect the individual needs and rights to confidentiality of people in healthcare settings. Relationships underpinned by trust can also be built between workplace colleagues if the same degree of confidentiality is also applied to collegial conversations.

Dealing with challenging communication situations in healthcare

Adjusting your communication style is particularly important when you are dealing with challenging communication situations. In interactions with colleagues, patients, clients and carers, many difficulties and challenges can arise. Some of the most challenging situations include:

- talking with people who have trouble communicating
- talking with upset or angry people
- delivering bad news
- communicating across cultures
- being assertive
- delivering or receiving negative feedback.

The first three of these situations are discussed here; others are the focus of other chapters.

Talking with people who have trouble communicating

The need to adapt your communication style is particularly obvious when you are dealing with patients or carers who have communication impairments. Approximately one person in seven has a communication impairment (Speech Pathology Australia, 2011); so, as a healthcare professional, you need strategies to communicate with people who have problems hearing, speaking, reading or writing. Many people with communication impairments can communicate using speech, if they receive some basic consideration and assistance from their communication partner. Some strategies to adopt when talking with people with a disability are listed in Handy Hint 18.1.

TALKING WITH SOMEONE WHO HAS A DISABILITY

- Speak directly to the person with the disability rather than to any companion or sign language interpreter.

- Ensure that you are on the same eye level when speaking to someone in bed or in a chair.

- Identify yourself and the others accompanying you when meeting someone with a visual impairment. Call the person you are speaking to by his or her name (to alert the client to who is being spoken to).

- Use a first name only if everyone is on first-name terms.

- Treat people in an age-appropriate way.

- Do not patronise people in wheelchairs by patting them on the head or shoulder.

- Do not lean against or hang on someone's wheelchair. People usually view their wheelchairs as an extension of themselves.

- Offer to shake hands when introduced—even if the person has limited hand use or an artificial limb.

- If you offer assistance, wait until the offer has been accepted (or not), then listen or ask for instructions.

- Try to relax.

(Adapted from De Vito, 2001)

/ AUGMENTATIVE COMMUNICATION /
Augmentative communication involves combined approaches and devices to improve the communication of people who cannot speak or be understood.

Some people lack understandable speech, or are unable to speak. These people often use **augmentative** or *alternative* **communication** (AAC), which involves the combining of approaches and devices to improve the communication of people who cannot talk or be understood. There are two types of AAC:

- *Unaided communication:* this includes body language, facial expressions, 'pointing' with one's eyes, fingers, hands or body, gestures and formal signs.
- *Aided communication:* this can be low-tech, using objects mounted on boards, charts and books containing photos, drawings, symbols, words or letters (depending on the person's intellectual and physical impairments), which the person looks at, points to or in some way selects to create a message; or high-tech, such as specialised computers and keyboards, or voice synthesisers.

Most people who communicate using AAC use a combination of low- and high-tech AAC. Using an AAC system tailored to their needs and physical and intellectual abilities can help people with a communication disability to achieve the same goals of communication as other people.

CASE STUDY 18.2
'HELLO': TALKING WITH SOMEONE WHO USES AAC (AUGMENTATIVE OR ALTERNATIVE COMMUNICATION)

Allowing adequate time to establish rapport is important for talking with someone using an AAC device. Healthcare professionals need to focus on the person using the AAC device rather than just talking to the carer.

Gary takes a deep breath to relax and slow down as he approaches Marie, a young woman with an acquired head injury who has come into hospital for investigation of abdominal pain. Marie has come into the ward with her carer. Gary introduces himself to Marie first and then to her carer. The carer tells Gary that Marie uses an augmentative speech device (it is sitting on the table in front of her) which requires her to type in words that the unit then 'speaks'. Gary first pops his head around the curtain and asks the next patient if they would mind turning their television down so that he and Marie can concentrate better. He then sits down beside Marie, and reaches towards her to shake her hand first and then that of her carer. He asks Marie about her device and how it works. She gives him an information sheet about the device, which he quickly reads. The carer pulls the device closer and Marie types in 'Hello'. A rather computerised voice issues from the box-like device: 'Hello'. Gary starts a bit but then smiles at Marie. She smiles back. They have begun their conversation.

This case study gives an idea of the different approaches that may be needed when AAC devices are used to conduct conversation with a person who has a communication difficulty. In the hurried and busy world of a hospital or clinic, it can be difficult for healthcare professionals to slow down sufficiently to allow a person with a communication difficulty time to understand and respond to speech approaches. The practitioner needs to try not to let anxiety about the unfamiliar situation interfere with the communication. Sometimes a carer familiar to the client may be present, but it is important to orient the talking to and with the person using the AAC device. Practitioners need to be careful not to slip into the habit of talking over the head of the person with the communication difficulty, or around them to their carer. Do not anticipate what the AAC user will say, jump in, or finish their turn for them unless they have previously indicated that this is OK (e.g. in their 'How I communicate' materials). AAC users often have a lot to say. People using AAC value social communication opportunities, so allow plenty of time for your conversation with them.

COMMUNICATING WITH PEOPLE WHO HAVE PROBLEMS TALKING OR UNDERSTANDING

- Get on the same level as your client; if they are seated, sit at their level. This empowers them, and allows you both to see and use body language.

- Learn to both read and use eye gaze, facial expressions and gestures to communicate more effectively.

- Have a pen and paper close at hand to draw or write key words, depending on what is easiest for your client to understand and use.

- Use yes and no questions to check their message (e.g. 'Did you say you want lunch?').

- Use open questions rather than closed questions to engage in conversation and keep it going (e.g. 'How was your weekend?' rather than 'Did you have a good weekend?').

- Tell your client when you have not understood; let the client rephrase the message. (This is especially important for AAC users.)

- If the person cannot 'converse', give choices to elicit a response (e.g. 'Do you want water or fruit juice?').

- Take turns in the conversation, but remember that AAC users may not be able to signal easily that their turn is finished, so watch their body language.

- Pause often, give the person time to formulate and communicate responses.
- Allow time, and learn to be comfortable with silence. For some clients with developmental disability or acquired brain injury, it might take 20–30 seconds to respond. AAC users may need up to three minutes to compose a simple response to what you have said. ●

Talking with upset or angry people

People who are upset or angry often need to have their concerns or grievances listened to before problem-solving can begin. The listening process can help them to clarify their emotions and separate them from the issues that need to be addressed. Being heard and respected can enable people to move towards possible solutions. Avoid expressing personal judgments; stay focused on the problem, not the personality. Jointly identify a solution to the problem; an imposed solution might be disregarded and cause further concern.

If you are the one who is upset or angry, consider whether it is appropriate to express your feelings. If you do express your emotions, refer to the issue or behaviour that upset you, not to personal characteristics. For example, it is not helpful to say, 'You are hopeless—you never write the results in the patients' notes'. A better way of approaching the situation could be to find out more about the context so you can better understand the person's behaviour and situation: 'I'm getting a bit frustrated with not knowing the patient's results. Can we discuss what we can do about it?' Chapter 15 provides further ideas on giving feedback, having difficult conversations with people, and assertive communication.

Difficult interactions can cause emotional distress. Taking some quiet time to wash your hands slowly, for example, can help you to settle and become calm again before going on to the next job or interpersonal interaction. Overall levels of work stress can then be managed in a more careful way. It can also be helpful to discuss a difficult interaction afterwards with a trusted colleague. Practitioners, as well as clients and carers, can benefit from reflective and supportive talk.

Unexpected issues may be identified when talking with upset people. These issues may need to be referred to other healthcare professionals for continued consideration. Case study 18.3 gives an example where further matters to be addressed are raised when a health practitioner deals sensitively with a client's recall of a distressing event.

CASE STUDY 18.3

IT IS OK TO TALK ABOUT DISTRESSING EVENTS

Getting on the same wavelength by sensitively talking with someone about distressing events can lead to the identification of other care areas that need further assistance.

Denise was chatting to her young client, Maxine. As they shared some reminiscences, Maxine confided to Denise that she had often been bullied at school and that she still got flashbacks about some of these situations. Her eating disorder had commenced soon after these events. Maxine became quite tearful as she talked. Denise listened and reassured her that it was OK to talk about this difficult issue if she wanted. She then waited as Maxine washed her face to settle herself and asked Maxine's mother (who was in the waiting room) to come in and join their conversation. Maxine seemed relieved to have shared her confidence. Denise advised Maxine and her mother to seek some advice from the clinic's psychologist and helped them to make an appointment by finding the phone number and letting them use the office phone.

Talking about bad news

Delivering unwelcome information and talking about bad news can be difficult but important tasks. Do not try to predict people's reactions to news; what we think of as bad news might not be viewed the same way by patients. For example, some patients might see 'bad news' test results as permission to stop fighting terminal illness and begin to plan their dying process. It is important to assess the person's awareness of and reactions to the information. Use this to decide the best way to talk about the news. Individuals use a variety of coping styles. Be aware that relatives also need support, and may react very differently from the client. Although you may refer patients or clients to professional colleagues, support group information—online or brochures in appropriate languages—can also help people cope with bad news.

Developing capability for meaningful talk

Healthcare professionals talk to clients, carers and colleagues as part of their everyday life and professional practice. Their work can be significantly assisted by a sensitive and well-developed ability to talk. Research has shown that it is possible to improve such skills (Harrington, Noble, & Newman, 2004). Strategies to improve communication can be practised and improved. Rehearsing or role-playing, and receiving constructive feedback in a supportive learning environment is a powerful process to improve your communication skills. Record (with appropriate consent) interactions with colleagues, patients, carers or fellow students, and then evaluate your talking style, observing its impact on your communication partner. Ask a peer to review the tapes, alone or with you, and give you feedback on the effectiveness of your communication. Write a journal to examine good or poor interactions. Seek feedback informally or as a planned part of a performance appraisal.

Reflection on talking

In the day-to-day flow of clinical practice, healthcare professionals can improve the way they talk to the people they deal with by spending some time in quiet review of what they have just done and how they talked with the people they worked with. Asking yourself questions about a conversation that has just passed (see Handy Hint 18.3) can highlight areas of particular difficulty, which can then be worked on by using some of the above strategies and techniques to improve your communication style and skill. Taking those reflections into subsequent clinical conversations helps practitioners to build their experience in talking with people in healthcare situations.

PERSONAL CHECKLIST FOR TALKING WITH COLLEAGUES, CLIENTS, PATIENTS AND CARERS

- Why am I talking? (e.g. to inform or to support)

- Is this the best time and place to talk?

- What level of technical language (lay or technical language) should I choose?

- How direct should I be? (e.g. when informing someone of bad news, you may need to use an indirect style to 'soften the blow')

- Am I balancing my talk with that of others? (talk turns should usually be kept short, and this can be especially important in some cases)

- Am I actively listening?

- Am I allowing appropriate silences?
- Am I keeping sentences suitably simple? (give preference to simple sentences without embedded clauses)
- Can I get my message across more clearly? (consider the mode of delivery of the message, such as oral, written, or using an alternative communication strategy, such as interpreted sign language, pictureboard or voice synthesiser)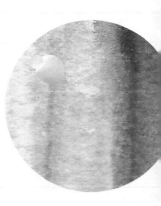

conclusion

In this chapter we have discussed ways in which healthcare practitioners can develop meaningful and effective talk for people, by people and with people, to better promote the healthcare process. These strategies can be practised, and we encourage you to do so, as good communication skills are the foundation of successful healthcare.

references

Concise Oxford Dictionary. (2008). Rapport. Retrieved from www.wordreference.com/definition/rapport

De Vito, J. A. (2001). *Human communication: The basic course* (9th edn). New York: Longman.

Edwards, I., Jones, M., Higgs, J., Trede, F., & Jensen, G. (2004). What is collaborative reasoning? *Advances in Physiotherapy, 6*, 70–83. doi: 10.1080/14038190410018938

Encyclopaedia of Nursing and Allied Health. (2011). Patient confidentiality. Retrieved from www.enotes.com/nursing-encyclopedia

Harrington, J., Noble, L. M., & Newman, S. P. (2004). *Patient education and counselling, 52*, pp. 7–16. doi:10.1016/S0738-399(03)00017-X

Speech Pathology Australia. *What is a communication disability?* Retrieved from www.speechpathologyaustralia.org.au/library/1.3_What_is_a_Communication_Disability.pdf

further reading

Lugton, J. (2003). *Communicating with dying people and their relatives*. Ascot Vale, VIC: Ausmed. This practical book provides assistance for dealing with practical and emotional aspects related to palliative care.

Robertson, K. (2005). Active listening: More than just paying attention. *Australian Family Physician, 34*(12), 1053–5. This is a useful guide to understand listening skills.

useful web resources

For useful tips to develop effective and active listening skills, see powertochange.
com/students/people/listen/

For definitions, information and further resources for AAC, see www.isaac-online.
org/english/home

For support for people affected by cancer, see cancerconnections.com.au/

Interviewing patients and clients

Stephen **LOFTUS** | Sandra **MACKEY**

key topics

This chapter covers the following topics:

- the purpose of interviewing

- interview structures, protocols and heuristics

- interviews as dialogue

key terms

PROTOCOLS

DIALOGUE

MNEMONICS

HEURISTICS

Introduction

Interviewing patients and clients (in this chapter called *interviewees*) is a skill that most professionals need to master. Strong interviewing skills are crucial for planning effective care. Professional interviewing is not something that comes naturally to anybody; it is a skill that has to be learned and practised. In this chapter we explore some of the key aspects of interviewing in healthcare settings.

The purpose of interviewing

Most interviewing in the health sciences is carried out to inform decision-making. The decisions can range from making a diagnosis to planning treatment, or determining the nature and extent of interviewee education. Good decision-making is only as good as the information on which it is based. Much of the important information needed for decision-making in the health sciences comes from interviews.

In many health professions the interview forms the first part of a comprehensive assessment, and can be followed by a physical examination, and perhaps by special investigations such as radiographs or blood tests. The interview is crucial to the establishment of rapport between the interviewee and the health practitioner, which is the foundation for the development of a therapeutic relationship.

Planning and preparation

Before the interview commences, the health professional needs to ensure that arrangements are in place to maximise comprehensive data collection. Consider:

- *Preparation:* If there are records available, read them first and make a note of the questions you want to ask. The culture of the patient needs to be taken into account. For example, women from some cultures may prefer to be interviewed by another woman or might want a chaperone to be present. If the interviewee is from a non English-speaking background, arrangements may need to be made for an interpreter to be present. Although family members are sometimes acceptable as interpreters, their presence can constrain what the interviewee is prepared to reveal. Some institutions insist that a qualified and independent interpreter is used (e.g. NSW Government, 2006). This can take some time to arrange, so plan ahead if you are able. Consider where you will seat the interpreter in relation to yourself and the interviewee, and brief the interpreter on your expectations; for example, that everything will be interpreted, not just summarised.

- *Children and adolescents:* Children should normally be interviewed in the presence of a parent or legal guardian. Where possible, the child should be involved and asked to answer the questions he or she is capable of answering. Most children can point to a source of pain, for example. Interviewing adolescents can be more problematic. Younger adolescents are legally children and you may be required to interview them in the same way as you would a child, with a parent or guardian present. But some adolescents may prefer to be interviewed alone, especially for delicate subjects.

- *Disclosure:* It is worth finding out beforehand what your institution and profession require about disclosure. Normally, any information given to you by an interviewee is regarded as confidential. Occasionally, certain information must be notified to others; for example, if it emerges that a patient has a disease such as typhoid or cholera then public health authorities must be notified. What do you do if a patient gives you information that incriminates the patient or someone else? Do parents have the right to know what emerges in an interview with their adolescent child? There are both legal and ethical issues here, and it is worth finding out what guidelines are provided by your institution or professional body.

- *Timing:* Schedule the interview to ensure that it can be completed without interruption. Consider the interviewee's condition and age in determining the length of interview. It may be necessary to collect your interview data in a number of sittings.

- *Setting:* Privacy is crucial to the disclosure of personal information. It is also important to remember that although the setting may be a normal environment for you, for the interviewee it can be quite threatening, especially if the interview has to occur in a place like an intensive care unit or a busy emergency department, with other people close by and where the client is surrounded by strange and noisy machinery. If the interview must take place in such a setting, be sensitive to the feelings of the interviewee. If 'delicate' personal information is needed, it is best to ask for this in a quiet and private setting, if at all possible.

- *Comfort:* Ensure that the area in which the interview will be carried out is at a comfortable temperature for both you and the interviewee. Adequate lighting and appropriate seating will also facilitate the interview process.

- *Equipment:* Make sure you have all the necessary documentation and a pen that works, before you begin the interview. If you are using electronic equipment to document interview findings, ensure it is in working order. Check that the interviewee's visual or hearing aids are in place and working.

Phases of an interview

Most interviews can be divided into three simple phases. First is the *introductory phase*, during which interviewer and interviewee establish who they are, what they are doing and the purpose of the interview. Always introduce yourself to the interviewee and tell the person who you are. Seek permission from the interviewee to conduct the interview and to make the necessary documentation; this is particularly important if you are a student. Ensure that you address the client appropriately; do not use the interviewee's first name until you are invited to do so. Make sure that you use the interviewee's correct title. For instance, an elderly single woman may not take kindly to being addressed as *Mrs* rather than *Miss*. Our experience has shown that making what may seem to be this simple mistake can result in a most uncooperative interviewee.

Second is the *working phase*, which normally takes up the bulk of the time, and in which the interviewer gathers most of the information needed. This phase in particular requires the use of a range of verbal and non-verbal communication skills, such as:

- using clear and concise speech and language, avoiding jargon and clinical terms
- using open-ended questions to encourage free-flowing dialogue
- using closed questions when you need specific information or to contain the length of the interview
- making effective use of prompts to encourage elaboration and precision of information
- asking for clarification when necessary
- appropriately using eye contact, gesture, posture and touch (Jarvis, 2012).

Third, is the *termination phase*, in which the interviewer may summarise information for clarification, outline further steps arising from the interview if needed, and then draw the interview to a close.

Protocols for interviewing

A typical interview has to cover a lot of different information. A logical, systematic structure is needed for the interview, so that no important information is missed. Fortunately for beginners, most professions have developed well-known and formal **protocols** that interviewers are expected to follow. Whatever the protocols for your profession, you need to learn them by heart at an early stage, so that you can use them as soon as you start meeting interviewees in a professional setting. Most protocols break the interview process up into a series of stages, with questions that focus on particular aspects (or categories) of the problem with which your interviewee needs you to deal. It is useful to think of a professional interview as a process of progressive working through these categories and their questions.

/ **PROTOCOLS** /
Protocols break the interview process up into a series of stages.

Start at the beginning—determine the reason for seeking care

In the health professions, after checking the identity of the interviewee and introducing yourself, the first category of information to work through usually deals with the presenting problem or chief complaint of the interviewee; that is, the reason the interviewee is seeking healthcare. 'What's the problem you're here for today?' could be a typical opening question designed to elicit this information. This would then be followed by questions that encourage the interviewee to tell the story of the chief complaint. If the interviewee's chief complaint is pain, for example, this cues the professional to ask a series of questions that can prompt for important information, such as: Where exactly is the pain? Does it come and go? How long does it last? Does anything make it worse? Does anything make it better? The answers to any of these questions can provide crucial information in helping you to establish a diagnosis and treatment plan. Even if the answers to many questions do not seem significant in themselves, they can still provide important background information.

Knowing what to cover in the interview

In a health setting, these opening stages are followed by questions that explore different aspects or categories of the interviewee's life and health status. The depth and breadth of the categories explored at interview are determined by the reason for seeking care. For instance, if the interviewee has pain from a toothache, the information you collect will have an emphasis different from that of an interviewee who complains of chest pain.

The interviewee's health history is one typical category of information; others include the social and family history. Some of these topic areas, such as the health history, can be quite large, and it is convenient to subdivide them further into subcategories. In a medical setting, the health history can be subdivided into a systems review, with questions about the interviewee's respiratory system, the cardiovascular system, the nervous system and so on. The social history typically includes questions about lifestyle factors such as smoking and alcohol consumption, and the family history covers information about the health of other members of the interviewee's family. If you suspect an interviewee might be diabetic, for example, then knowing that many members of the immediate family are diabetic will increase the likelihood that the person in front of you is suffering from that problem.

In many cases, the interview focuses on a particular aspect of the interviewee's health status. This is usually the situation when the interviewee has been receiving treatment for a particular problem (e.g., surgical repair of a broken arm), and in the interview you just want to get an update on the condition and the effectiveness of the treatment. Screening for risk factors associated with specific health problems is another situation in which focused interviews are carried out. For example, in screening for cervical cancer, the interviewer focuses on gathering information about the interviewee's exposure to risk factors for this condition, rather than information about the person's whole health status. Focused interviews are commonly carried out in the emergency or outpatients department of hospitals, and in community-based general medical practice.

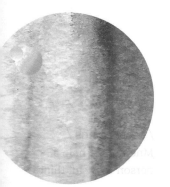

interview need to be interpreted with care. Consider when to apply a particular maxim and when to apply its opposite—but this judgment only comes with practice and experience of many cases.

conclusion

Professional interviewing is an important and sophisticated skill for anybody working in the health sciences. Proficiency can come with experience and practice. Many professions provide protocols that can help to make the process more routine. However, whether you are using protocols or not, interviews always need to be conducted with sensitivity and an awareness that every person is different. Each interview is a unique dialogue in which interviewer and interviewee jointly construct the story of the interviewee's health. A well-conducted interview provides health professionals with much of the information they need to help interviewees, and to reassure those same interviewees that they are receiving the attention of a competent and caring professional.

references

Charon, R. (2006). *Narrative medicine: Honoring the stories of illness*. Oxford: Oxford University Press.

Jarvis, C. (2012). *Physical examination and health assessment* (6th edn). St Louis: Saunders.

Montgomery, K. (2006). *How doctors think: Clinical judgment and the practice of medicine*. Oxford: Oxford University Press.

NSW Government. (2006). *Standard procedures for working with health care interpreters*. Retrieved from http://www.health.nsw.gov.au/policies/pd/2006/PD2006_053.html

Touhy, T., & Jett, K. (2011). *Ebersole & Hess' toward healthy aging* (8th edn). St Louis: Mosby.

Intercultural communication

Franziska **TREDE** | Barbara **HILL**

key topics

This chapter covers the following topics:

- culture and intercultural communication

- the need for cultural competence

- communicating across culturally and linguistically diverse groups

- strategies for intercultural communication

- working with interpreters

key terms

INTERCULTURAL COMMUNICATION

CULTURAL COMPETENCE

Introduction

International patterns of globalisation, migration and mobility require effective intercultural communication. The people of Australia make up one of the most culturally and linguistically diverse nations in the world. They speak hundreds of languages and most of the world's religions are worshipped here, with 27 per cent of Australians having been born overseas (ABS, 2010). In an increasingly globalised world and mobile workforce, competence in intercultural communication is an important ingredient for harmonious workplaces, as well as for accessible, safe and appropriate professional service delivery (Australian Government NHMRC, 2006). Culturally competent interpersonal communications reduce misunderstandings, misdiagnoses and time wasted; they increase access to and compliance with management plans, boost staff and patient satisfaction, and encourage ethical practices (Le Roux, 2002).

It is a universal human right to have access to high-quality services (Australian Government NHMRC, 2006). A recent quality and safety report identified miscommunication as a crucial factor that led to 25 per cent of all critical incidents in New South Wales (NSW Health, 2005). People-centred approaches to communicating with clients are prominently taught in undergraduate education and professional development, and relate well to good intercultural communication practices. Their common key features are valuing clients' perceptions, expectations, fears and hopes and, at the same time, appreciating your own perspectives, encouraging involved participation of clients, and focusing on practical, functional and appropriate goals. In this chapter we discuss theories of intercultural communication, and consider key principles and skills that prepare health scientists for working effectively in culturally diverse workplaces and ensuring that services are accessible, acceptable, safe and appropriate for the diverse needs of clients.

Theories of intercultural communications

/ **INTERCULTURAL COMMUNICATION** /
Intercultural communication involves working effectively and relating appropriately to others in diverse cultural contexts.

Study of **intercultural communication** can be categorised into three frameworks: cross-cultural, intercultural, and interdiscursive communication. The *cross-cultural* communication framework is based on the assumption that there are distinctive cultures that are directly comparable (Piller, 2007). People are identified as belonging to a particular cultural group according to country of birth, language, ethnicity and religion. It is assumed that particular communication and language skills can be used when interacting with people from any cultural group. There is an assumption that cultures are homogeneous, and that one communication style will fit each and every culture.

The *intercultural* communication framework is based on the assumption that communication styles need to be adapted to each distinctive culture. Kleinman and Benson (2006) suggest that an ethnographic methodology, non-verbal observations and verbal competency provide professionals with an intensive and imaginative empathy for the experience of the people from other cultures. Intercultural communication studies provide insights into other cultures and how to interact appropriately with members of particular cultural groups (Hofstede, 2001). When one of the authors is invited to conduct workshops on cultural competence with other healthcare professionals, she is often asked to discuss, say, Greek or Japanese culture, so that staff can work better with patients from these backgrounds. These requests are based on the assumption that better knowledge of a culture's religious customs and national traits improves communication with people from that culture. Avoiding sweeping assumptions, you can make recommendations such as: Japanese people consider a cancer diagnosis to be a death sentence, so replace the word 'cancer' with 'growth' or 'tumour' to maintain hope and the will to live; you should not judge or make assumptions about Indigenous Australians for avoiding eye contact, but also consider avoiding eye contact if given the appropriate non-verbal clues; Muslim women are usually accompanied by their husbands when seeking medical services. Although it is useful to recognise the behaviours and customs of cultural groups, it is important to remember that not all members who identify with these groups share the same beliefs, experiences, expectations and behaviours.

The *interdiscursive* communication framework challenges the notion of rigid, static and singular cultural membership (Piller, 2007). Instead, it places emphasis on interpersonal communication and professional relationships. This framework moves the focus from cultural groups towards individuals. It suggests that people create their own cultures in the way they choose to engage with one another: how they negotiate who is allowed to talk, what is allowed to be talked about and what is not, how people agree on care plans, when to refer patients to other services and what to do next. Interdiscursive communication emphasises the importance of not prejudging people according to their appearance, accent, gender, religious belief, disability or any other distinguishing features. Clinicians adopting an interdiscursive framework work well with individuals to address their needs.

Defining culture

People may identify with a cultural group on the basis of language, religion, ethnicity and country of birth. However, they may not all share the same views. Not all Australians love rugby or barbecues. There is no one accepted definition of culture. A commonality seems to be the acceptance of culture as a process of learning values, being involved in collective rituals, role-modelling and understanding symbols like myths, legends, dress, jargon and lingo. Hofstede (2001, p. 4) suggests that culture is 'mental programming ... patterns of thinking and feeling and potential acting', and Jones (2007, p. 3) reminds us that 'ingredients of culture are acquired from birth. They are influenced by family, school, religion, workplace, friends, television, newspapers and books, and many other sources'. Culture manifests itself in our routine activities: how we greet each other, dress, talk or raise children. Culture does not exist independently; we construct it ourselves. Culture can be understood as a *lens* through which we make sense of the world. Culture can influence, but not necessarily predict, how people think, feel and behave. Cultural values are dynamic, and can change with life experiences and other external events. It might be more useful to consider economic, educational, social, gender, political, ethnic and language influences on health rather than lumping them all under the umbrella of culture.

ASPECTS OF DEFINING CULTURE

- There are different interpretations of culture that go beyond nation and ethnicity.
- Culture is an abstract model.
- Culture includes shared knowledge, values, meanings, beliefs and experiences.
- Cultural backgrounds do not necessarily predict behaviour and expectations.

In healthcare settings, culture is often simplistically understood as ethnicity, religion, country of birth and language. This perspective is reinforced through patient record systems with labels for country of birth, language and religion. People may have mixed cultural heritage; within any 'cultural' group there is a range of differing values. There can be a difference between first- or second-generation Australians, between remote, rural and urban Australians. Not all second-generation Australians identify with their parents' cultural backgrounds. Some Greek migrants are seen to be more Greek than people back in Greece, but others do not want their Greek heritage to be known. Furthermore, people may identify with different cultures in different contexts. There are work cultures, family cultures, eating cultures and sport cultures. It is difficult to put people into one cultural box. Professionals who use the traditional definition of *culture* as denoting religion, language and ethnicity run the risk of racist behaviour by patronising and dominating others, and reducing them to single identities. They may unintentionally label cultural differences as a cause of miscommunication, when in fact the issue might be about gender, power or other factors. Broader definitions of *culture* include culture as a product of technology, arts, education, economy and science. Cultural values denote what is important to individuals. These values are not rigid and can change with life experiences. Appreciating values helps us to assess individual needs that might be overlooked because of differing social, physical, sexual, political, environmental, economic, spiritual, linguistic or mental backgrounds. These broader dimensions of culture can help professionals to appreciate different interpretations in relation to health and illness and, in particular, can raise awareness of different interpretations of pain, illness behaviour, disability, spirituality (including fatalistic beliefs about life and death) and disclosure.

/ CULTURAL COMPETENCE /
Cultural competence is the ability to engage appropriately and effectively with people across different cultures.

Cultural competence

From our discussion of culture, it is evident that the concept of **cultural competence** is not a technical skill acquired through training (Kleinman & Benson, 2006). Cultural competence involves a set of skills and dispositions that enable people to work well across cultures. It is generally recognised that all health science professionals need to be on the journey to becoming culturally competent. In New Zealand, Maori nurses instigated the notion of *cultural safety*, which is often used in preference to and instead of *cultural competence*. Cultural safety means that 'there is no assault, challenge or denial of their [people's] personal identity, of who they are and what they need. It is about shared respect, shared meaning, and shared knowledge and experience, of learning together with dignity, and truly listening' (Williams, 1999, pp. 213–14). Cultural safety has been closely linked to patient safety and quality services.

Although there is no universally accepted definition of *cultural competence* many definitions share key elements. These include: valuing diversity, having the capacity for cultural self-assessment, being conscious of the dynamics inherent in cross-cultural interactions, and institutions embedding the importance of cultural knowledge in policies and making adaptations to service delivery that reflect cultural understanding. These measures can go some way towards helping to redress power imbalances that influence healthcare communication (see Chapter 2). It is important to note that cultural competence needs to be viewed as a process or an ideal to strive for, rather than a destination.

A contemporary culturally competent practitioner is someone who is competent in applying a set of principles to ensure accessible, effective, quality, acceptable, safe, appropriate and equitable services. These principles include:

- critical self-awareness and assessment of a person's own values, biases and assumptions
- respect for a variety of interpretations and their impact on health
- use of inclusive dialogue that allows patients to express their particular needs.

These principles develop knowledge, attitudes and skills of effective communication with *all* people, and therefore also ensure appropriate and accessible services for culturally and linguistically diverse people. Cultural competence embodies the same principles as people-centred approaches to practice and communication, which include awareness of personal and professional values, respect for diverse perspectives, and an understanding that communication is not only about telling and explaining but also includes deep listening, which entails not interrupting. Becoming culturally competent involves observing, learning, being curious and being inclusive by checking that you understand and are being understood. Handy Hint 20.2 is adapted from the *Diversity Health Kit* (SESIAHS, 2007).

handy hint 20.2

TOWARDS CULTURAL COMPETENCE

- Avoid stereotyping.
- Treat others as you want to be treated.
- Do not assume—ask.

- Develop personal ethics statements that include values of inclusiveness, respect and access.
- Show your colleagues you value them.
- Be respectful.
- Be kind and caring.
- Reflect on your communication experiences in order to learn from them.

Cultural competence in intercultural communication saves time, avoids complaints and reduces miscommunication that can lead to misdiagnosis, malpractice and poor health outcomes (Williams, 1999). Cultural competence also ensures shared understanding, increased treatment adherence, patient satisfaction and cultural safety (Johnstone & Kanitsaki, 2005). Intercultural communication is a challenge because people do not all share the same:

- communication styles and preferences
- understanding of who is responsible for health, disease and recovery
- expectations of the roles of patients and human service professionals
- interpretations of pain, disability and gender roles.

These are just some examples of the many differences people bring to a professional consultation. They show why it is vital to appreciate a variety of interpretations when communicating with others. However, having discussed the challenges of communicating effectively with patients from diverse backgrounds, we emphasise that working effectively with people from different linguistic backgrounds can be facilitated when we use interpreters to bridge language barriers.

Working with interpreters

The need to understand and be understood is fundamental in the provision of safe professional services. It is incumbent on health professionals to use professional healthcare interpreters when people are not proficient in English, to ensure equal access to knowledge and quality of services. Interpreting involves translating what is said in one language into another language; for example, interpreting what is said by an English-speaking health professional into Cantonese for a Cantonese-speaking patient, and then interpreting the patient's replies from Cantonese into English for the health professional. Simultaneous or consecutive interpretation may be used. With *simultaneous interpretation*, the interpreter translates while the speaker continues to deliver the message for translation. This is a difficult task for the interpreter, requiring high-level skills, such as those seen in diplomatic missions. More commonly, *consecutive interpreting* is used: the speaker delivers a sentence or two, pauses for the interpreter to interpret, and then continues with the next part of the message.

Working as a speech pathologist sometimes requires word-for-word interpretation to assess a client's communication skills. This is called *literal interpretation* (Isaac, 2002). Literal interpretation is not required in all contexts; the health professional should brief the interpreter before client contact about the degree of literalness required.

Effective interpreting requires a qualified and accredited interpreter who is conversant with the health or social services setting, with professional terminology (such as medical and social work) and with the culture of the patient. An interpreter may speak the same language as a patient but not be familiar with his or her particular culture (think of the many countries in which Spanish is spoken), so check the cultural background of both patient and interpreter when booking an interpreter. Sometimes a qualified interpreter is not available. It might be possible to use a telephone interpreter service, or you might, as a last resort, use an untrained interpreter; perhaps a family member, a member of staff at the healthcare facility or a community member. Be aware that there are many potential problems with using untrained interpreters, and it may contravene health institution policies. Familiarise yourself with the language and healthcare interpreter policies of your workplace when working with people from non-English-speaking backgrounds. Most organisations have language cards or ward words to help communication about daily ward matters. You must use a professional interpreter in your practice when a client asks for one, or when you are not confident that you understand or can be understood by clients.

Consider the following issues when working with people from non English-speaking backgrounds (adapted from SESIAHS, 2007):

- All patients, their families and their carers have the right to a professional interpreter. Patients need to understand and be understood. This is a prerequisite for providing competent healthcare.
- As staff are legally liable for the information they provide, it is *strongly recommended* that a professional interpreter is always used when obtaining consent. A face-to-face or telephone interpreter must be used for pre-admission, admission, discharge, assessment and treatment plans (including referrals and explanation of medication), mental health review tribunals and magistrate hearings, reportable incidents, health education and health promotion programs.
- Staff should not be removed from their usual duties to interpret.
- Use your professional judgment to determine if a person is *fully* able to understand you and be understood in return. Remember that the stresses associated with illness, injury and exposure to the hospital system can affect language skills, particularly for people who have learned English

recently as a second or third language. Language proficiency also decreases as we age. Be aware that basic functional English is very different from the terminology used to discuss medical conditions, treatment options and Western health concepts.

- If you use family members as interpreters you cannot ensure accuracy and control over the interpretations; you cannot determine what they censor, misunderstand or even deliberately mistranslate, or whether they have refrained from interpreting all of what you or the client says. Further, patients may not feel comfortable discussing sensitive or personal information in front of people they know, or who differ from them in age, gender or social class. You could end up with incomplete or inaccurate information.

KEY ISSUES ABOUT INTERPRETERS

- Healthcare interpreter service (in public hospitals in Australia) is a free, confidential and professional service.
- Patients have a right to an interpreter.
- Family members and staff are not professional interpreters.
- Staff have a responsibility to use interpreters when they are not confident that patients are proficient in English.
- It is a legal requirement to use interpreters when you seek consent for treatment, and especially for invasive procedures.

Effective interpreting requires adequate briefing between practitioner and interpreter (Isaac, 2002). Because of the time taken to interpret, a session with a client requiring interpretation will take longer than a normal interaction. You need to schedule more time for the appointment, and maybe more than one session to complete the task (e.g. to complete a thorough assessment or to provide adequate counselling).

WORKING WITH AN INTERPRETER

When working with an interpreter, make time for a briefing before the client arrives and for debriefing afterwards.

In the briefing session, share with your interpreter:

- the purpose of the interview
- the patient history that is relevant for the interpreter to know to be able to interpret in context
- any hints from the interpreter that you should be aware of

- the type of interpretation you require; for example, literal interpretation (word for word).

In the debriefing session:

- discuss with your interpreter your impression of how the session went

- invite the interpreter to contribute comment.

Use of healthcare interpreters requires you to remain in control of your consultation. Start with a formal introduction to the patient and interpreter; explain that everything said will be translated and that there might be time afterwards for a social chat. Many patients use the interpreter as a social outlet because the language barrier isolates them. Consider where people sit, and maintain eye contact with your patient, not the interpreter. The interpreter is only there to bridge the language barrier. Book the interpreter to arrive early for briefing and allow time after the session with the interpreter for debriefing.

Post-session debriefing allows you to discuss interaction problems, identify communication breakdowns and agree on strategies for improving future interactions. Use the interpreter as a 'cultural informant'. Debriefing is especially important if you work regularly with a particular interpreter or cultural group.

conclusion

Culture is a complex and dynamic concept. It means more than country of birth, religion, language and ethnicity, and it can change over time. Effective intercultural communication is essential wherever we work. In this chapter we have highlighted aspects of communication that enhance equality and access, and suggested strategies for effective intercultural communication and working with interpreters.

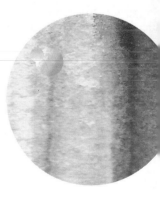

references

ABS. (2010). *Migration, Australia 2008-9*. Cat. No. 3412.0. Canberra: Australian Bureau of Statistics, Commonwealth of Australia.

Australian Government NHMRC. (2006). *Cultural competency in health: A guide for policy, partnership and participation*. Canberra: Australian Government and National Health and Medical Research Council.

Hofstede, G. (2001). *Culture's consequences: Comparing values, behaviors, institutions and organizations across nations* (2nd edn). Thousand Oaks, CA: Sage.

Isaac, K. (2002). *Speech pathology in cultural and linguistic diversity*. London: Whurr.

Johnstone, M. J., & Kanitsaki, O. (2005). *Cultural safety and cultural competence in health care and nursing: An Australian study*. Retrieved from www.rmit.edu.au/nursing/cultural-safety

Jones, M. (2007). Hofstede—Culturally questionable? Oxford Business & Economics Conference. Oxford, UK, 24–26 June, 2007.

Kleinman, A., & Benson, P. (2006). Anthropology in the clinic: The problem of cultural competency and how to fix it. *PLoS Med, 3*(10), e294. doi:10.1371/journal.pmed.0030294.

Le Roux, J. (2002). Effective educators are culturally competent communicators. *Intercultural Education, 13*(1), 37–48.

NSW Health. (2005). *Patient safety and clinical quality program: First report of incident management in the NSW Public Health Care System 2003–2004,* Publication SHPN (QBS) 040262, NSW Department of Health.

Piller, I. (2007). Linguistics and intercultural communication. *Language and Linguistic Compass, 1*(3), 208–26.

SESIAHS. (2007). *The diversity health kit*. South East Sydney and Illawarra Area Health Service: NSW Health.

Williams, R. (1999). Cultural safety: What does it mean for our work practice? *Australian and New Zealand Journal of Public Health, 23*(2), 213–14.

further reading

Du Pre, A. (2005). *Communicating about health: Current issues and perspectives* (2nd edn). Boston: McGraw Hill. This book outlines the research and theory of health communication and offers practical advice and examples that allow students to further develop skills in health communication.

The National Translating and Interpreting Service (TIS). The Australian Government, through TIS National, provides free interpreting services to non-English-speaking Australian citizens and permanent residents. See www.immi.gov.au/living-in-australia/help-with-english/help_with_translating/free-services.htm

The Diversity Health Institute Clearinghouse. This is a central access point for Australian multicultural health services, resources, research and projects, training, and events. See http://203.32.142.106/clearinghouse/default.htm

acknowledgments

We acknowledge Lindy McAllister and Annette Street who authored the chapter on this topic in the second edition of this book. Our chapter has revised and updated their earlier version.

Communicating clinical reasoning

Rola AJJAWI | Joy HIGGS | Lindy MᶜALLISTER

key topics

This chapter covers the following topics:

- the nature of clinical reasoning

- types of clinical reasoning

- how to communicate reasoning

key terms

CLINICAL REASONING

Introduction

/ CLINICAL
REASONING /

Clinical reasoning is a broad term denoting the thinking, judgments and decision-making involved in clinical practice.

Clinical reasoning is central to clinical practice. Health professionals often need to make decisions based on their professional knowledge and judgment in situations where there are no right answers, and where textbook and research knowledge is insufficient, or needs to be adapted to the particular client (or patient). This is a key aspect of being a professional. The process of reasoning drives practice decisions and actions. Clear communication of reasoning enables clients and clinicians to work together and helps teams to function effectively.

Clinical reasoning includes *micro* decisions, such as: What questions do I need to ask this client? What assessments are appropriate for this client?; and *macro* (or major) decisions, such as: What are this client's major problems? What is this client's diagnosis and prognosis? How does this client envisage her future after this accident? What is the best management plan for this client? Clinical reasoning also includes the *meta*-thinking and decision-making that you will constantly undertake during practice as you monitor your thinking. For instance, you will ask yourself: How do I know if the answer the client just gave me is complete? Did he understand my question? How well can I do that test, and can I trust my findings? Do I understand enough about this person and this condition to make a sound decision about care? Do I need help here?

The nature of clinical reasoning

Clinical reasoning is a broad term denoting the thinking, judgments and decision-making involved in clinical practice. At times, for instance when the setting is more community-based than clinical, it is preferable to speak of *professional decision-making*. Clinical reasoning is not a readily observable phenomenon, even though you can see and hear people talking about it, and see the results of their decisions. For this reason, researchers and clinicians have sought to understand clinical reasoning through research and theoretical models (see Higgs, Jones, Loftus, & Christensen, 2008).

The *hypothetico-deductive reasoning* model (Elstein, Shulman, & Sprafka, 1978, 1990) portrays clinical reasoning as a process of establishing hypotheses (provisional diagnoses and ideas for treatment), testing them by gathering data (during history-taking, physical examination, medical tests and treatment), and analysing these data (see Figure 21.1). Hypothetico-deductive reasoning occurs in a number of professions, including medicine, physiotherapy, occupational therapy, speech pathology, dentistry and nursing. It is a thorough, careful process, frequently used by novices and by more experienced practitioners working with unusual or difficult cases.

Pattern recognition (Groen & Patel, 1985) is a more rapid process, by which experienced clinicians directly retrieve existing knowledge from their rich, discipline-specific knowledge base when they are in situations where they are familiar with the type of case or condition being considered. Novices have been found to use pattern recognition. However, the likelihood of making diagnostic errors is greater when based on a knowledge base that is not well developed (Eva, 2004). In reality, clinicians frequently utilise pattern recognition as a component of or in combination with hypothesis testing and evaluation.

Other models of clinical reasoning have been proposed, particularly in nursing, occupational therapy and physiotherapy, to reflect the growing emphasis on client-centred care and the 'wellness' model (e.g. Fleming 1991; Jones 1992; Fonteyn, 1995). These approaches include (Higgs, 2003):

- *Interactive reasoning*–occurs when dialogue in the form of social exchange is used to enhance or facilitate the assessment-management process. This reasoning provides an effective way of understanding the context of the client's problem and creating a relationship of interest and trust.

- *Narrative reasoning*–involves the use by practitioners of stories of past or present clients to help themselves and their clients further understand and manage a clinical situation. Practitioners can use such real-life scenarios to enhance the credibility of the advice or explanations they give to clients. Narrative reasoning can also involve the practitioner and/or the client constructing a story of the client's future life after an illness or with a disability, as well as reconnecting the client to his or her life story. Narrative reasoning is used in some fields to facilitate ethical reasoning (see e.g. Charon & Montello, 2002).

- *Ethical* or *pragmatic reasoning*–is used by practitioners to make decisions regarding moral, political and economic dilemmas, such as deciding how long to continue a client's treatment. Body and McAllister (2009) have provided many case studies of ethical reasoning which considers such dimensions.

- *Shared decision-making*–involves respecting the self-knowledge of clients and their capacity to share in decision-making about their health, and encouraging their collaboration in genuinely client-centred care that is person- and situation-specific.

It can be seen from the range of models presented here that to reason effectively, health professionals need cognitive capabilities and the necessary underpinning knowledge, metacognitive (monitoring thinking), social and interactive, and emotional capabilities (Smith, Higgs, & Ellis, 2008).

Communicating reasoning is inherent in the various models of clinical reasoning identified here (to collect data in the hypothetico-deductive model, to construct a client narrative, or for informing and empowering clients to share in the decision-making process). Recent research into clinical reasoning has further emphasised the interactive and collaborative nature of reasoning (Ajjawi, 2009; Loftus, 2009). Clinical reasoning requires the development of language skills, including learning a shared language among members of multidisciplinary health teams (Loftus & Higgs, 2006). Learning this shared language provides you with access to the relevant professional community. The key message is to recognise the complexity involved in your clinical reasoning, and to know that flexibility in thinking based on the demands of the situation is important. Thus there are no simple steps to follow that will facilitate communication of reasoning. The suggestions in Handy Hint 21.1 will help you to reflect on and develop your clinical reasoning and communication skills.

FIGURE **21.1** | HYPOTHETICO-DEDUCTIVE REASONING

```
                    ┌─────────────────┐
                    │   Information   │
                    │   perception    │
                    │      and        │
                    │ interpretation  │
                    └─────────────────┘
                             │
                    ┌─────────────────┐        ┌─────────────────┐
                    │ Initial concept │        │      Data       │
                    │      and        │  More  │   collection    │
                    │    multiple     │  info  │ • Subjective    │
                    │   hypotheses    │ needed │   interview     │
                    └─────────────────┘        │ • Physical      │
                             │                 │   examination   │
                    ┌─────────────────┐        └─────────────────┘
  • Knowledge base  │    Evolving     │
  • Cognitive skills│    concept      │  More information
  • Metacognitive   │  of the problem │  needed
    skills          │(hypotheses      │
                    │   modified)     │
                    └─────────────────┘
                             │
                    ┌─────────────────┐
                    │    Decision     │
                    │  • Diagnostic   │
                    │  • Management   │
                    └─────────────────┘
                             │
                    ┌─────────────────┐
                    │ Physical therapy│
                    │  intervention   │
                    └─────────────────┘
                             │
                    ┌─────────────────┐
                    │  Reassessment   │
                    └─────────────────┘
```

Source: Jones, Jensen & Rothstein 1995. Reproduced with the permission of M. Jones.

IMPROVING YOUR CLINICAL REASONING

- Spend some time thinking about how you make clinical decisions.
- Listen to how experienced practitioners justify and explain their decisions.
- Seek feedback on your clinical reasoning from peers and teachers.
- Practise explaining your decisions with your peers or students, and discussing the knowledge you are using to justify your decisions. Challenge each other to provide credible rationales. For example, ask 'How do you know that this knowledge is true?' and 'How credible is that theory as the basis for your treatment decisions?'.

Communicating your clinical reasoning

Communicating reasoning does not necessarily reflect actual reasoning processes, because reasoning is rapid, situated, and involves tacit knowledge. Instead, communication of reasoning represents a reconstruction of the main processes perceived as most relevant to the co-communicator; that is, it is framed and delivered to match the audience. In her research examining how experienced physiotherapists communicated their reasoning, Ajjawi (2009) found that communication of clinical reasoning is a complex, dynamic skill that becomes mostly habitual; it is context-dependent, and fluid in content and style. Five key components of effective communication of clinical reasoning were identified in that research (Ajjawi & Higgs, 2011):

- *Active listening* entails an open and flexible attitude towards the other person's thoughts and reasoning.
- *Framing and presenting the message* involves having practitioners deconstruct or systematically break down their thinking processes, and reconstruct messages in ways that suit the situation. Framing and presenting the message is a complex process of 'unbundling' rapid and, at times, subconscious thought processes so that they can be presented in a way that the message can be understood.
- *Matching the audience* requires evaluating, judging and matching the co-communicator's frame of reference, and being aware of specialist language and jargon that might not be part of the co-communicator's vocabulary or common language. Therefore, communicating reasoning requires making judgments about the co-communicator's frame of reference, cognitive ability, communication skills, language comprehension and knowledge base.
- *Self-monitoring* involves checking that the spoken message was what was intended, that the language chosen was appropriate and that the message was understood as intended.
- *Awareness, capability and clarity in reasoning* require knowledge of the reasoning or message content to be communicated. It would be difficult to communicate something that is unknown, ill-formed or poorly understood.

Considering the audience

From this discussion of communication of clinical reasoning, it is evident that the first person you actually communicate with in clinical reasoning is yourself. This is a good place to start, because thinking occurs at a rapid rate, in ideas rather than sentences, often in a rather subconscious way. By reflecting on your clinical reasoning you can regulate your thinking and become sensitive to possible errors and so avoid them in practice (by making the wrong diagnosis, or providing inappropriate intervention or care).

In comparison, when you communicate with your colleagues, you are seeking to explain something clearly, justify your decisions or get feedback about your reasoning (such as what you are thinking about doing for, and with, this client). This reasoning therefore needs to be clear, in sentence form, supported by credible evidence, and relevant to the task and audience. Practitioners often use professional jargon and abbreviations (such as *BP* and *CVP*) when talking with colleagues. Remember that such jargon is a tool when talking with peers, a useful shorthand or common language, but it can create a confusing and distancing barrier if used when you are talking with clients or other professionals who do not speak the same language. When you are presenting a case at a staff seminar you would use different language (such as more formal and more detailed explanations) than when you are conversing in a ward with a colleague to share information about a client.

Your language and communication style will vary again when you are talking with a client, or with family members or caregivers. It is often helpful to put yourself in their place. Questions they might want to ask include: 'What do I need to know about my condition or my care? Why do they want me to do this? What aren't they telling me: do I have some terrible condition? Do they think I know nothing about my own health? Why can't they ask me what I think?' Reflect on these questions and you will see that you are not the only one who is reasoning or thinking, or making decisions. Your clients are doing those things too. If you are trying to provide client-centred care, or if that is what your client is expecting or demanding, what does it mean for your communication? It means recognising that you might know more about your profession and what it can offer than your clients and their family or carers do, but they know more about their bodies, their children, their health and healthcare needs than you do. It means that sometimes you need to teach people or provide them with enough information so they can be actively involved in decision-making. It means talking *with* clients, making decisions *with* them, and working *with* them to achieve the goals you both agree on for their wellbeing. This collaboration obviously varies in level and style, depending on the age, mental capacity, cultural expectations and wishes of your client. Remember that communication is a two-way activity; it is not just you telling people what you have decided is best for them and expecting them to comply.

COMMUNICATING REASONING

- Understand the purpose of your communication. What reasoning are you trying to convey or share?
- Recognise the needs and background of your audience and adjust your communication accordingly.
- Think about the context (such as formal, informal, emergency, scholarly debate) and tailor your communication to that context.
- Remember, communication is all about human interaction.

Being credible—articulating and providing evidence for your reasoning

If you communicate your reasoning, you will persuade others of the credibility of your decisions. Apart from using a language style that is appropriate for your audience, being credible requires giving an explanation of the reasoning behind your decisions. This is a challenging task for several reasons.

First, reasoning can happen rapidly, at a subconscious level. Our minds process many pieces of information quickly, and we often do not articulate all the connections we make in thinking (such as which of the many factors in the clinical situation make it preferable to choose one treatment option over another). In the classroom and during clinical education, students are encouraged to slow down and scrutinise their thinking so that they can explain the decisions they are making and the basis for these decisions. When they do this, students are often surprised at how much they actually know about their professional role and the rationales for proposed actions. They can also find out how much they still need to learn about people, their conditions and their healthcare needs.

Second, you need to provide evidence to justify your clinical decisions. This fits with the requirement of evidence-based practice in the broad, rather than narrow, sense of evidence focusing explicitly on quantitative research findings. Evidence for practice can be equated to knowledge, but there are many forms of knowledge generation, including but not limited to research. It is important to understand that credible knowledge, or evidence for practice, can be derived from practice as well as from research. Higgs and colleagues (2004, p. ix) argue that 'knowing how practice knowledge is created, used and developed [further] should become an explicit dimension of the core, the regularity and the expectation of professional practice'.

Evidence includes:

- *Professional craft knowledge.* Tested knowledge arising from practice experience (e.g. knowledge of the effectiveness of treatment strategies).

- *Propositional knowledge*. Knowledge from both quantitative and qualitative research into the effectiveness of clinical interventions; systematic reviews of the research literature can help you to collate and critique research-based evidence of best practice.
- *Theoretical knowledge*. Knowledge that provides a rationale for treatments or actions.
- *Applied science knowledge*. For example, how the body works, how people interact, and how cultural influences affect behaviour.
- *Data gained from interaction with the client*. Data on matters such as pain levels, needs and preferences, capacity to participate in treatment, and fears and concerns.

All these forms of evidence can be used in clinical reasoning to make decisions that facilitate best practice for the client in the particular situation.

handy hint 21.3

IMPROVING YOUR COMMUNICATION OF CLINICAL REASONING

To analyse how well you communicate your reasoning, think through the following matters:

- What approaches do you recognise in your reasoning (e.g. hypothetico-deductive or narrative)?
- What ethical issues do you face in your clinical practice? How do you deal with them?
- What do you think is important to say when talking to clients or colleagues about your clinical or professional decisions?
- What difference does it make if you are talking to adults or to children, to clients in hospitals or in community settings, to clients or to their carers?

conclusion

As a health professional, you are accountable for your decisions and service provision to various stakeholders, including clients, caregivers, health sector managers, policy-makers and colleagues. An important aspect of this accountability is the ability to clearly articulate and justify your management decisions in a manner appropriate to the audience. Communicating reasoning is also an essential aspect of shared decision-making with your clients. However, because of its rapid, complex and often subconscious nature, clinical reasoning is not a skill that can be simply explained, understood and recalled. To improve the communication of your clinical reasoning, you need to learn to become aware of your thinking and seek feedback on your communication from patients, students, peers and teachers.

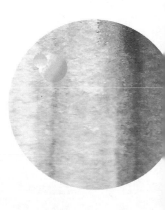

references

Ajjawi, R. (2009). *Learning clinical reasoning and its communication: In physiotherapy practice*. Saarbrücken, Germany: VDM Verlag Dr. Müller.

Ajjawi, R., & Higgs, J. (2011). Core processes of communication of clinical reasoning: A qualitative study with experienced Australian physiotherapists. *Advances in Health Sciences Education*. doi: 10.1007/s10459-011-9302-7.

Body, R., & McAllister L. (2009). *Ethics in speech and language therapy*. Chichester, UK: Wiley & Sons.

Charon, R., & Montello, M. (Eds.) (2002). *Stories matter: The role of narrative in medical ethics*. New York: Routledge.

Elstein, A. S., Shulman, L. S., & Sprafka, S. A. (1978). *Medical problem solving: An analysis of clinical reasoning*. Cambridge, MA: Harvard University Press.

Elstein, A. S., Shulman, L. S., & Sprafka, S. A. (1990). Medical problem solving: A ten year retrospective. *Evaluation and the Health Professions, 13*, 5–36.

Eva, K. W. (2004). What every teacher needs to know about clinical reasoning. *Medical Education, 39*, 98–106.

Fleming, M. H. (1991). The therapist with the three track mind. *American Journal of Occupational Therapy, 45*, 1007–14.

Fonteyn, M. E. (1995). Clinical reasoning in nursing. In J. Higgs & M. Jones (Eds.), *Clinical reasoning in the health professions* (pp. 60–71). Oxford: Butterworth Heinemann.

Groen, G. J., & Patel, V. L. (1985). Medical problem-solving: Some questionable assumptions. *Medical Education, 19*, 95–100.

Higgs, J. (2003). Do you reason like a (health) professional? In G. Brown, S. Esdaile & S. Ryan (Eds.), *Becoming an advanced healthcare practitioner* (pp. 145–60). Edinburgh: Butterworth Heinemann.

Higgs, J., Jones, M., Loftus S., & Christensen N. (Eds.) (2008). *Clinical reasoning in the health professions* (3rd ed.). Oxford: Butterworth Heinemann.

Higgs, J., Richardson, B., & Abrandt Dahlgren, M. (2004). Preface. In J. Higgs, B. Richardson & M. Abrandt Dahlgren (Eds.), *Developing practice knowledge for health professionals* (p. ix). Oxford: Butterworth Heinemann.

Jones, M. A. (1992). Clinical reasoning in manual therapy. *Physical Therapy, 72*, 875–84.

Jones, M., Jensen, G., & Rothstein, J. (1995). Clinical reasoning in physiotherapy. In J. Higgs & M. Jones (Eds.), *Clinical reasoning in the health professions* (pp. 72–87). Oxford: Butterworth Heinemann.

Loftus, S., & Higgs, J. (2006). Clinical decision making in multidisciplinary clinics. In H. Flor, E. Kalso & J. O. Dostrovsky (Eds.), *Proceedings of the 11th world congress on pain* (pp. 755–60). International Association for the Study of Pain, Seattle: IASP Press.

Loftus, S. (2009). *Language in clinical reasoning: Towards a new understanding.* Saarbrücken, Germany: VDM Verlag Dr. Müller.

Smith, M., Higgs, J., & Ellis, E. (2008). Characteristics and processes of physiotherapy clinical decision making: A study of acute care cardiorespiratory physiotherapy. *Physiotherapy Research International, 13*(4), 209–22.

further reading

Ajjawi, R., & Higgs, J. (2008). Learning to communicate clinical reasoning. In J. Higgs, M. Jones, S. Loftus & N. Christensen (Eds.), *Clinical reasoning in the health professions*, (3rd ed., pp. 331–8). Edinburgh: Elsevier.

Writing records, reports and referrals in professional practice

Lindy M^cALLISTER | Shazia NASER-UD-DIN

key topics

This chapter covers the following topics:

- writing professional documents

- purposes and types of reports, records and referrals

- writing for different audiences

key terms

CLINICAL REPORTS

PATIENT RECORDS

MEDICO–LEGAL REPORTS

REFERRALS

CONFIDENTIALITY

/ CLINICAL REPORTS /
Clinical reports have a number of different purposes in patient care, including keeping records and handing over client information.

Introduction

A key communication skill for health professionals is the ability to write high-quality reports, records and referrals. These need to be clear, succinct and informative, and satisfy the practitioner's duty of care responsibilities, while avoiding ethical and legal pitfalls. In this chapter we provide advice on a range of formats and practices for writing effective professional reports, with a focus on **clinical reports**.

Purposes and types of clinical reports

Clinical reports have a number of different purposes in patient care, including keeping records, handing over client information, reporting on needs assessments and professional consultations, documenting progress, providing advice to others, requesting information or advice from other providers, and supporting clients' service requests. Table 22.1 lists different types of reports commonly used in the health sciences, and describes key features of each report type. Clinical reports may also serve audit, research, medico-legal, practice management and forensic functions (Arotiba et al., 2006).

Increasingly, reports and records are maintained digitally, offering both advantages and disadvantages. Advantages include reduced resource costs with a paperless office, easier transfer and access to information as patients move around, and improved record-keeping (Spicer, 2008). Entries are dated and locked in; this reduces overwriting and tampering, an asset in medico-legal cases. Disadvantages include the challenge for staff of learning to use the software involved, and the time required to produce error-free records. Once errors are placed into a record, often the only way to correct them is to put in another entry with errata. Hence, it is paramount to correctly enter and cross-check before hitting the 'save' button.

TABLE 22.1 | TYPES OF CLINICAL REPORTS IN HEALTH PROFESSIONS

TYPE OF REPORT	DESCRIPTION
Assessments, initial evaluations, diagnostic reports	Record results of initial assessments of clients' needs, concerns or presenting problems, together with professionals' judgments (e.g. diagnosis, prognosis), recommendations, options for action (e.g. program or management plan), requests for input by or referral to other professionals to obtain additional relevant information or advice. May be sent to referring agent or summary may be provided in a letter back to referring agent.
Summaries, interim reports, progress reports	Record intervention and/or progress to date, issues or concerns arising, recommendations for future action. Often written for team meetings or case conferences, or government departments or insurers to inform on services provided and progress made, and to request ongoing funding for services.

< cont. >

< cont. >

TYPE OF REPORT	DESCRIPTION
Client records, progress notes	Record results of daily, weekly or intermittent treatment sessions; may form part of the main medical record or patient file, centrally located but accessible to all service providers so that all providers are kept up-to-date and can coordinate care. May be kept within departmental file (e.g. allied health departments in hospitals may maintain separate files containing details about treatment programs, with written summaries in clients' main records or charts).
	Typically kept in point form; may include diagrams, charts (e.g. see Figure 22.1), X-ray images, photographs (e.g. see Figure 22.2), virtual 3-D models (in lieu of plaster models in orthodontics); increasingly, records are digitised (e.g. see Figure 22.3).
Discharge or final reports	Record the content and outcomes of treatment and/or services to clients, reasons for discharge, recommendations for future management if required, forming part of a main record. May be sent to insurer or given to clients and their families for future reference by them or other professionals; should provide evidence that discharge has been discussed with and understood by the patient and/or family (Hersh, 2003).
Referrals	Written to another professional to request assessment and recommendations for management of client, or request a second opinion.
Medico-legal reports	Requested by insurers, courts (by subpoena) or government departments to provide independent assessment of a person's current and potential future capacity, or professional judgment of another professional's work. If requested to provide one, consult your supervisor or manager for advice. Your organisation's lawyers should review the report; justify every statement made; include quantitative measurement data; remove opinions, impressions and observations; state inferences or generalisations drawn from data carefully (e.g. 'Mr M. reported that he can …' (rather than 'Mr M. is able to …').
Prescriptions	Common form of communication between health professional (usually doctor or dentist) and pharmacist, or provider of specific services or appliances. Information includes name of the therapeutic agent, dosage, timing instructions, specific usage instructions and warnings in case of problems arising. Podiatrists, optometrists and orthotists also provide prescriptions for aids and/or equipment for clients.

/ PATIENT RECORDS /
Patient records record results of daily, weekly or intermittent treatment sessions; may form part of the main medical record or patient file, centrally located but accessible to all service providers so that all providers are kept up-to-date and can coordinate care.

/ REFERRALS /
Referrals are written to another professional to request assessment and recommendations for management of client, or request a second opinion.

/ MEDICO-LEGAL REPORTS /
Medico-legal reports may be requested by insurers, courts (by subpoena) or government departments to provide independent assessment of a person's current and potential future capacity, or professional judgment of another professional's work.

FIGURE 22.1 | EXAMPLE OF A NURSE'S ENTRY IN A PATIENT CHART

30/5/11 10.15 a.m. Nursing entry

Patient complained of feeling hot and sweaty.

Day 2 post right hip replacement.

Temp: 38.5°C orally. Flushed appearance to face and neck, diaphoretic.

Wound—no sign of redness or oozing. Chest—no cough, normal breath sounds.

IV site—no redness. Indwelling urinary catheter draining cloudy, dark-yellow urine.

Dip-stix urine test—ph 7, + blood, ++ protein, +++ nitrites, +++ leucocytes.

No abdominal pain.

RMO notified. Will come to see patient. Catheter specimen of urine collected and sent to lab.

Increase oral fluids to 200 ml per hour if tolerated.

FIGURE 22.2 | PATIENT RECORDS WITH PHOTOS AND X-RAYS
(DOLPHIN VERSION 11.5 USA).

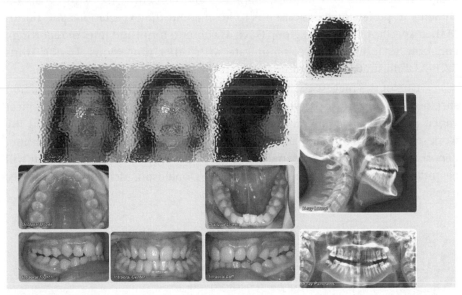

Artistic glass effect to protect patient identity.

FIGURE 22.3 | EXAMPLE OF DIGITAL NOTE ENTRY IN ORTHODONTICS WITH BRIEF SUMMARY OF PAST, PRESENT AND FUTURE TREATMENT OBJECTIVES

Entry Date	17/12/2010
Entry Time	01:56pm
Entered By	UQSNASER
Notes	

Kirsty has CTB for over a year and was advised to activate the midline palatal screw 2x a week. On examinations is presenting as Class III incisor relationship tendency with increased lower face height. The patient believes she has made an improvement and she can bite better. OHI provided along with disclosing tablets and instructions given.Keen for Fixed Appliance treatment. Kirsty has cerebral palsy and that needs to be addressed in any treatment plan provided.

NB: CTB is a commonly used abbreviation for Clark Twin Block.

Formats of clinical reports

The format of a report or record depends on its type and function. Reports from different professionals and in different situations (such as a health promotion program) have different formats, emphases and content. One of the goals for students in professional education is to learn about the expectations and norms of their specific professional group (such as content, form, and lines of reporting), and how to interact and communicate with other professions. Handy Hints 22.1–22.4 illustrate some common formats.

One of the biggest challenges in writing reports is to provide information succinctly. You need to be able to write both short and long reports to meet varied professional requirements, and to adapt to the intended reader and the work setting. Acronyms and abbreviations need to be explained at first mention. Reports for non-professionals and clients need to be written in language that will be understood by those who read or use them (Donaldson, McDermott, Hollands, Copley, & Davidson, 2004).

SAMPLE FORMAT FOR ASSESSMENT, INITIAL EVALUATION OR DIAGNOSTIC REPORTS

- Relevant history and background
- The results of formal assessment
- The results of informal assessment
- Clinical observations or impressions
- Summary
- Statement of the problem and a provisional diagnosis

- Tests to be ordered (if relevant)
- Prognosis (if possible and appropriate)
- Goals of management
- Recommendations for immediate treatment or longer-term management of the patient ●

SAMPLE FORMAT FOR SUMMARIES OF CARE AND/OR SERVICES, INTERIM REPORTS AND PROGRESS REPORTS OF SERVICES

- Diagnosis, or statement of problem requiring treatment, intervention or service
- Summary of previous treatment or services (if applicable)
- Description of or rationale for current services being provided or program being implemented
- Outcomes and/or feedback from client
- Factors facilitating and/or impeding progress
- Strategies found to be effective
- Recommendations (and rationales) for: continued management, discharge, alternative management or referral ●

SAMPLE FORMAT FOR DISCHARGE OR FINAL REPORTS

- Management/treatment goals (including rationales)
- Outcomes
- Issues in management
- Reasons for discharge
- Ongoing needs and problems
- Recommendations for future management, resources
- Statements of ongoing needs, problems and recommendations should incorporate patient perspectives ●

WHAT TO INCLUDE IN A REFERRAL LETTER

- Nature of the referrer's current contact with the client
- Summary of evaluations and treatment or services received to date (if any)

- Test results or evaluation findings if available
- Referring practitioner's professional judgment, opinion or assessment of the situation
- Reason for referral
- Intended use for any information requested: confirm a provisional diagnosis, assist in treatment planning, request a takeover of patient management, or request client services ●

Ethical and legal issues

/ **CONFIDENTIALITY** /
Confidentiality entails that we keep *information* about clients private. To safeguard clients' confidentiality, share information only with those authorised to access it.

Many professions have a code of ethics that states how their members should behave toward clients, colleagues and students, with due consideration of duty of care, informed consent, **confidentiality** and ethical principles. Ethical principles apply to what we write, as well as to what we say and how we behave. There are also legal constraints on what professionals can write or do with documents about clients. For example, privacy legislation provides tight safeguards for *who* can know *what* about clients, and who can gain access to or be shown client reports without their consent. Freedom of Information (FOI) legislation stipulates that, under certain conditions, clients can have access to their files. These legal safeguards help to ensure that what is written about clients is valid and fair. Legislation differs from state to state, so check what is relevant to your workplace. Legal action and complaints to ethics boards often point to inadequate record-keeping or inappropriate content in records. Good record-keeping is essential, and attention should be drawn in records to any miscommunications with the patient, idiosyncratic behaviour or reluctance of the patient to share previous medical records.

Duty of care

Implicit in professional codes of ethics, and explicit in some legislation, is the concept of duty of care. Duty of care implies not writing anything about clients that might cause them harm or deny them access to services (see Chapter 3). We have a duty of care to provide correct and relevant information in client documents within our area of expertise. We are expected to maintain the confidentiality of information disclosed to us by patients and to keep sensitive documents secure.

Information management and security

In response to legislation, most human service organisations have established policies on how information about clients is to be managed. In each new setting in which you work, you need to understand the organisation's information management policies. In particular, these policies identify who has access to documents across six major stakeholder groups (patients/clients, human service professionals, human service managers, government and policy-makers, researchers, educators and students) and when. The use of digital record-keeping makes information management an even more important consideration for health professionals. Files must be stored in places accessible only to those authorised to access them. Paper files should be kept in locked file drawers or cupboards; digital records should be stored in password protected files. There are additional ethical and legal risks involved with digital records; they must be kept secure and confidential in transmission, as well as storage (Denton, 2003). In Australia, the law requires that records be kept for a minimum of 7 years from last contact, or until the age of 25 in the case of children.

Informed consent and confidentiality

You may only access and share information about clients if you have obtained their informed consent to do so as part of the provision of services. Informed consent is obtained during a client's first contact with a healthcare service or provider. Ensure that such consent *is* truly informed; that the client or the guardian understands the nature of the investigations and services proposed. Obtaining informed consent from people who are seriously ill or mentally, linguistically or cognitively impaired (e.g. because of aphasia following a stroke, or intellectual impairment) is a challenge. Adapted consent forms that use pictures or symbols as well as text can help in obtaining informed consent (Hersh & Braunack-Mayer, 2000).

Ownership of information

It is not always clear who owns a client's file. Is it the client, the professional, the hospital, workplace, health services agency, community centre or someone else? In some cases, if a report has been requested and paid for by a third party, that party is generally understood to own the report. For example, a medico-legal report commissioned by an insurer may be owned by the insurer; the client and other healthcare providers may not have access to the report (even though it may be in the client's file) without permission from the insurer. As a general rule, documents about clients in public facilities are owned by the facilities, but clients are entitled to consult them. Sometimes organisations consider that unfettered access to documents might not be in a client's best interest; for example, reports on mental health status may be considered unsettling to a client. If clients ask to see their file, you need to ascertain why they wish to do so and seek advice from a supervisor before handing it over. In some facilities, clients need to fill out a 'Request for file access' form. Clients can, of course, use Freedom of Information legislation to gain access to documents pertaining to them, should organisations restrict access.

WRITING EFFECTIVE CLINICAL REPORTS

- Use the accepted structure for the type of report in question.
- Write clearly, legibly and succinctly.
- Use short sentences and write in plain English.
- Provide adequate and accurate information.
- Write at the language level of the intended reader.
- Write for the average reading level of adults—in the Western world this is 10–14 years (Vahabi & Ferris, 1995).
- Avoid jargon.
- Use only accepted abbreviations.
- Use correct spelling and grammar.
- Proofread what you write.
- Sign and date reports.

Tips and strategies for successful report writing

Good reports are well structured and provide sufficient detail without containing redundant information. The formats for different documents provided earlier in this chapter will help you produce an appropriate report. Reports should provide all the necessary identifying and contact information of the client and the person preparing the report, and must contain the dates of contact with the client and the date the report is written. Reports should be written as soon as possible after contact with the client, to ensure that accurate and current information is recorded. The vocabulary should be appropriate to the target audience. Although technical vocabulary may be appropriate when you are writing to professionals in your field, it is not appropriate when you are writing a report for the parents or family members of a client. Successful report writing shows evidence of attention to matters of content and style. Use short sentences and 'plain English' (use the plain English website in the Further Reading section as a guide). Table 22.2 shows some key report-writing strategies and provides good and poor examples of each.

TABLE 22.2 | KEY STRATEGIES IN REPORT WRITING

STRATEGY	POOR EXAMPLE	GOOD EXAMPLE
Distinguish between opinion and fact.	Susan is a loner.	Susan appears to have a limited social network (or) Mrs M. reported Susan is a 'loner'.
Use definite, specific, concrete language; give examples.	Peter has no social skills.	Peter does not maintain eye contact, take turns in conversation, or stay on topic. He stands too close to the person with whom he is talking.
Use positive rather than negative language.	Eating a normal meal is not permitted until …	Patients can eat a normal meal when …
Avoid sweeping statements and over-generalisations.	Like most teenage mothers, Kate is a poor parent.	Kate reports she lacks confidence in her skills as a parent.
Use commands if writing instructions (such as for medication or exercises).	These exercises should be done prior to meal times.	Do these exercises before eating.
Do not use abbreviations or acronyms without first using terms in full and/or supplying a glossary.	The CELF and the PPVT were administered.	The Clinical Evaluation of Language Functions (X edition, year of publication) and the Peabody Picture Vocabulary Test (Y edition, year of publication) were administered.
Use vocabulary suited to the reader.	(In a report to the parents of a child with a head injury) John sustained damage to the inferior sulcus of the medial edge of the left parietal lobe.	John's head injury has damaged the left side of his brain in the area that controls …
Do not criticise other people or the client.	The doctor who delivered this baby obviously allowed the labour to proceed too quickly.	Mrs B. reported that Emma's birth was 'very quick'.
Coordinate ideas.	Jenny said her first words at 12 months of age. She began to use two-word combinations at 18 months of age. By two years she was using small sentences.	Mrs F. reported that Jenny began using single words at 12 months, two-word combinations at 18 months, and three- to four-word combinations at two years of age.
Use personal pronouns appropriately.	(a) The examiner noted that … (b) The client said …	(a) I noted that Michael … (b) He said that …
Do not use colloquial expressions.	Janie wore a groovy coat to the interview.	(If it is appropriate, comment on the client's clothing.) Janie wore clothes that indicated her interest in fashion.

< cont. >

< cont. >

STRATEGY	POOR EXAMPLE	GOOD EXAMPLE
Do not use qualifiers.	(a) Mrs W. was very weepy. (b) Susie was rather withdrawn.	(a) Mrs W. cried frequently during the interview. (b) Susie did not initiate interaction with me, nor did she respond when I attempted to engage her in conversation.
Choose short, familiar words.	We will commence this consultation by …	We will start your consultation by …
Use tense appropriately. Use past tense:		
(a) for all past events	(a) Six years ago David is injured	(a) David sustained a right frontal lobe injury in 1998
(b) for indicating information that was reported to you	(b) David tells me he has memory problems	(b) David reported that he still had difficulty remembering the names of friends
(c) for reporting performance in testing.	(c) David names all the items	(c) David named all the items
(d) for indicating your interpretation or inference.	(d) When I test him, David seems confused	(d) David seemed confused
Use present tense for ongoing conditions.	David did not read	David does not read

Drafting, proofreading and obtaining feedback on your reports

Writing professional reports can be challenging. It requires the ability to interpret, critique, synthesise and summarise a wide array of information, and combine it into a readable whole. Draft and proofread your report, and obtain feedback on its content and appropriateness, perhaps several times, to ensure that it meets the needs of the intended audience. Lovatt (2002) advises health professionals to tailor the readability of their reports to the language levels of the intended readers. Given that the average reading age of adults in the Western world is 10–14 years (Vahabi & Ferris, 1995), the majority of professional reports would probably be difficult to read for many of our clients, even if jargon-free. A number of readability indices are available, including the Flesch readability test, which is incorporated into major word-processing packages. This test includes measures of sentence length, multisyllabic word use and grammatical features that add complexity to text.

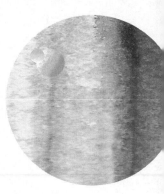

conclusion

A well-written report is a pleasure to produce and read. We hope the information and strategies in this chapter encourage you to develop your skills in this crucial aspect of professional practice.

references

Arotiba, J. T., Akinmoladun, V. I., & Okoje, V. N. (2006). An audit of medical record-keeping in maxillofacial surgery at the University College Hospital, Ibadan using the CRABEL scoring system. *African Journal of Medicine and Medical Sciences*, *3*, 93–5.

Denton, D. (2003). Ethical and legal issues related to telepractice. *Seminars in Speech and Language*, *24*(4), 313–22.

Donaldson, N., McDermott, A., Hollands, K., Copley, J., & Davidson, B. (2004). Clinical reporting by occupational therapists and speech pathologists: Therapists' intentions and parental satisfaction. *Advances in Speech-Language Pathology*, *6*(1), 23–38.

Hersh, D. (2003). 'Weaning' clients from aphasia therapy: Speech pathologists' strategies for discharge. *Aphasiology*, *17*(11), 1007–29.

Hersh, D., & Braunack-Mayer, A. (2000). Uninformed about informed consent? Ethical issues and informed consent in aphasia research. In C. Lind (Ed.), *Research, reflect, renew: Proceedings of the Annual Conference of Speech Pathology Australia* (pp. 176–81). Melbourne: Speech Pathology Australia.

Lovatt, C. (2002). Written communication. In M. Darley (Ed.), *Managing communication in health care* (pp. 165–203). Edinburgh: Bailliere Tindall.

Spicer, R. (2008). Bytes and bites—using computerized clinical records to improve patient safety in general dental practice. *Dental Update*, *35*, 614–16; 618–19.

Vahabi, M., & Ferris, L. (1995). Improving written patient education materials: A review of the evidence. *Health Education Journal*, *54*, 99–106.

further reading

Plain English at Work www.dest.gov.au/archive/publications/plain_en/homepage.htm

acknowledgments

We acknowledge Iain Hay and Annette Street, who authored the chapter on this topic in the second edition of this book. Our chapter has revised and updated this earlier version.

Case conferences and student case presentations

Ann **SEFTON** | Annette **STREET**

key topics

This chapter covers the following topics:

- what is a case conference?
- preparing for a case presentation
- getting to know the patient who is to be presented

key terms

CASE CONFERENCE

CASE PRESENTATION

Introduction

A **case conference** is a professional meeting in which a patient is discussed, often within a multidisciplinary team, in order to make decisions about patient management (especially diagnosis and treatment). The health circumstances of the patient or client are presented for discussion by the group. Students in the different health professions are expected, either individually or as part of a team, to make case presentations to different groups about patients and their problems. For student presenters, the scope of the presentation depends on their stage of development and the particular focus of the conference. The nature of the audience and local customs will determine the specific content and complexity of the presentation; the time available will govern how comprehensive it can be. Presenting a case is a sensitive task, and you must balance the needs of the patient with those of the audience of students and/or professionals.

What is a case presentation?

A **case presentation** is often the trigger for discussion by the participants in a case conference. Presentations can include interviews with and physical examinations of patients by practising professionals. These skills are essential for making a diagnosis, suggesting lines of investigation, determining progress and negotiating management. An essential part of professional practice is the presentation of key features of interviews, and examinations of patients or clients to a tutor, fellow students, examiners or a professional team participating in a case conference. A case presentation demonstrates the processes of clinical reasoning within your discipline.

/ **CASE PRESENTATION** /
A case presentation is an interview and/or clinical assessment to provide information for the case conference.

Presentations range from brief statements that present a diagnostic or management decision, or report on specific aspects of recent progress, to the presentation of information accumulated in more prolonged encounters. Relatively brief oral presentations, increasingly supported by online resources, are widely used to provide concise information to members of the health team who are not familiar with a particular patient or client (e.g. in a team meeting, at a change of shift or in a class tutorial). Written presentations are particularly important for referrals and reports to other health professionals. Because of their central importance in clinical practice, case presentations, oral or written, are often used to assess students.

Preparing for a case presentation

Each health profession has its established patterns for case conferences, emphasising different issues. Furthermore, there are often local rules about the structure of presentations, and there can be strict time limits. Before starting to interview and examine the patient you are to present, you must be clear on what is expected of you in the case presentation. Most teachers offer guidelines or models to assist you in developing the relevant skills, and provide you with opportunities to practise. The time allocated determines the depth and breadth of your presentation, and it is essential to organise the presentation to fit the time available.

You should also think about the following factors:

- Is the case to be presented orally or in writing?
- How much time is available for the prior interview, clinical examination or family discussion, and for the presentation or conference itself?
- Is it to be based on a single interview or does it reflect a longer association?
- What is the emphasis—diagnosis, immediate management, assessing ongoing progress or reporting on the negotiation of long-term treatment planning?

- Will the audience or conference members be your tutorial group, a whole class, a professional clinical team or examiners?
- Will your patient or client be there during the presentation and open to questions from the group?
- Will you be expected to elicit and demonstrate physical signs?
- Will you need to show images or include reports of clinical tests?
- Are you expected to use overhead or PowerPoint presentations?
- Are clinical demonstration aids available to assist you to illustrate your points?

Table 23.1 gives more guidance on how to prepare case presentations.

TABLE 23.1 | PREPARING A CASE PRESENTATION

ASPECT OF CASE	POSSIBILITIES AND CONSIDERATIONS
Purpose	Diagnostic, procedural, rehabilitative, review
Audience	Peers, senior staff, multidisciplinary team, examiners
Time allocated	Implications for depth and breadth
Resources available and permissible	Access to clinical notes, diagnostic or therapeutic data, or images
Presentation resources	Use of PowerPoint, online case information, overhead projector
Current evidence base	Systematic reviews, clinical guidelines, medication
Patient information available	Single interview, comprehensive workup, repeat interviews
Patient history	Past health, presenting problems
Diagnosis	Problem statement
Possible action	Active treatment, interventions or therapies; 'wait and see' approach; referral
Monitoring	Process, timing, plan for review
Outcome	Discharge, continue treatment, cease intervention, or refer on

The timing of the conference influences the nature of the information collected and reported. For example, at an initial encounter in a clinic or hospital setting, the initial focus is on assessment. This can involve taking a history of symptoms and eliciting signs, leading to a set of diagnostic possibilities that might require immediate management or indicate the need for further investigation. At later stages, health professionals engaged in applying diagnostic tests need to demonstrate skills in the acquisition and interpretation of data, and need to offer explanation and reassurance to the patient. Once a diagnosis is established, a plan of management must be negotiated. Negotiating the plan requires sensitivity to the patient's needs, values and constraints within the context of available resources.

Establish how much time is allocated for interviewing and for the presentation itself; plan carefully to ensure that the important points are included and are presented in a logical way. Find out whether you have access to current or previous clinical notes, and diagnostic or therapeutic data. Often, however, you must elicit the relevant clinical information from the patient or client without the help of clinical notes, particularly if you are to be assessed. You should take the opportunity to consult the relevant literature, including your texts and sources relating to evidence-based practice. See Case study 23.1 for an example of a specific case presentation plan.

CASE STUDY 23.1
EXAMPLE CASE PRESENTATION PLAN

A medical student presents a patient recently admitted to hospital complaining of severe abdominal pain.

Purpose	To demonstrate diagnostic and reasoning skills, based on a single interview and examination
Audience	Peers, tutor
Time	Presentation 8 minutes, class discussion 10 minutes
Resources	Student's notes of interview and examination
Presentation resources	Whiteboard for discussion, light box for images (if available)
Current evidence base	Evidence-based medicine resources on computer, accessible by student before presentation
Patient history	Report on interview and physical examination, summarising key issues
Diagnostic possibilities	Presented systematically, in order of probability or of urgency

< cont. >

< cont. >

Possible action	Systematic plan of investigations suggested to exclude key possibilities
Monitoring	Organisation logical, within time frame
Outcome	Initial diagnostic decision(s), immediate investigation to include/ exclude possibilities

Getting to know the patient who is to be presented

In a conference, you are expected to have a good understanding of the patient or client, and his or her problems. It is important to put patients at ease, even if you are nervous. After introducing yourself as a student, and seeking the patient's consent to be interviewed, you need to outline what will happen. Your patient may prefer to be addressed informally by given name at interview, but at the presentation a more formal title is often appropriate. If you are interviewing children, a parent needs to be present; and for some patients you may need to include a carer or relative. If communication in English is likely to prove difficult, you should arrange an interpreter beforehand, and you will need to brief the interpreter. If you are expected to review existing clinical notes and test results, be sure to read them thoroughly beforehand and cross-check important details with your patient.

EFFECTIVE CASE PRESENTATION INTERVIEWS

- Explain your status as a student and gain consent from the patient or client.
- Put the person at ease.
- Explain the purpose of the interview.
- Be systematic and focused in your questioning.
- Encourage the person to contribute personal information and views.
- Keep the language appropriate for the person.
- Explore the necessary contextual information about the person.
- Listen carefully to answers and use them to refocus the subsequent questions.
- Allow adequate time for a considered response from the person.
- Offer information or support if needed.

You may have adequate time to explore issues in depth with the patient. If this is the case, consider 'building' a case history instead of 'taking' it. Building a case history and presentation is based on an information-sharing approach, using a conversational mode to elicit information. You need to combine the emerging biomedical picture with the patient's view, incorporating psychosocial history into the developing assessment (Haidet & Paterniti, 2003). These collaborative processes allow patients to present their views and gain a better understanding of their health problems through explanation and discussion, in contrast with traditional assessments in which the clinician directs the interview and asks questions that can be answered simply by 'yes' or 'no'.

On the other hand, contact time is often limited, and you might not be able to conduct a leisurely, comprehensive and systematic review. That constraint creates particular problems in exploring questions relating to sensitive issues, such as the use of drugs or alcohol, and sexual practices. When time is short, you need to determine the key issues quickly, and efficiently acquire as much relevant information as possible. Learn to focus your questions on significant issues rather than aiming to cover every possible aspect of the case (Bannister, Hanson, Maloney, & Raszka, 2011), but keep in mind that narrowing too early can lead to errors if you miss relevant information (Maddow, Shah, Olsen, Cook, & Howes, 2003). In all cases, listen carefully to the patient's responses, systematically develop some hypotheses as you proceed, and think logically about whether each new piece of information refutes or supports these hypotheses. If you are sure that you have captured the major features, you can then explore additional issues.

You may be required to present a case study of a patient who is unconscious or unable to communicate because of age or disability. You may need to rely solely on written records and diagnostic tests. It is vital to cross-check important details with other health professionals, preferably those responsible for the test analyses or the clinical notes. You may also need to interview family members to gain a better understanding of clinical and psychosocial issues.

Preparing the presentation

It is important to set priorities so that the most important information is presented first, particularly if it is directly relevant to diagnosis or management. You will be able to supply more details, if requested, during or after your presentation.

Providing breadth (an overview of and some context to the patient's background) must be balanced with a more detailed review of the specific problems to be discussed. It is normal to state the patient's name, age, home address and reason for presenting. The patient's background and occupation are usually included also, as they are often relevant for diagnosis, to understanding the implications of the clinical problem and for effective management. If you have strictly limited time for presentation, you need to be well organised to ensure that you have clearly and logically included the key elements. It is helpful to practise with your tutor or with colleagues before you give a major presentation.

Presenting and discussing the case

After preparation, the next task is to give an effective case presentation. Arrive at the venue early and make sure it is set up in the way you need. Often, case presentations and conferences are held in multipurpose clinical rooms that are rearranged frequently. The seats may be in an unexpected configuration, or the equipment moved to a new position. Check that the necessary equipment functions properly with your material. If you are anxious about the use of equipment, ask for assistance to test it before the event, or arrange for a technician to help you set up.

You need to know whether your audience will expect to interrupt you and whether you have a defined time to present. At the outset, briefly explain what you will cover. Set out the sequence of topics, making sure that you link important pieces of information and explain their relationship to each other. Make your clinical reasoning and decision-making processes as transparent as possible. Whether you recommend referral or intervention, your audience needs to be able to follow your reasoning. Make clear distinctions between *the evidence* and *your opinion*. Repetition or rephrasing of your key points assists comprehension, as does a clear summary.

handy hint 23.2

INTERACTING WITH YOUR AUDIENCE

- Be aware of local expectations and rules.
- Arrive early and check the room set-up.
- Briefly explain what you will cover.
- Present your material in a logical sequence.
- Maintain good eye contact with your audience.
- Pace your presentation.
- Watch for audience non-verbal reactions.
- Stand straight and do not fidget.
- Speak clearly and slowly.
- Link important pieces of information together.
- Explain the relationships between pieces of evidence.
- Distinguish between evidence and opinion.

- Repeat and rephrase your main points.
- Provide a clear concluding summary.
- Treat each questioner and each question with equal respect.
- Repeat complex questions to check your comprehension. ●

As you speak, maintain good eye contact with all the people in the room. You can adjust the speed or content of what you say in response to the non-verbal reactions of audience members. Always stand straight, and avoid fidgeting and other distracting behaviour. Speak clearly and slowly, especially if you are nervous.

In the discussion phase of a conference, be prepared to handle questions and to intervene if there are misconceptions or errors. Think beforehand about likely issues that might be raised, and decide how you will respond. Treat each questioner and each question with equal respect. If a question has more than one part, it is a good idea to list the parts before answering. If you are nervous, jot down a few words to help you remember the various parts of the question. If you are unclear about the meaning of a question, reword it and repeat it, to check that you have understood it.

references

Bannister, S. L., Hanson, J. L., Maloney, C. G., & Raszka Jr, W. V. (2011). Using the student case presentation to enhance diagnostic reasoning. *Pediatrics, 128*(2), 211–13.

Haidet, P., & Paterniti, D. A. (2003). 'Building' a history rather than 'taking' one. *Archives of Internal Medicine, 163*(10), 1134–40.

Maddow, C. L., Shah, M. N., Olsen, J., Cook, S., & Howes, D. S. (2003). Efficient communication: Assessment-oriented oral case presentation. *Academic Emergency Medicine, 10*(8), 842–6.

useful web resources

http://libraries.umdnj.edu/camlbweb/patient/presentation.html. This site provides clear information about clinical case presentations with preparation strategies, a template for guidance and some final tips.

Preparing a community health proposal

Lucie SHANAHAN | Lindy McALLISTER

key topics

This chapter covers the following key topics:

- structuring a community health proposal

- profiling a community

- planning and conducting a needs assessment

key terms

COMMUNITY HEALTH

FUNDING PROPOSAL

COMMUNITY PROFILE

NEEDS ASSESSMENT

Introduction

Hospital-based health services tend to focus on care of individual patients, whereas community health services focus more on promoting and maintaining the health of people living within their communities. As governments gradually shift funding from hospitals to community health organisations (Baum, 2008; Keleher, MacDougall, & Murphy, 2007; McMurray & Clendon, 2011), those in the health professions must become adept at writing funding proposals to finance the design, development, delivery and evaluation of new community services and health promotion projects. In this chapter we outline common sections of community health proposals and funding applications, and offer suggestions for writing successful applications. An example of a successful community health proposal prepared by one of the authors is included.

Why write a community health proposal?

Staff in the hospital, **community health**, and not-for-profit sectors in community service agencies are all involved in attempting to secure funds for community health programs. Government initiatives such as the extended Medicare items for multidisciplinary care for people with chronic conditions and 'GP Super Clinics' are driving the development of new models of care, but access to funds is dependent on high-quality **funding proposals**. Proposal writing has become a core skill for professionals at all levels. There are many possible reasons for writing a community health proposal; for example:

- to improve the quality of a service
- to address an unmet need in your community
- to gain more staff and resources
- to develop networks with key stakeholders
- to position your service for increased resources, roles and funding in the future
- to diversify your work role
- to improve your career prospects (e.g. by building a track record in obtaining funding).

/ COMMUNITY HEALTH /
Community health services focus more on promoting and maintaining the health of people living within their communities.

/ FUNDING PROPOSALS /
Funding proposals must be written to finance the design, development, delivery and evaluation of new community services and health promotion projects.

Structuring a community health proposal

Proposals for funds to develop and implement a community service program use similar headings to other funding proposals (see Handy Hint 24.1). Here, we focus on how to make an argument for your proposal. This requires specialised skills compared, for example, to the skills required for a literature review for a research grant.

STRUCTURE OF A COMMUNITY HEALTH PROPOSAL
- Executive summary
- Name, details and track record of organisation applying
- Title of project
- Goals and objectives
- Rationale—need for the project, literature review

- Community profile
- Description of project
- Participants and/or stakeholders
- Strategies and activities
- Budget
- Timeframe
- Evaluation procedures
- Dissemination strategies

Note: Not all funding bodies require all these sections.
Check their guidelines for applications. ◑

Making an argument for your proposal

First, review the literature for projects similar to the one you are proposing. Take note of the methods of evaluation that were used, the credibility and appropriateness of those methods, and the reported outcomes of those projects. Critiquing the literature along these lines allows you to argue for a particular approach to the implementation of your project.

You also need to convince the assessors of funding organisations that your target community requires the service you are proposing. For example, you would be unlikely to receive funds for a health promotion project addressing the prevention of falls in the elderly if the target community already has appropriate services in this area, or if the group you are targeting is not highly represented in the community in question (say a new suburb full of young families). To convince funders, you need to conduct a community assessment. This task involves two processes: developing a **community profile** and conducting a **needs assessment**.

Developing a community profile

Creating a community profile is a dynamic process. Communities change constantly, and the information you want to gain from a profile also changes, depending on the purpose of your project. An up-to-date community profile helps you determine and describe the demographic and social issues shaping the community; the values, health needs, resources and potential project partnerships within the community; and the power and leadership within it (e.g. the local government structure, key organisations and influential people within these groups). You may need to consult community members through interviews or focus groups to obtain their perspectives on existing needs. Developing a community

/ **COMMUNITY PROFILE** /
A community profile helps you determine and describe the demographic and social issues shaping the community; the values, health needs, resources, potential project partnerships within the community; and the power and leadership within the community.

/ **NEEDS ASSESSMENT** /
A needs assessment assesses and describes the needs of the community of interest.

profile involves the collection and analysis of data from a variety of national, state and local sources. You must consider all the aspects of a community that are relevant to your proposal, including what constitutes health and wellbeing for that community (Hodges & Videto, 2011). The purpose of the profile is to provide a context for your proposal and to educate funding assessors about the merits and feasibility of your proposed program. With the wealth of information available on the internet, and the growing number of strategic documents and policies that could contribute to a profile, it is easy to become sidetracked. In Table 24.1 we list some typical areas of research needed in preparing your report, and indicate where information in these areas can be obtained.

TABLE 24.1 | FIELDS AND LOCATIONS OF INFORMATION TO BE INCLUDED IN A COMMUNITY PROFILE

KEY AREA	WHERE INFORMATION CAN BE OBTAINED
Demographics	• Australian Bureau of Statistics (census data) www.abs.gov.au • Local centre of public health • State health department website • Echidna (Victorian demographics information only; other states and territories will have similar databases) www.med.monash.edu.au/srh/resources/echidna/ • Completed community profiles (such as local Division of General Practice)
Epidemiological data	• Australian Bureau of Statistics • Australian Institute of Health and Welfare www.aihw.gov.au • Local centre for public health • Local Division of General Practice • Burden-of-disease databases, such as www.health.sa.gov.au/burdenofdisease/DesktopDefault.aspx
Environment Local government Recreation and leisure services Health services Education services Industry and key employers Transport	For all these areas: • general internet searches using Google, Alta Vista, etc. will help you locate relevant specific websites or contact details (for example the shire council website, local hospital website, sporting club websites); plan the search terms to use before commencing • review key policies

Planning and conducting a needs assessment

Early work by Bradshaw (1972) is still used as a definitive guide to needs assessment; that is, assessing and describing the needs of the community of interest. Bradshaw identified four types of need: felt need, expressed need, normative need and comparative need. *Felt* and *expressed needs* are most commonly service gaps or problems identified by the community. *Normative need* is a need determined by experts (i.e. what would normally be considered 'right' or adequate for a community). *Comparative need* refers to past responses to similar issues, or analysis of a similar community's response to the same issues.

It is imperative to determine the type(s) and extent of need in a community and to present this information in your proposal. If a need does not exist or cannot be argued for, the community will not engage with your program and funding bodies will not fund it. Similarly, if a community's high-priority needs are not addressed, community members might not participate in the program, because they do not think it meets their most important needs. It is strongly recommended that programs not be developed based only on one type of need. Each of Bradshaw's need categories, if used alone, has inherent limitations. Types of need, the constraints of each and ways to measure needs are outlined in Table 24.2.

TABLE 24.2 | TYPES OF, CONSTRAINTS ON AND WAYS TO MEASURE COMMUNITY NEEDS

TYPE	CONSTRAINTS IN EXPRESSING OR INTERPRETING THIS NEED	MEASUREMENT
Felt	• People might not ask for exactly what they want for fear it will be 'too much'. • Needs identified may be 'self-based' rather than community-based. • The same problem may be repeatedly raised by the same people. • Opinions can be influenced by media campaigns and social media, so that participants report what they think the researcher wants to hear.	People say what they need, through the use of interviews, surveys, focus groups.
Expressed	• Data can be misinterpreted; for instance, waiting list data could reflect a policy decision or a real inability to provide services to all those seeking assistance. • People's beliefs about their 'rights' affect their actions.	Demonstrated by use of services or demand for them: waiting lists, petitions, letters to directors and politicians.

< cont. >

< cont. >

TYPE	CONSTRAINTS IN EXPRESSING OR INTERPRETING THIS NEED	MEASUREMENT
Normative	• This approach is not sensitive to the needs of specific communities. • Professional opinions can change over time. • Epidemiological data can be limited. • Professional opinion can be influenced by political or policy constraints.	Research, professional opinion.
Comparative	• To compare your program with another program, review the parameters (such as target group, goals and activities) of the two programs and the demographics and relevant needs of the two communities. • Superficial knowledge of services in other communities might lead to the erroneous conclusion that these services are superior; a more thorough investigation is necessary.	Investigate programs that have been developed to meet your identified need. Use health promotion databases such as Knowledge Hub www.anpha.gov.au/internet/anpha/publishing.nsf/Content/knowledgehub-lp

Developing a budget proposal

One problem noted by reviewers of funding applications is that budgets commonly either overestimate or underestimate what is required. Funding bodies will not fund a proposal that is suggestive of 'empire-building' or has been padded to obtain more resources than are actually needed. Nor will they fund projects that are likely to be under-resourced and could possibly fail, as judged by the stated goals, desired outcomes and sustainability. Developing an appropriate budget is a matter of balancing the quality of planning inputs and outcomes with the quantity of resources available.

When preparing a budget, you must realistically estimate the time and resources needed, and obtain accurate costings for all items. Remember that the salary paid to an individual is only one part of the wages cost for an organisation. On-costs ranging from 10 to 33 per cent (depending on the sector, and full-time or part-time status) need to be added to cover superannuation, leave loadings, long-service leave entitlements and workers' compensation. Another hidden expense can be transport costs for staff to travel to meet with clients of the project or for clients to travel to a program centre. Consider whether you will use an existing car pool, purchase a car(s) (perhaps using fleet purchasing arrangements), hire cars, reimburse staff for mileage in private vehicles or use public transport. Your manager and staff in your employing organisation's pay office, human resources department or finance office should be able to help you obtain costings and develop a realistic budget. Items included in a typical budget are shown in Handy Hint 24.2.

Start working on your proposal well in advance of the due date, so that you can obtain the details you need and can write multiple drafts to achieve a clear, succinct style that sells your idea. The chances of your proposal succeeding will increase if you ask experienced colleagues to review drafts. See Handy Hint 24.3 for more tips on proposal writing.

An example of a successful proposal

Case Study 24.1 shows excerpts of a successful proposal developed by Lucie Shanahan. Guidelines and application forms were provided on the funding organisation's website. As you read the example proposal, note the definite and positive language used regarding the benefits of this proposed program for the identified community. Aspects of the proposal that made it successful include linking it to existing government-funded initiatives, grounding it in existing literature, and highlighting outcomes across a range of skills and settings. Further, the proposal clearly identifies collaborative networks that will ensure the product is sustainable.

CASE STUDY **24.1**

A SUCCESSFUL COMMUNITY HEALTH FUNDING PROPOSAL

HEALTH DEPARTMENT—SUBMISSION FOR PROJECT FUNDING

1. TITLE OF PROJECT

We're all in this together—an information folder for families living with acquired brain injury.

2. DESCRIPTION OF PROJECT

2.1 Brief description of project (200 words max.)

Traumatic brain injury (TBI) is the largest cause of long-term disability in children and young adults (references). When acquired in childhood, TBI also results in significant levels of stress and burden for families (references). This project will finalise the collation of practical, user-friendly resources that have previously been demonstrated to be helpful to families learning to live with TBI. The material has been developed by a multidisciplinary team of health professionals and implemented with specific families over the past decade. Piloting material in this way has allowed the team to refine and focus information so that it is most relevant, useable and accessible to families. Literature in the field of TBI rehabilitation has documented that families require educational information to be provided on an ongoing basis, as different issues and challenges arise, children move through developmental stages, and families develop skills in negotiating life post-injury. This folder provides key information, creates a space for essential documents to be stored and serves as a lasting resource for families learning to live with lasting changes.

2.2 Objectives (desired outcomes)

To develop a resource folder containing a range of referenced, user-friendly fact sheets, strategies and ideas addressing common sequelae of TBI and common rehabilitation options, that can be used in conjunction with support provided by TBI health professionals.

Strategies

- That relevant and practical information be collated for use by families living with children with TBI.
- That relevant and practical information be collated for use by health professionals working with children with TBI.
- That the resources be formatted in a uniform manner so to achieve a publishable state.
- That the practical application of the booklets be piloted and evaluated by a selected reference group.
- That the product be refined to a marketable state.
- That the product is published and introduced to the TBI service network as a current and clinically applicable tool.

2.3 Rationale/background

This project will develop and evaluate a range of tools (functional and educational) that can be used by staff working with children with TBI and their families. The tools will improve the quality and equity of services, as well as developing resources for parents aimed at empowering them to proactively manage their child's social reintegration following injury. The development of literature and functional tools, based on a combination of clinical and familial experiences, will further increase the equity of service. This tool will enable rehabilitation clinicians to resource families with relevant information at key transition, growth and development periods.

Clinical experience of our team has confirmed the value of a family information folder. The folder brings together a variety of easily read information sheets, useful and proven strategies, real-life scenarios and practical solutions that demonstrate how to apply a variety of cognitive, behavioural and educational tactics in the everyday setting. Our team has found the folder to be an effective measure in providing a well-resourced consultative service. Our team has been able to recommend a particular approach, knowing that support people can draw further information and resources from the folder. In its current form, the folder has been very well received by the intended audience and the team has received requests from other organisations wishing to purchase copies. However, we have been unable to adequately reference all material and circulate draft versions for final preparation and printing due to other work commitments. Use of the folder will result in significant cost savings, with the reduction of the number of visits to schools and service providers (references). The folder will enable an organisation to increase the equity of its service provision, as all people supporting a child will be able to use this resource, thereby working from a common platform.

2.4 Proposed timetable

STRATEGY	KEY PERFORMANCE INDICATOR	TIMEFRAME
Appoint Project Officer	Officer appointed	April 2010
Collation of booklet material	Folder follows cohesive plan	June 2010
Develop feedback form	Feedback form printed	July 2010
Folder distributed to reference group	Reference group members receive copies of folder	July 2010
Feedback sought from reference group	Feedback forms distributed to and returned from reference group	September 2010
Feedback evaluated and feasible suggestions adopted	Revision of folder	October 2010
Folder uniformly formatted	Folder produced in copy form for publishing	November 2010
Folder disseminated to service units	Paediatric service workers report receipt of folders	January 2011
Folder available to service network	Marketing of folder at service forum	March 2011

2.5 Impact

A feedback form will be distributed to all reference group members. It will enable quantitative and qualitative data to be obtained. Quantitative data will be collected via 5-point Likert scale ratings assessing the content, format, readability and usability of the folder. Qualitative data will be collected via open-ended questions as well as digital recordings of reflective discussions held at a reference group meeting. The feedback form will be used again, following refinement of the trial product, to gather evaluative feedback from service workers six months post dissemination of the final product. While the first data set will be used initially to identify necessary refinements to the document, both data sets will be used to ultimately establish the impact of this product.

3. BUDGET

3.1 Total amount sought and proportion of actual cost this represents

- Total amount: $19,472.00   Proportion of actual cost: 100%

3.2 Detailed budget breakdown and explanation

ITEM	COST $	COMMENT
Capital		
Desktop publishing accessories	800.00	
Colour laser printer	6,000.00	To be used for production of trial folder
Salaries		
Project Officer	10,500.00	Health Education Officer (pro rata 1 day/wk for 10/12)
On-costs		Calculated at 14.5% annually
Project Officer	1,522.00	
Other costs		
Publishing consumables	650.00	Paper, covers etc. for initial 500 folders produced.
Total	19,472.00	

conclusion

Changes in population demographics and health funding in Western societies have increasingly led health professionals to provide services to communities outside of traditional healthcare institutions. Professionals need to understand their communities' needs and preferences for services. This requires skill in needs assessment, networking and teamwork, to develop funding proposals in order to deliver and evaluate community health and health promotion programs.

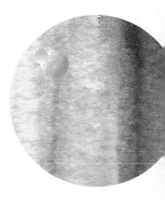

references

Baum, F. (2008). *The new public health* (3rd edn). Melbourne: Oxford University Press.

Bradshaw, J. (1972). The concept of social need. *New Society, 19*(496), 640–3.

Galbally, R. (2001). *How to win a philanthropic grant: The essential guide.* Melbourne: Our Community.

Hodges, B., & Videto, D. (2011). *Assessment and planning in health programs.* Sudbury, MA: Jones & Bartlett Learning.

Keleher, H., MacDougall, C., & Murphy, B. (2007). *Understanding health promotion.* Melbourne: Oxford University Press.

McMurray, A., & Clendon, J. (2011). *Community health and wellness: Primary health care in practice* (4th edn). Chatswood, NSW: Elsevier.

CHAPTER
25

Communicating with the community about health

Linda **PORTSMOUTH** | Franziska **TREDE** | Marissa **OLSEN**

key topics

This chapter covers the following topics:

- community
- health communication
- social marketing
- community engagement
- community development

key terms

COMMUNITY

HEALTH COMMUNICATION

SOCIAL MARKETING

COMMUNITY ENGAGEMENT

COMMUNITY DEVELOPMENT

Introduction

As a health practitioner, you may need to communicate about health with an entire community. In this chapter we define what a **community** is and how you can engage with members of the community to communicate with them about health. We also consider how communities learn and how they can take control of their own health. Advice is given on how to develop effective dialogues with communities.

/ **COMMUNITY ENGAGEMENT** /
Community engagement is the communication, cooperation and collaboration with a community undertaken by health professionals to improve or maintain that community's health.

professionals can foster **community engagement**. It is vital that health programs are based on what the community sees as its priorities, rather than on how health professionals interpret health statistics. A program shaped by interacting with the various stakeholders in a community is far more likely to succeed in improving health in that community than one planned exclusively by a group of health professionals.

handy hint 25.2

DEVELOPING DIALOGUE WITH A COMMUNITY

Take a partnership approach

- Remember that while you may be an expert in your area of health, community members are experts in their own community's health. The person with the health problem or disability is the ultimate expert. The people who live with them represent the next level of expertise. Involve them wherever possible.

- Seek out and get to know community opinion leaders and decision-makers, and involve them as much as you can, but also give voice to the least powerful people in the community.

- Respect everyone's opinion, and try to find out why various people hold particular opinions. Try to see things from the community's point of view, and ask for feedback from members of the community on the accuracy of your views.

Learn about the community

- The more you know about a community, the better you can communicate with the people. They will also feel respected, and appreciate that you took the time to get to know them.

- Ask open questions that allow community members to answer as they choose. Ask 'What do you think needs changing?' rather than 'Do you want this or that?'

- Try to find out as much as you can about the history of the health issue. What has been done before? What worked? What did not work? How did the community feel about it at the time? How do they feel about it now?

- Try not to have any preconceptions about what the community might want, need or be experiencing.

Overcome communication and partnership barriers

- Be consistent and honest. Trust will develop if you are honest and your motives are clear and unchanging.

- Lose your professional jargon. Learn how to say everything that you need to say in simple, straightforward language, especially if what you say is being translated into another language.

- Be curious and listen, especially when you communicate with people who are not of your culture, religion, language, class, age or gender. Learn from them and help them learn from you.

- Work out, as best you can, what is appropriate for you to do and say, but be true to yourself. Do not pretend to be someone you are not.

- It might be better for community members, rather than health professionals, to communicate about health with their peers.

- Pass on skills and knowledge whenever you can, to whomever you can, in a way that respects the other person. Such generosity is rewarded in many ways.

- Give everybody continual feedback about what is happening. Health team members need to know what other team members are doing. Let team supervisors know about the team's communication with the community, and let the community know what the people in the health organisation are thinking. Convey what you learn from community groups to other sections of the community—unless what you have been told is confidential.

- Be flexible with your timeline for the project. Some communities may be able to communicate exactly what they need immediately; others take more time. ●

Community organisation and community development

Community organisation is 'the process by which community groups are helped to identify common problems or goals, mobilize resources, and develop and implement strategies for reaching the goals they have collectively set' (Minkler & Wallerstein, 2005, p. 26). Health professionals recognise that a health problem exists within a community, and work with the community to improve the situation. **Community development** is a form of community organisation that also aims to empower the community. Health professionals working to develop communities need to be free to work with the health issues identified by the community, in ways chosen by the community, and in the timeframe that the community requires. For this approach to work, health organisations and funding agencies need to cede control to the community itself. The role of the health professionals is to enhance problem-solving capacity while acting as coordinator, catalyst and advocate (Fleming & Parker, 2007). The challenge of community development is to deal effectively with conflicting values and with the uncertainty of outcomes, while the benefits include fostering community ownership and responsibility for health.

/ **COMMUNITY DEVELOPMENT** /
Community development is a form of community organisation that also aims to empower the community.

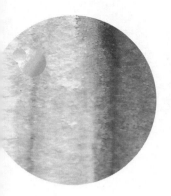

conclusion

The key to successful health communication with communities is remembering that communication is a two-way process. When developing health communication strategies and methods, it is essential that health professionals work at every stage of the communication process with members of their intended audience. Developing dialogue with communities is vital for the success of health programs; it can empower communities to assume control over their own health.

references

Australian Medical Association. (2010). *Social media and the medical profession—A guide to online professionalism for medical practitioners and medical students.* Retrieved from www.ama.com.au/node/6231

Baum, F. (2008). *The new public health* (3rd edn). Melbourne: Oxford University Press.

Donovan, R., & Henley, N. (2010). *Principles and practice of social marketing: An international perspective* (2nd edn). Melbourne: IP Communications.

Fleming, M. L., & Parker, E. (2007). *Health promotion: Principles and practice in the Australian context* (3rd edn). Crows Nest, NSW: Allen & Unwin.

Freire, P. (1970). *Pedagogy of the oppressed.* Harmondsworth, Middlesex: Penguin Education.

Kolb, D. A. (1984). *Experiential learning: Experience as the source of learning and development.* Englewood, NJ: Prentice-Hall.

Minkler, M., & Wallerstein, N. (2005). Improving health through community organizing and community health: A health education perspective. In M. Minkler (Ed.), *Community organising and community building for health* (2nd edn) (pp. 26–50). New Brunswick, NJ: University Press.

Piotrow, P. T., Kincaid, D. L., Rimon, J. G., & Rinehart, W. (1997). *Health communication: Lessons from family planning and reproductive health.* Westport, CT: Praeger.

World Health Organization. (1986). *Ottawa charter for health promotion.* Retrieved from http://www.who.int/hpr/NPH/docs/ottawa_charter_hp.pdf

World Health Organization. (1997). *The Jakarta Declaration on leading health promotion into the 21st Century.* Retrieved from http://www.who.int/hpr/NPH/docs/jakarta_declaration_en.pdf

further reading

Portsmouth, L. (2012). Health and the media. In P. Liamputtong, R. Fanany & G. Verrinder (Eds.), *Health, illness and wellbeing: Perspectives and social determinants* (p. 257). South Melbourne: Oxford University Press. This book chapter discusses the impact of the mass media on health and how the mass media can communicate health to the community.

Taylor, J., Wilkinson, D., & Cheers, B. (Eds.). (2007). *Working with communities in health and human services*. South Melbourne: Oxford University Press. This book provides an excellent exploration of working with communities.

useful web resources

For a successful social marketing intervention that has increased fruit and vegetable consumption in the community, see www.gofor2and5.com.au

For an interesting new social marketing intervention working to improve mental health in the community, see actbelongcommit.org.au/

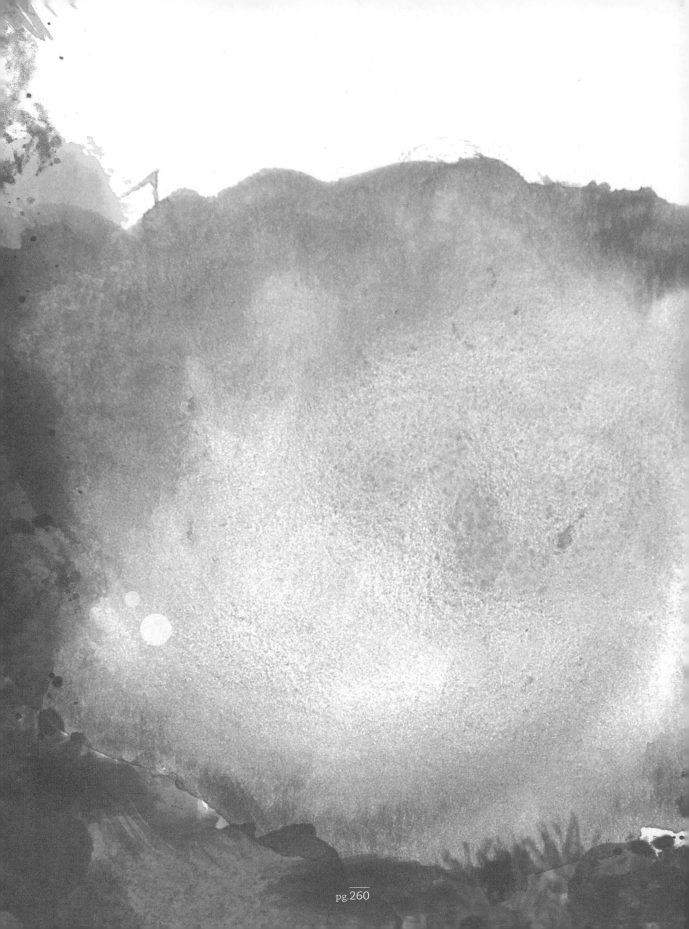

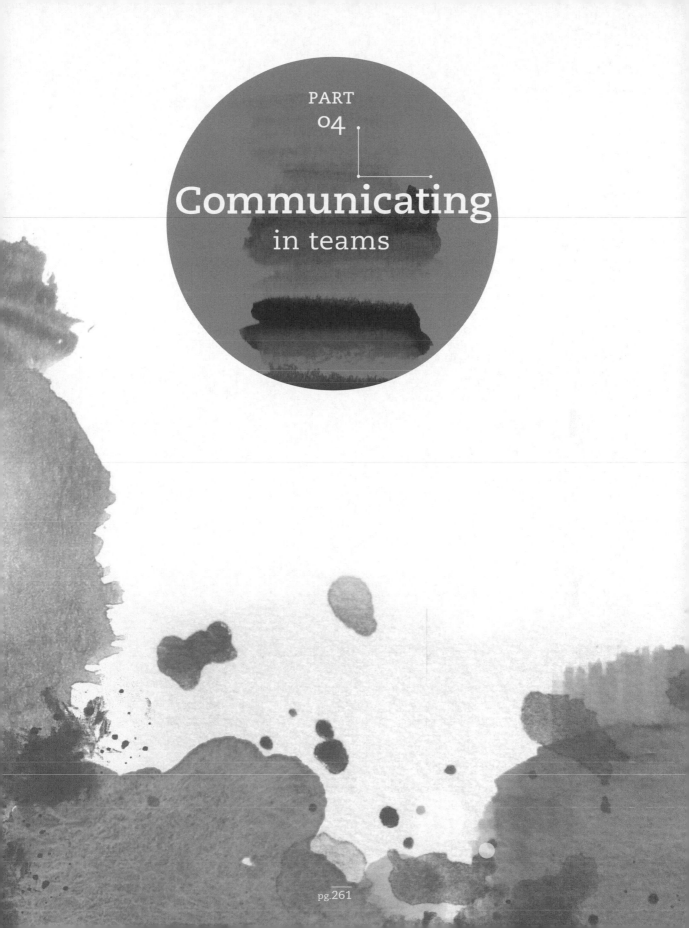

PART
04

Communicating
in teams

Working with groups: consulting, advocating, mediating and negotiating

Ann **SEFTON** | Lyndal **TREVENA** | Stephen **LOFTUS** | Jill **HUMMELL**

key topics

This chapter covers the following topics:

- basic strategies for working with groups or teams

- asking for and delivering consultative advice

- advocacy on behalf of patients and clients

key terms

ADVOCACY

CONSULTING

MEDIATION

NEGOTIATION

Introduction

Although many interactions with clients are one-to-one, few practitioners in the health professions work entirely on their own. Particularly in institutional settings, it is common to practise as a member of a team, either small or large. Your working group or team is likely to consist of health practitioners and colleagues with a wide range of different but complementary skills and knowledge. You may be a member of a number of formal and informal groups. Specific individual and group responsibilities (such as tasks and actions to pursue between meetings) must be clearly determined, whereas many general group responsibilities (such as following the group 'rules' of behaviour) will be progressively established, both explicitly and implicitly, as the group sets up its norms and patterns of working together.

Asking for and delivering consultative advice

Health professionals are often called upon to share their expertise through consultations. Obtaining advice from, and **consulting** with, other professionals may occur formally or informally between peers and work colleagues, between supervisors and junior staff, or between a particular group and an external source such as a government agency or welfare group.

/ **CONSULTING** /
Consulting with other professionals means seeking their advice or information, and exchanging opinions.

When you recognise the need for consultation, it is important to define your problem or issue accurately and to prepare before engaging in the consultation. This might involve listing the key issues you are seeking advice about, prioritising them and possibly grouping them into categories (such as problem identification, goal, action or intervention strategies).

Working in a multidisciplinary team utilises particular skills that enable you to work collaboratively and consultatively with other team members. For example, a patient might be assessed by a number of different health professionals, who then meet to discuss their findings. Rather than simply repeating information that others have also found, the team will expect you to present only the important findings relevant to your professional expertise or role, and that add to the emerging picture of the patient. It is also important to develop negotiation skills so that differences of opinion are managed diplomatically and client outcomes are optimised. Differences of opinion can be viewed as opportunities to learn from each other rather than confrontations. If you are leading a team, you need to develop further skills in team management; for example, it is important to ensure that all team members feel that their opinions have been heard and taken seriously.

Larger groups or organisations may need the consultative skills of external agencies to conduct surveys or interviews, or to produce reports. It is important to provide such organisations with a clear statement of your requirements, or you risk not obtaining the type of advice and information you seek. If there is a problem in your team concerning an interpersonal relationship, you might need advice from a more senior or experienced person, or a counsellor.

It is important to consider the degree to which you can trust the advice you receive, to determine whether advice comes from a trustworthy source. Consider if the advice:

- is independent or comes from someone with a vested interest
- has the endorsement of a higher authority (such as a government department or specialist)
- is consistent with widely accepted professional ethics and standards
- contains information collected using valid methods.

Whether advice is trustworthy, credible and sound also depends on the context of its application. What works successfully in some settings might not work in others. You will often need to make judgments about whether the advice you have received applies to your own situation. Sharing decisions with your team (while maintaining client confidentiality) about the benefits and limitations of using the advice is often a good strategy.

For those who are requested to give advice through consultation, there are important issues to consider. It is essential to listen carefully to what is required. Summarise what you understand to be the advice that the person or group is seeking. Be honest about your ability to meet these requirements, taking into account your expertise, your resources (including time) and potential conflicts of interest. Offer to involve other experts, if appropriate. The way you deliver your advice should be appropriate to the context in which it is sought. Informal oral advice could be the most appropriate form of delivery for an interpersonal matter between colleagues, whereas a written report or letter is best for matters of expertise. It is generally wise to document the advice you give.

CASE STUDY 26.1
DEFINING THE PROBLEM AND DUTY OF CARE

Jill is a social worker at a charitable organisation in a large city. The agency has become concerned about the safety of one of its intellectually disabled female clients, who appears to be the victim of physical abuse by her boyfriend. The client is reluctant to talk about her boyfriend with staff, but the agency is worried because she met her boyfriend while attending its service. At a staff meeting everyone agrees that outside advice is needed. How might the staff define their problem? Is it identifying the legal rights of the client in case advice is needed? Is it identifying appropriate services for client support? Do the agency staff members need further training in this area? Does the agency need clarification about its duty of care to clients? Do they need advice on more than one of these issues?

Advocacy on behalf of clients

Individual professionals, or service organisations or agencies may act as advocates. Taking on the role of advocate for clients generally means speaking up for them, supporting them, or interceding for them with a higher authority. People with illnesses, disabilities and social disadvantages are often in a position of diminished power. In contrast, as a professional practitioner you are often in a position of authority, and may be able to act on their behalf in a number of ways. Students should consult their clinical educator, fieldwork supervisor or teacher before taking on an **advocacy** role; it might be more appropriate for the senior staff member to take action. Advocacy requires some level of assertiveness to ensure that your message is clear to all parties (Tyler, Kossen, & Ryan, 2005).

/ **ADVOCACY** /

Advocacy is presenting the cause of another individual or group. Clients may need advocacy of a political, social, legal, personal or health nature.

CASE STUDY 26.2
ADVOCACY OPTIONS

Jill gathered information on the living conditions of several of the organisation's intellectually disabled clients, and found that many of those with mild or borderline disabilities did not qualify for a government case worker, despite the fact that a number of them struggled to live independently. What are her options for advocacy in this case? She can advocate as an individual by writing letters to politicians and raising public awareness through the media, or she can look for organisations that might be able to act on behalf of the organisation's intellectually disabled clients. To what extent do the clients want her advocacy? If so, how could they be involved? How would you approach this situation?

Advocacy for groups of clients can occur at political, legal and socio-economic level (e.g. improving the legal rights and living conditions of vulnerable groups through government or non-government agencies). It can also involve influencing community attitudes through the media, a potentially powerful avenue for advocacy. Professionals often advocate at this broader level to improve the health, wellbeing and safety of the general community. Examples of this approach include advocating for smoke-free workplaces and the use of cyclists' helmets. Individual advocacy by human service professionals on behalf of clients may include vouching for their identity on an application, or supporting their claim for housing assistance, legal support or welfare benefits.

Professionals can find themselves in direct conflict with their employers if their client advocacy challenges or questions the quality of service or management of the organisation. For this reason, many hospitals and consumer advocacy groups (such as breast cancer support groups) act independently on behalf of individuals and groups of clients. It is often best to refer clients to such independent advocates, particularly if you envisage a potential for conflict with your employer. Independent advocates will usually be able to provide an experienced and independent voice on behalf of the client.

It is also important to consider the attitude and role of your clients. Do they desire and accept your advocacy? It is important to gain clients' permission to act on their behalf, or your altruism may end up doing more harm than good. To what extent do they want to be involved? Self-advocacy can be empowering, and some would argue that all clients should be involved in advocacy on their own behalf. In some cases, however, this is neither feasible nor appropriate, particularly for vulnerable groups without resources. Your clients' autonomy and self-respect might be seriously damaged if their advocate appears to be taking control of their situation without their consent, albeit with good intentions.

Mediation between individuals and groups

Differences of opinion or more serious conflicts are almost inevitable between members of human services teams, and between clients and/or their families or carers. The role of mediator is a difficult one, and it is not possible to prescribe a set of strategies that will always be successful. The general principles in Handy Hint 26.1 are a useful guide.

GENERAL PRINCIPLES FOR MEDIATION

- Use an independent mediator who is perceived not to have a vested interest in the issues or outcomes.
- Provide opportunities for all interested parties to express their views, separately and together.
- Clarify the interested parties' values and beliefs.
- Focus on issues and events rather than on individuals.
- Identify areas of agreement.
- Avoid blaming people if possible, and encourage openness.
- Use an empathic approach (try to understand the different viewpoints).

You can usually resolve differences that arise, such as in the interpretation of a key clinical observation or in determination of the most appropriate intervention strategy, by seeking additional information. Issues that appear to involve personality clashes, or opinions without a strong basis in evidence, are much harder to resolve. Probably the most difficult are those in which deeply held cultural values or religious beliefs are at stake.

The first step in **mediation** is to identify the nature and seriousness of the conflict or disagreement, and to determine where they are arising and who is involved. Once the participants and issues have been identified, it is necessary to gain an understanding of the specific details of the dispute or disagreement. That is often best done by interviewing separately the individuals or groups involved, to gain an understanding of each of their perspectives. It is important to separate actual data from perceptions and interpretations. If the differences have arisen because of misconceptions or ignorance, then agreement may be achieved by providing clear, straightforward explanations or relevant data. If significant issues cannot be resolved simply, it is usually necessary to invite the interested parties to participate in mediation. The mediator is often a senior member of the healthcare team but, for serious conflicts, an experienced outsider may be needed. The mediator must have a clear understanding of the history of the situation. He or she must consider whether compromise is likely or possible, or whether the situation is bitterly adversarial, making it probable that there will be no mutually satisfactory solution, but rather perceived 'winner(s)' and 'loser(s)'. If there are potentially serious legal issues involved, the mediator needs to have the required legal training and experience.

/ **MEDIATION** /

Mediation involves an independent party seeking to resolve disagreements or disputes between people.

CASE STUDY **26.3**
MEDIATION IN ACTION

Barbara Bates, who is 84 years old, suffered a stroke that left her with significant disability. She has been moved for rehabilitation to a residential unit at the hospital, under the care of a multidisciplinary team. Her husband, aged 87, is alone at home and is adamant that his wife should be discharged to return home in the next few weeks, a view endorsed by some other relatives. The patient herself is unwilling to return home at this stage, and is worried about her husband's ability to cope in the short and longer term if she is discharged home. The team believes that she is some weeks away from the level of mobility required for her home environment. Also, home assessment has revealed that some significant alterations need to be made to the home prior to Barbara being able to return there, and that these will take some time to address, should the client and family agree to complete them. A mediator in this situation would first establish the facts and perceptions, identifying the key issues by consulting the interested parties separately, and then attempt to negotiate a compromise acceptable to all parties.

If you are asked to fulfil (or assist in) the role of mediator, seek advice on appropriate procedures from an experienced colleague. Be sure you understand the issues clearly and keep accurate records of meetings. One approach, when you are acting as a mediator with all parties present, is to set the scene briefly, outlining your understanding of what has happened. Ensure that the parties agree about the key issues, concerns and disagreements. Everyone involved needs to be given an opportunity to express their particular perspectives and recollections. The mediator summarises what appear to be the key concerns, encouraging discussion with the intent that common ground is reached. A useful strategy is to engage in a process of question and answer, gaining agreement from the parties on important events, interpretations and points of principle. It might be possible to negotiate an acceptable compromise, but in some cases it will become clear that one side has a stronger case. Once an agreement has been reached, it must be made specific, endorsed by all parties, and documented.

A mediator requires considerable tact and understanding; it is important to treat all people with respect, regardless of their behaviour or viewpoint; those who emerge as 'losers' need to be able to accept that the process itself was fair and reasonable.

Negotiation to achieve optimal outcomes

/ NEGOTIATION /
Negotiation involves seeking agreement about matters people are concerned about or interested in changing.

Negotiation is closely related to mediation, although it need not involve a dispute or conflict. In negotiation there is some give and take in agreeing on outcomes and how best to achieve them. In some situations, a client negotiates with one or more members of a human services team. In other circumstances, negotiation is needed between team members to ensure that there is agreement on specific issues. Negotiation relies on discussion, flexibility and willingness to compromise; you must listen to all parties and consider a range of options and ideas.

Similar skills are needed in negotiation, as in mediation. For example, clients (and their families) might be unwilling to undertake recommended treatments or to adopt biomedical strategies to ameliorate their situations. To negotiate agreement with these strategies, you would need to be flexible, to make compromises and to accept that some of your goals might not be fully met. There may also be external barriers (e.g. financial concerns) or inherent limitations (e.g. language barriers) that restrict a client's options. Such obstacles need to be made explicit (sensitively) and considered, so that the client and the family or carer can achieve their goals.

In the simplest model of negotiation, an individual client discusses his or her problems with a single professional and negotiates with the professional to achieve an acceptable outcome. When several professionals are involved with a client, the practitioner with primary responsibility for the client usually organises other necessary consultations and advice. Effective communication is essential between this primary professional and others who provide specialist advice. It may be necessary for the primary practitioner to negotiate specific issues in the process of referring the client to colleagues.

In complex situations it may be that outcomes seen as ideal by some professionals in the team are not considered desirable by the other team members. Negotiation will be successful if the team members are prepared to compromise and consider the best overall outcome for the client, rather than perfect individual (discipline-specific) outcomes. One strategy is to establish realistic goals or outcomes, and to gain agreement on priorities from each team member. It may be necessary to negotiate each goal, setting intermediate targets to provide encouragement to the client.

Negotiation occurs between the team leader and the client, and with all members of the team, who each contribute their expertise. Occasionally, an expert (such as a radiologist) will be consulted without the direct involvement of the client. Although the team leader carries the overall responsibility, other members of the team also communicate directly with the client. Those diverse interactions assist the team to achieve the collaboratively determined client goals. Some clients, however, may try to negotiate with individual team members, hoping to gain special information or some perceived advantage. Effective open communication within the team is essential to ensure that all members adopt an agreed approach. Negotiation is possible only when all those involved are prepared to make concessions in order to achieve optimal client outcomes.

conclusion

Working with others in workplace groups or informal groups has the potential to integrate the strengths and expertise of team members and to optimise client outcomes. It can also create problems if differences of opinion arise. The skills of consulting, advocating, mediating and negotiating are important in preventing and managing these problems.

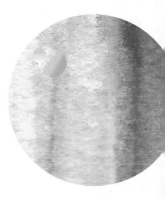

reference

Tyler, S., Kossen, C., & Ryan, C. (2005). *Communication: A foundation course* (2nd edn). Frenchs Forest, NSW: Pearson Education.

further reading

Freegard, H. (Ed.) (2007). *Ethical practice for health professionals.* Sydney: Thomson Learning.

Reeves, S., Lewin, S., Espin, S., & Zwarenstein, M. (2010). *Interprofessional teamwork in health and social care.* Oxford: Wiley-Blackwell.

World Health Organization. (2010). *Framework for action on interprofessional education and collaborative practice.* Geneva: World Health Organization, Department of Human Resources for Health.

Working as a member of a health team

Linda **PORTSMOUTH** | Julia **COYLE** | Franziska **TREDE**

key topics

This chapter covers the following topics:

- health teams—what, who and why

- collaborative practice

- models of health teamwork

- communication to enhance teamwork

key terms

HEALTH TEAM

CLIENT

Introduction

Health teams are found across the spectrum of health services, from hospitals to the community, and are recognised as a vehicle for health practitioners to work together to provide **client** services. There is considerable variation in team structure, size, and model of team practice, as these factors are dependent upon the health outcomes required, the availability of staff, and team practice capabilities of individual members. This chapter explores team composition, purpose and importance, as well as models of teamwork in health and methods of team communication.

What is a team?

A team is a group of people who work together interdependently, commonly employing a shared set of rules, guidelines or professional ethics. Manion and colleagues (1996, p. 5) define a *team* as a 'specific structural unit in the organisation' and *teamwork* as 'the way people work together cooperatively and effectively'. A successful team works in a collaborative environment based on trust, respect, and open and honest communication among its members.

Health practitioners rarely work in isolation from other practitioners. Even if they see clients on a one-to-one basis, they communicate with other health practitioners involved with clients and their families and work together as part of a team. In these contexts, communication involves a mix of informal and formal methods, including consultations, referrals, reports, letters, phone calls and emails, and must be founded on principles of client confidentiality, which require appropriate communication of client information within (but not outside of) professional team member and colleague relationships.

Ideally, health practitioners work in a collaborative team in order to optimise health outcomes, taking into account multiple aspects of a client's requirements, and balancing practitioner needs with the full complexity of services provided. All team members bring their personal perspectives and contribute through provision of their clinical and disciplinary expertise. True collaborative practice results in team delivery of the highest quality care in partnership with clients, families, carers and communities (World Health Organization, 2010, p. 7).

Who are members of the health team?

/ **HEALTH TEAM** /
A health team is a team of practitioners who work together to prevent health problems or disability, maintain good health, improve health and/or maximise ability.

As **health team** composition is dependent upon the needs of the client, teams are not necessarily composed solely of health practitioners. Descriptions of health teams frequently focus on the allied health, nursing and medical professions but, in reality, teams include many other workers who are vital to the successful integration and implementation of health services. In hospitals, teams include health workers from the service arm of the organisation, such as administrative staff, cleaners and orderlies; palliative care teams may have members of the clergy involved; paediatric teams are likely to involve teachers.

Community-based health teams may work from community health centres or disability service organisations. Their practice may involve both care for clients in the centre and services in clients' homes or workplaces. Such teams can include community services providers from workplaces, schools, childcare, day care, seniors' centres, recreation activities and home help or meals on wheels. Population and public health teams work on a community or population-wide basis, and thus need to consult widely across all sectors of society. For example, the provision of clean water and safe waste disposal requires environmental health officers to work closely with local government planners, engineers and laboratory technicians; the development of a mass media campaign to communicate health messages requires health promotion professionals to work in collaboration with marketing and media professionals.

Clients, their families and their carers play a vital health team role (Poulton, 1999). Clients (i.e. individuals, communities and populations) have the right to ask for or refuse interventions. They also have a responsibility to inform the team of relevant information. Client participation is critical for effective, high-quality health service delivery. The involvement of community members in the planning, implementation and evaluation of community and population-wide interventions is also fundamental to their success. Through the community working in partnership with health practitioners, interventions may be modified to better meet needs, and communities are empowered as they actively take responsibility for their own health (WHO, 1986).

/ **CLIENT** /

The term *client* in this book refers to all people receiving team services—including consumers, patients, communities and populations.

Why have health teams?

Team practice is integral to health service delivery due to increasing specialisation, the emergence of new and para-professions, changes in healthcare practices (e.g. increased emphasis on primary healthcare), greater client health literacy and technological advances. As health knowledge expands, the education of health professionals has become increasingly more specialised. The World Health Organization (2010) has responded with a call for increased interprofessional education, which 'occurs when two or more professions learn about, from and with each other to enable effective collaboration' (p. 13) in order to better prepare practitioners for an environment now dependent upon teams.

Healthcare teams that work well and consider clients' needs are important from the clients' perspective. For clients, navigating clinical services across multiple, separate specialties can hamper their capacity to effectively access adequate healthcare and to be able to manage their own health.

Clients come from diverse backgrounds, and can present with numerous concurrent and multi-faceted problems. Teams that are able to draw on the expertise of multiple practitioners and integrate their approach such that they alleviate the burden on clients can deliver high-quality, comprehensive health services. Public health teams must work in collaborative inter-sectoral contexts (e.g. with government and industry) to achieve outcomes that extend beyond individuals to encompass populations through policy and legislative change.

Models of team practice

Many different labels have been used to describe how health teams work. Three key classifications predominate; they use the prefixes *multi-, inter-* and *trans-*. The *Oxford advanced learner's dictionary of current English* (2005) defines *multi-* as 'more than one; many', *inter-* as 'between; from one to another'; and *trans-* as 'across; beyond'. The prefixes *multi-* and *inter-* are sometimes used interchangeably. Commonly, *multi-* is used for different health workers working separately (parallel practice) and reporting or sharing information. The prefix *multi-* thus reflects the retention of role boundaries by the professions. Greater confusion surrounds the use of the prefix *inter-*. For example, professionals may share roles (Masterson, 2002) or work separately (Stepans, Thompson, & Buchanan, 2002), retain boundaries (Paul & Petersen, 2001) or traverse them. There is consensus that the prefix *trans-* implies an emphasis on shared roles, role blurring and even role exchange.

The three terms *multidisciplinary* or *multi-professional, interdisciplinary* or *interprofessional* and *transdisciplinary* or *transprofessional* thus form a continuum that describes team process, with *multi-* at one end and *trans-* at the other. Consider the three hypothetical teams in Case Study 27.1. These community-based health teams all provide services to preschool children with developmental delays. They function in ways that place them at different points on the continuum. Each team consists of an audiologist, a clinical psychologist, a doctor, an occupational therapist, a physiotherapist, a social worker and a speech pathologist.

CASE STUDY 27.1
HEALTH TEAMS PROVIDING SERVICES TO PRESCHOOL CHILDREN WITH DEVELOPMENTAL DELAY

TEAM A, A MULTIDISCIPLINARY/MULTIPROFESSIONAL TEAM: PARALLEL PRACTICE

Robert, a 2-year-old boy with Down's syndrome, is referred to the team. He is assessed separately by each practitioner. Robert and his parents, Carl and Rebecca, attend seven appointments in the community clinic over 2 weeks. They are asked many of the same questions at each appointment. It is difficult for them to get time off work, and they find the whole experience stressful. They haven't found anyone who can answer all of their questions, and they struggle to decide what issue to discuss with each different practitioner. Robert gets bored during the repetitive assessment sessions and stops performing at his best. Rebecca becomes anxious that some of the practitioners are not seeing him do all that he can.

After all assessments are complete, the team members meet to discuss their findings. Robert is in good health, and has hearing within normal limits. The family is coping well, with no particular difficulty. The clinical psychologist finds that Robert has a moderate intellectual delay. The doctor, social worker and psychologist decide to review his progress after 6 months. The physiotherapist, occupational therapist and speech pathologist decide to offer regular appointments. They give Carl and Rebecca ideas for home activities to help him develop gross motor, fine motor, play and communication skills. They each draw up a plan of intervention, arranging separate sessions at the clinic over the next 6 months. They each visit Robert's childcare centre to give the childcare workers ideas to help him to develop targeted skills. At the end of the 6-month period, team members reassess Robert individually, and meet to discuss their findings. Carl and Rebecca are invited to this meeting.

TEAM B, AN INTERDISCIPLINARY/INTERPROFESSIONAL TEAM: MORE INTERDEPENDENT PRACTICE

Kara, a 3-year-old with a developmental delay, is assessed during two visits at home; one from the psychologist and speech pathologist and one from the physiotherapist and occupational therapist. Kara's parents, John and Michelle, are asked only a few of the same questions twice. The team members pool their assessment results, noting that the GP has found Kara to be in good health before referral to the team. They arrange for Kara to see an audiologist for a hearing test and no hearing difficulties are found. The whole team meets with the parents to set Kara's priorities.

Kara attends fortnightly sessions with the occupational therapist and speech pathologist that incorporate some ideas from the physiotherapist and psychologist. The sessions combine activities that promote gross motor skills, fine motor skills, play skills and the communication that arises naturally during these activities. John and Michelle participate, and encourage Kara to do similar activities with them at home. After a few weeks, Kara joins a series of weekly group sessions with three other children of similar age and needs. She enjoys being with the other children, and John and Michelle gain much from their interaction with the other parents. The occupational therapist and physiotherapist run these groups, and incorporate ideas provided by the speech pathologist for encouraging communication.

TEAM C, A TRANSDISCIPLINARY/TRANSPROFESSIONAL TEAM: INTEGRATED AND MERGED PRACTICE

Cooper is a 2-year-old boy with developmental delay. The team normally appoints one of its members to be the family's case coordinator. This is the member who they predict, based on the referral information, would be the main person (or one of the main people) involved with Cooper on an ongoing basis. The case coordinator in this case is Janet, the occupational therapist. She visits Cooper and his mother, Charlene, to carry out an initial assessment, asking one set of questions. The answers are shared with the rest of the team later. Janet is an experienced professional who has learned a great deal from the other members of the team, both informally and during formal training sessions. She can answer most of Charlene's questions, and gets back to her with any answers that need to be checked with other team members. Following consultation with the other team members, Janet and Charlene identify priorities and decide on further assessment.

Cooper visits the audiologist, and is found to have a hearing problem; he is referred to the ear, nose and throat specialist. The physiotherapist and speech pathologist visit Cooper and Charlene at home at the same time as the case coordinator. They provide Charlene and Cooper with extra program ideas. Janet and Charlene plan Cooper's interventions. They are arranged and monitored by the case coordinator, who involves different members of the team at different times. Initially, the speech pathologist and the case coordinator visit weekly. They help Charlene to develop Cooper's communication, play and fine motor skills. As Cooper's communication skills improve and his hearing problem is resolved, the speech pathologist ceases to visit. The physiotherapist then begins to visit once a month. Charlene feels she understands and is in control of what is happening at all times.

Collaboration and interdependence in teams

Collaborative teamwork does not necessarily come easily or naturally. Effective teamwork takes time; members need training to develop interdependence (Heinemann & Zeiss, 2002). Without daily contact among team members, preferably face-to-face, effective teamwork becomes more difficult. Health professionals need to plan ways to ensure that they are working collaboratively towards common team goals on a day-to-day basis. Detailed joint planning, clear delineation of roles and responsibilities, action statements for named team members and set dates for progress reviews will assist in this process. Achievement of interdependent and collaborative client-centred practice requires all members of a health team to collectively monitor, develop and adjust their work practices. Collaborative teamwork can give team members great job satisfaction and a heightened sense of wellbeing (Mickan, 2005).

COMMUNICATION SKILLS AND IDEAS TO BUILD AND ENHANCE TEAMWORK

Share goals, expectations and philosophy to develop greater understanding among team members, resolve and avoid communication problems, and transcend boundaries and work more effectively together:

- Shared goals assist teams.
- Put the client first and make it clear to your colleagues that you do.
- Communicate your reasoning to colleagues.
- Discuss your expectations and be flexible.
- Develop a shared understanding of the philosophy of client care.

Prioritise teamwork:

- Help new team members to settle in.
- Help team members who leave to hand over to their successors and to the rest of the team.
- Know how the team needs to work.
- Respect the roles of every team member.
- Develop greater understanding of your fellow team members.
- Include absent team members: be flexible in your use of communication tools to include absent team members.

Develop and maintain clarity of purpose and shared understanding:

- Listen and read carefully, and check that your impressions are accurate.
- Try to appreciate others' points of view.
- Don't be afraid to ask questions or say when you don't understand or agree with something.
- Seek opportunities for face-to-face communication.
- Express yourself clearly and avoid unhelpful and unfamiliar jargon.
- Communicate in a variety of ways.
- Keep copies, and document verbal communication in the client file.
- Prepare for communication and take time to communicate well (including in emails).
- Communicate in a timely manner.
- Pay attention to deadlines.
- Be honest and discuss issues that are disrupting good teamwork.

Reflect on your teamwork:

- Think about what you have done: take time to reflect on decisions and outcomes, teamwork practices and team communication. Encourage the team to reflect as a group on its impact on clients. Learning from experience will develop your professional skills and help build an effective health team.

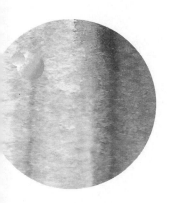

conclusion

Successful collaboration and communication between team members is vital for the successful functioning of health teams and the provision of excellent client care.

references

Heinemann, G. D., & Zeiss, A. M. (2002). A model of team performance. In G. D. Heinemann & A. M. Zeiss (Eds.), *Team performance in health care: Assessment and development* (pp. 29–42). New York: Kluwer Academic/Plenum.

Manion, J., Lorimer, W., & Leander, W. J. (1996). *Team-based health care organizations: Blueprint for success.* Gaithersburg, MD: Aspen Press.

Masterson, A. (2002). Cross boundary working: A macro political analysis of the impact on professional roles. *Journal of Clinical Nursing, 11*(3), 331–9.

Mickan, S. (2005). Evaluating the effectiveness of health care teams. *Australian Health Review, 29*(2), 211–17.

Oxford advanced learner's dictionary of current English (7th edn) (2005). Oxford: Oxford University Press.

Paul, S., & Petersen, C. Q. (2001). Interprofessional collaboration: Issues for practice and research. *Occupational Therapy in Health Care, 15*(3/4), 1–12.

Poulton, B. C. (1999). User involvement in identifying health needs and shaping and evaluating services: Is it being realised? *Journal of Advanced Nursing, 30*(6), 1289–96.

Stepans, M. B., Thompson, C. L., & Buchanan, M. L. (2002). The role of the nurse on a transdisciplinary early intervention assessment team. *Public Health Nursing, 19*(4), 238–45.

World Health Organization. (1986). *Ottawa charter for health promotion.* Retrieved from http://www.who.int/hpr/NPH/docs/ottawa_charter_hp.pdf

World Health Organization. (2010). *Framework for action on interprofessional education and collaborative practice.* WHO/HRH/HPN/10.3, Geneva, Switzerland. Retrieved from http://whqlibdoc.who.int/hq/2010/WHO_HRH_HPN_10.3_eng.pdf

further reading

Ontario Ministry of Health and Long Term Care. (2005). *Guide to collaborative team practice.* http://www.health.gov.on.ca/transformation/fht/guides/fht_collab_team.pdf. This document describes how to provide high-quality collaborative care as part of a program to increase access to primary healthcare via the development of family health teams. The advice for team development is excellent and the team performance checklist is invaluable.

useful web resource

For information about the Australasian Interprofessional Practice and Education Network, see www.aippen.net/index.html

Communicating in teams

Anne **CROKER** | Julia **COYLE**

key topics

This chapter covers the following topics:

- situational influences on communicating in teams
- motivation for communicating in teams
- nature of interactions when communicating in teams
- capability for communicating in teams

key terms

COMMUNICATING

TEAM MEMBERS

Introduction

There is no 'one size fits all' approach to **communicating** in teams. Not only is each team situation unique, but so too are the people within the teams. For example, structures and processes vary between teams (some are hierarchical whereas others seek to share authority), and **team members** often demonstrate different capabilities for communicating (some might be wonderful communicators whereas others might be described as less capable, or 'tricky', individuals). Further, what works well for communicating in one team might not work as well in another team and, as people come and go in a team, the nature of team communication usually alters.

Communicating effectively with a range of people in different teams does not necessarily just happen. Health professionals commonly need to develop their capabilities for this. Understanding influences on communicating in teams (as shown in Figure 28.1) is a suitable starting point. In this chapter, influences on communicating in teams are discussed in four sections:

1. the situation in which the communication takes place;
2. people's motivation for working together;
3. the nature of interactions within the team; and
4. an individual's capability to communicate effectively.

This discussion presupposes that team communication is inherently client-centred and that team members are capable of developing their communication capability through critical reflection on team experiences. To facilitate reflection, this chapter includes a case study, with reflection prompts, presented in two parts.

FIGURE 28.1 | FACTORS INFLUENCING HOW TEAM MEMBERS COMMUNICATE

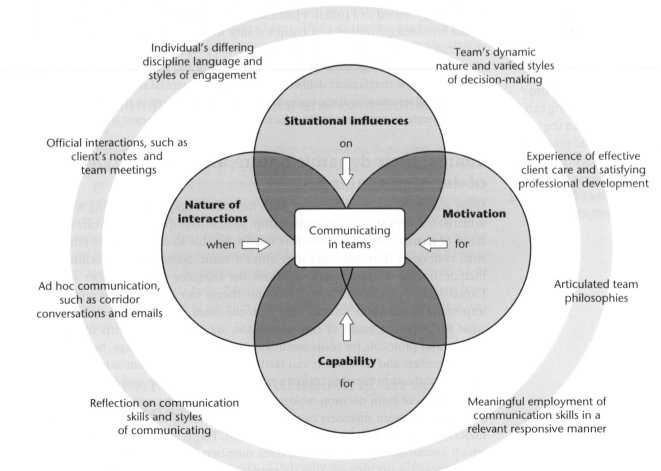

support. Team members share perspectives and knowledge about clients' problems and situations in order to formulate goals and evaluate progress. Effective client care is mediated through team communication; role overlaps are clarified and negotiated, and appointments are appropriately scheduled. Team communication can provide a rich source of learning about a person's role in healthcare and the roles of others. Professionals involved in teams need to be proficient in their own discipline roles and to have a sound understanding of the roles of others. Such understanding, developed in part through team participation, provides an important basis for establishing role clarity and negotiating professional boundaries.

Once teams develop understanding and expertise through ongoing interaction, and are seen to generate new knowledge, they may shift from being simply a collection of people who identify with each other and work together to become a community of practice (Wenger, McDermott, & Snyder, 2002). An important aspect of a community of practice is that members can learn together and support each other's ongoing professional development, providing an important dimension to team membership and sense of identity. Ongoing professional development may be formalised through regular educational sessions such as journal clubs, or learning may be opportunistic, when team members access each other's knowledge and skills as needed.

Motivation for teams

It can be useful for members to articulate and document a team's collective vision, values and objectives. This can be referred to as the *team philosophy*; it clarifies what the team is all about and the reasons they need to communicate. For example, a simple philosophy is articulated below, based on the values of high-quality person-centred collaborative care:

- the team values and respects input from all team members (including clients and carers)
- the team establishes goals that are meaningful to clients and carers
- all team members work towards these goals
- members share roles and blur discipline boundaries in response to client needs
- the team advocates for clients' needs
- team members value ongoing professional development.

Although healthcare teams are care-focused, they also benefit from time and opportunities to socialise and become more cohesive. Effective communication is supported by creating and maintaining the social glue that holds a team together. Regular events, such as morning teas to welcome new members or acknowledge significant occasions, provide opportunities for members to get to know each other and interact socially. These interactions can help establish a supportive climate and develop a sense of belonging, which in turn provides motivation for effective communication.

CASE STUDY 28.1
COMMUNICATING IN TEAMS

The team was gathering for the weekly rehabilitation case conference. Halimah and Mark were organising clients' medical records. As they sorted records in the order which discussion would follow, they talked about Mrs Roberts' cognition problems. Hearing the discussion, Sam joined the debate about whether the problems were transient or permanent. Jenny, a student, hovered nearby; she seemed uncertain whether she should be there. Explosive laughing marked the entrance of Jamilah and Emma. They sat down opposite Wulan, who was quietly reading. Sarah strode in with Julie in tow, saying 'Let's get started'. Julie sat down, was handed the first client file by Mark, and started the summary of the client's history. Six minutes into the meeting a harried-looking Liz crept in, sat next to Wulan, who whispered where they were up to.

REFLECTION PROMPTS

- What different types of communication are you able to identify?
- No professional affiliations have been used. Does this make a difference to your perspective on the individuals? Try allocating a professional affiliation to each person in the team and consider why you chose a profession for a specific individual. What does this say about your own perspectives? Compare your perspectives with another person's. What challenges does this present to effective communication?
- What challenges to effective communication occur with the team's processes and context?

The nature of team communication

There are basically two types of team communication: official and ad hoc. Examples of *official* team communication are clients' records and formal case meetings. Examples of *ad hoc* communication are handover notes and the so-called 'corridor chat'. To make either type of communication truly effective, it is important to understand their differences.

Official interactions commonly reflect organisational and legislative requirements of health service delivery, and predominantly relate to documentation in clients' notes and what occurs in official meetings. Although these provide clarity around expectations, such official interactions do not always allow for the uncertainties, subtleties and negotiations needed in real-world clinical practice. However, the official interactions set the scene for more ad hoc forms of interaction. For example, in an official meeting, new members can learn to understand the preferred communication styles of fellow team members. These face-to-face events also provide valuable opportunities to get to know other team members.

However, team members usually find the need to add to official interactions through innumerable ad hoc interactions, such as corridor conversations, whiteboard messages, handover notes, emails, diaries and mobile phone texting. Grasping opportunities to discuss client issues outside the more formal prescribed interactions is commonplace in healthcare. Learning how to manage these informal interactions so that they enhance rather than hamper effective teamwork is important. For example, health workers should ensure that they share new information appropriately across the team while maintaining client confidentiality. It is also important to note that ad hoc meetings are not the setting in which to make key decisions that should be made in more official meetings and involve the rest of the team. If key decision-making is undermined in this way then the cohesion of the whole team is threatened.

As we move into an era which increasingly relies upon technology for communication, it is critical that clients' confidentiality be protected. For instance, sharing interesting cases or photos on Facebook, uploading snippets into Twitter, or texting messages with client details to colleagues can all violate clients' confidentiality. Using technology for team communication can enhance client care, but should always be informed by a client-centred approach.

Capability for communicating in teams

Team members need to bring a readiness to communicate to their teams. Such readiness is evidenced in being proficient in their own roles, being positively attuned to others, respecting other people's diversity, valuing different contributions and really 'hearing' others. Having and making time to communicate is important, as it presents a clear demonstration of commitment, which is important to both client outcomes and team coherence.

Communicating in teams is underpinned by a number of skills, including attentive listening (to encourage speakers and hear their messages), questioning (to elicit information and understand the perspectives of others), providing information (explaining and informing through clear verbal explanations or written reports), responding (providing feedback about messages received), clarifying (to check understanding and highlight areas of tension) and empathising (to create an appropriate communication climate). The challenge of communicating meaningfully in teams is to reliably employ these skills in a timely, efficient and flexible manner that is relevant to the rest of the team and responsive to the situation. There is also a need to reflect critically on the team's collective experience so that all may learn. As reflection is a broad topic beyond the scope of this chapter, the reader is directed to Brown and Ryan (2003). Another way of developing capability for effective team communication is the use of role models and mentors. Mentors can help us develop awareness of many aspects of our practice, including the capability to interact and communicate with other team members.

CASE STUDY 28.1 (CONTINUED)

Discussion moves on to Mr Petrie. All team members are present except the speech pathologist.

Julie: It says here he's on a soft diet, but isn't he on a normal one?

Mark: Yes

Halimah: Does it say in his notes?

Julie looks at the notes and comments: Can't see anything.

Mark leaves to check the main patient record.

Wulan: I hope it's normal, as his friend fed him fried takeaway chicken when he was in bed the other day!

They all laugh.

Liz: So do I, we're giving him normal food in therapy.

Continued laughter and chat.

Mark returns and with a triumphant grin, saying: Soft diet.

There is a stunned silence, sheepish grins.

Liz: Oops (pauses), then: So speech pathology to review the soft diet.

All laugh.

Emma: This is why we have case conferences!

(Coyle 2008, p. 189)

REFLECTION PROMPTS

- One discipline representative is absent from the meeting. What are the implications of this for effective communication and client care? What are the different types of communication used to overcome this deficit? How might communication be improved in this situation?

- What communication capabilities do the speakers demonstrate? What are your thoughts on the timing of this conversation?

- How broad should team communication be? Who should be included in communication in this situation?

- In relation to communication, what should the team do next?

THINGS TO THINK ABOUT ...
BASE YOUR CONTRIBUTIONS ON SOUND INFORMATION AND JUDGMENT

Understand the purpose behind each team interaction. Make sure that you have all the required information. Be prepared to articulate your reasoning when communicating your needs. Be honest with yourself and others about your proficiency in your role.

BE AWARE OF DIFFERENT PERSPECTIVES AND SITUATIONS

Welcome different perspectives that might challenge your assumptions, as they can lead to different ways of viewing situations and new understandings. Try to understand your fellow team members' contexts and constraints.

SHOW THAT YOU VALUE OTHERS THROUGH YOUR COMMUNICATION STYLE

Give people your full attention. Respect others' rights to voice their opinion; make the effort to understand their perspectives. Understand that others have a variety of styles of communication and respect these differences. For example, don't demand instant input into decisions from team members who prefer time to contemplate issues.

BE ABLE TO ADAPT COMMUNICATION TO SUIT DIFFERENT NEEDS

Be flexible in the way you convey information and explain your views. For example, anecdotes or stories can generate discussions or lead to elaborations on particular points in case conferences, whereas quick corridor interactions may require concise information and brief rationales for requests. Use non-judgmental language to maintain an objective focus on issues under discussion, rather than allow the issues to be obscured by emotion.

DO WHAT YOU SAY YOU WILL DO, AND TELL IT LIKE IT IS

Acknowledge the constraints in your own context. Efficient teamwork is founded on the capacity of others to rely on you. Failure to meet expectations can lead to conflict, or to duplication should others lack faith in you. Tell other team members if you can't meet a deadline. This gives them the opportunity to renegotiate needs or to undertake the task themselves. It also helps others to have realistic expectations of you.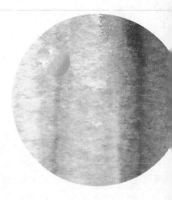

conclusion

Team communication is multifaceted and complex, and influenced by a range of factors. This complexity requires team members to critically reflect on their own and their team's capacity for effective communication. Realising capability for communicating should be a focus for health professionals. Developing good communication capability is a critical ongoing objective for quality client care.

references

Brown, G., & Ryan S. (2003). Enhancing reflective abilities: Interweaving reflective abilities. In G. Brown, A. Esdaile & S. Ryan (Eds.), *Becoming an advanced health care practitioner* (pp. 118–44). Oxford: Butterworth-Heinemann.

Coyle, J. (2008). *Being a member of a health care team: Physiotherapists' perspectives and experiences*. Unpublished doctoral thesis, Charles Sturt University, Albury, Australia.

Dwyer, J. (2003). *The business communication handbook*. Frenchs Forest, NSW: Prentice Hall.

Rehling, L. (2004). Improving teamwork through awareness of conversational styles. *Business Communication Quarterly, 67*(4), 475–82.

Stephenson, J. (1994). Capability and competence: Are they the same and does it matter? *Capability, 1*(1), 3–4.

Wenger, E., McDermott, R., & Snyder, W. M. (2002). *Cultivating communities of practice: A guide to managing knowledge*. Boston: Harvard Business School Press.

further reading

Kitto, S., Chesters, J., Thistlethwaite, J., & Reeves, S. (2010). *Sociology of interprofessional healthcare practice: Critical reflections and concrete solutions*. New York: Nova Science. This book critically analyses issues in interprofessional practice to facilitate understanding of successful practice in teams.

useful web resources

For information and resources about team practice, see SARRAH Education and Training website www.sarrahtraining.com.au/site/index.cfm?display=144985

Being assertive in teams and workplaces

Franziska **TREDE** | Megan **SMITH**

key topics

This chapter covers the following topics:

- defining and demystifying assertiveness

- dimensions that influence assertiveness

- discussing advantages of assertive behaviour for self, profession, team and clients

key terms

AGGRESSIVE BEHAVIOUR

ASSERTIVE BEHAVIOUR

CONFIDENCE

EMOTIONAL INTELLIGENCE

Introduction

Being assertive is often seen as a positive behaviour for members of teams. Chapters 27 and 28 cover team dynamics. In this chapter we focus on what **assertive behaviour** is and what it is not, and how it relates to effective teamwork and communication among team members. Being appropriately assertive in teams and workplaces is a crucial aspect of effective and satisfying work. If you want to be a respected team member whose opinion is recognised and valued, rather than just being told what to do, you require assertiveness. Being assertive ensures that your rights and responsibilities, as well as those of others, are respected and honoured. We discuss how assertive behaviour is influenced by various external and internal dimensions. Assertive behaviour in the workplace has advantages for you, your profession and the team, as well as your clients.

Demystifying assertiveness

Assertiveness is about making use of the right to express yourself and be heard and, at the same time, respecting other people's right to express themselves. Being assertive means standing up for your rights and ensuring that others are not taking advantage of you. Being assertive instils control, confidence and a sense of wellbeing. You are being assertive when you articulate your thinking, decisions, emotions and arguments in a manner that observes other people's dignity and rights, as well as maintaining your own. **Assertive behaviour** is underpinned by clear, polite, direct language, and it creates an environment of constructiveness with a focus on solutions.

Being assertive is often contrasted with being submissive, when your opinions and wishes are not expressed; being aggressive, when your opinions are expressed in a way that is perceived as hostile by others and may disregard others' points of view, dignity and rights; and being passive–aggressive, when passivity is interpreted by others as resisting communication and action and thus perceived as aggressive. Table 29.1 expands on the differences between assertive, submissive, passive–aggressive and **aggressive behaviour**.

/ ASSERTIVE BEHAVIOUR /
Assertive behaviour is taking actions that ensure that your rights and responsibilities, and those of others, are respected and honoured.

/ AGGRESSIVE BEHAVIOUR /
Aggressive behaviour is taking physical, mental or verbal action to increase your own dominance.

TABLE 29.1 | DIFFERENCES BETWEEN ASSERTIVE, AGGRESSIVE, PASSIVE–AGGRESSIVE AND SUBMISSIVE BEHAVIOUR

ASSERTIVE BEHAVIOUR	AGGRESSIVE BEHAVIOUR	PASSIVE–AGGRESSIVE BEHAVIOUR	SUBMISSIVE BEHAVIOUR
accountable	intimidating	resentful	defensive
responsible	threatening	stubborn	timid
respectful	coercive	sullen	sullen
trustworthy	minimising and reducing others	appearing to comply but actually resisting	agreeing with others without gaining trust
supportive	humiliating	procrastinating	indifferent
honest	denying, blaming others	indirectly negative	finding excuses
seeking partnerships	putting people down	resisting authority	fearing authority
fair	single minded, one-dimensional	resisting suggestions	not acting to promote fairness
self-confident	defensive	obstructive	lacking self-confidence
negotiating	ready to combat	hindering progress	unable to negotiate
giving and receiving compliments	making destructive comments	not commenting	not commenting

< cont. >

role. Workplaces that foster a culture of 'following orders' may encourage a passive–aggressive staff mentality of doing only those tasks that one has been told to do.

Workplace factors such as culture, and organisational structures that emphasise financial and technical aspects, can create an environment where authoritarian decisions prevail over the dialogues that focus on clients' needs and emotions. Lower priority might be given to team discussions about clients because of pressures to discharge and process people quickly. In these environments, particular skill and practice are needed to develop assertiveness strategies that achieve acceptable outcomes for clients and staff.

Although many books and courses offer strategies and resources for improving assertiveness, many people still confuse assertiveness with aggression, and do not want to impose themselves (Freeman & Adams, 1999). Some people think it inappropriate to display confidence or express feelings, and might find it easier to be submissive and accede to other people's wishes. These attitudes are often reinforced through gender perception, where it is assumed that assertiveness is a male behaviour. In some communities, assertive females may be viewed as less attractive.

Advantages of assertive behaviour for self, profession, team and clients

Assertive behaviour has advantages not just for your self-confidence but also for your profession, your multidisciplinary team and, last but not least, your clients. Assertive behaviour fosters effective communication skills, enhances effective teamwork and conflict resolution, and supports patient advocacy.

Effective communication

It is important to be clear about the assumptions and intentions that underpin communication behaviours. It is wise to be respectful, remain calm, and be clear about boundaries, no matter where people may be on the spectrum of passive-to-aggressive behaviours. You can contribute to good care by being assertive and asking team members to be assertive with you as well. You encourage positive assertiveness when you listen to people, take their questions seriously, and try to respond to them in a way that is meaningful to them.

Effective teamwork

Teamwork requires professionals to work together to achieve common goals. Assertiveness is an important attribute for team members, as it is the means by which all team members can have their professional contribution integrated into the team's functioning. Although all team members might desire to have their interests communicated and acknowledged, working in a team can also be associated with ineffective communication and potential conflict. In these situations, appropriate assertiveness is often linked with other concepts related to effective teamwork, including learning from each other, conflict resolution and collaboration. Effective collaboration is a means of working towards a point where members communicate their opinions and needs, and work together to determine an outcome that could achieve everybody's aims.

CASE STUDY 29.2
WHO SEES THE CLIENT FIRST?

You are the physiotherapist working on a rehabilitation ward. You have booked to see a stroke client at 9 a.m. You have chosen this time because the client should be less fatigued than at any other time of the day, and better able to participate fully in your treatment. The occupational therapist on the ward calls you, because he also wants to see the client at 9 a.m. You and the occupational therapist each feel that you are acting in the client's best interests. How might you resolve this situation using appropriate assertiveness?

Possible solution
You meet with the occupational therapist and consider the goals you are both trying to achieve. You agree to alternate your treatment sessions so that one day you see the client at 9 a.m. and the next day your colleague treats the client. After the discussion, you feel that you have managed to collaborate effectively to achieve an optimal outcome. Even though the outcome isn't exactly what you had planned, you can still achieve your objectives.

Assertiveness by team members and for patients is essential to ensure team effectiveness. Advocating on behalf of patients and their families, when their voices are not heard by all members of the team, is also being assertive.

CASE STUDY 29.3
OPTIONS FOR LONG-TERM CARE

An elderly patient and his family want him to be discharged home after a recent admission to hospital after a fall. Many members of the team feel it is in the patient's best interests to go to a nursing home. The family wish to explore other options, but feel they aren't being considered in the discussion. The patient and family have discussed their feelings with you. Assertiveness in this situation would involve advocating on the patient's behalf to have their voice added to the discussion.

Assertive professionals can empower their patients to be assertive

Clients might tell you about medical advice they have received, dropping hints that they do not agree, and ask you for your opinion. It is wise to ask further questions so you get a more complete picture of the context within which advice was given. You can thus encourage clients to reflect on the advice, and enable them to rethink their opinions. Conducting a dialogue about the advice in this manner fosters fair and respectful attitudes, and helps clients to become aware of their way of reasoning. It may confirm their beliefs, or it may enable them to rethink. By probing clients' comments you can facilitate assertiveness in your clients. If you simply took the hints and spoke against the medical advice to please a client, you would not have asserted your professional judgment but simply succumbed to your client's intent. Modelling assertive behaviour by showing respect, and being curious and honest instils trust, and also encourages assertiveness in your client.

SKILLS IN ASSERTIVE BEHAVIOUR

Here are some strategies you can use to facilitate and practise being assertive:

- Support assertive behaviour with body language and a tone of voice that expresses calmness, relaxedness and confidence.

- Ask questions when you are confused; for example, when people use acronyms you do not know.

- Contribute to discussions.

- Voice your concerns or ideas.

- Speak in the first person to assert yourself: 'I think …'. Relate directly to people and use a firm yet polite tone of voice.

- Make eye contact.

- Not only the words, but also the manner, make up assertiveness. Assertiveness is best learned by practising it. Read the sentence above aloud, and use a variety of tones of voice and body language: polite and firm, strong and aggressive, or soft and defensive. Although the language is the same, the message can be different and confusing when accompanied by various types of body language and tone of voice.

DEALING WITH PASSIVE–AGGRESSIVE COMMUNICATION

Here are some suggestions on how to respond to people who display passive–aggressive behaviour:

- 'When you said that, did you mean ...?'
- 'Have you considered viewing the situation from other people's perspective?'
- 'When you do ... it affects .... I would prefer it if you ...'

Be genuine with your questions and display a sense of curiosity. Try to understand (passive) aggressiveness together with the person displaying it.

Interactions with other team members can be more complex than simply responding assertively to situations where you feel uncomfortable. You cannot control the behaviour of others; you can only control your own actions. Challenges can arise even when you are being assertive (Davis, 2006):

- You cannot control other people's behaviour—you can only assert your point of view with respect to the other person's rights and feelings.
- Being assertive involves attention to non-verbal behaviours such as tone of voice, body position and eye contact.
- Assertiveness is about assessing the situation, being mindful of maintaining relationships, and determining the optimal course of action. This can include saying nothing or defusing the situation.
- You might need to repeat assertive statements more than once to resolve a situation.

conclusion

Effective communication in teams is underpinned by members' assertiveness. Through assertiveness, team members can express their views and opinions in a manner that also considers the rights of others. For effective team outcomes in the best interests of clients, assertiveness needs to be linked to collaboration and conflict resolution.

references

Davis, C. M. (2006). *Patient practitioner interaction: An experiential manual for developing the art of health care* (4th edn). Thorofare, NJ: Slack.

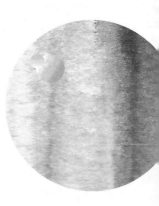

Freeman, L. H., & Adams, P. F. (1999). Comparative effectiveness of two training programs on assertive behaviour. *Nursing Standard, 13*(38), 32–5.

Goleman, D. (1996). *Emotional intelligence*. London: Bloomsbury.

Jordan, P., & Troth, A. (2002). Emotional intelligence and conflict resolution in nursing. *Contemporary Nurse, 13*, 94–100.

McCabe, C. (2003). Teaching assertiveness to undergraduate nursing students. *Nursing Education in Practice, 3*(1), 30–42.

Salovey, P., & Mayer, J. D. (1990). Emotional intelligence. *Imagination, Cognition and Personality, 9*, 185–211.

useful web resources

For useful tips in how to deal with difficult people at work, see http://hbr.org/web/management-tip/tips-on-managing-difficult-people

CHAPTER
30 /

Leadership in health practice

Maree **SIMPSON** | Narelle **PATTON**

key topics

This chapter covers the following topics:

- distributed leadership
- leading by participation
- leading by being an effective role model
- planning—avoiding the Guppy moment
- team participation—role and responsibilities

- negotiating and responding
- advocacy
- shared wisdom

key terms

ACCOUNTABLE

CONFLICT MANAGEMENT

DISTRIBUTED LEADERSHIP

ENGAGING LEADERSHIP

Introduction

Health professionals often choose their profession because they want to help people and make a difference in people's lives and health outcomes. To be effective as a health professional, every individual needs to be an appropriate role model for their profession: developing and maintaining competence, demonstrating integrity in their dealings with others, being held **accountable**—which means taking personal responsibility for their actions—and showing compassion and altruism in their interactions with others. These are expected professional behaviours and attributes, and we shall see in this chapter that they are also characteristic of distributed or engaged leadership.

/ ACCOUNTABLE /
Being held accountable involves taking personal responsibility.

pg.299

Leadership

Although health professionals are required to take personal responsibility for their own practice and outcomes, the majority will also work with or supervise other similarly qualified professionals, and many will supervise technicians or assistants to their profession. Furthermore, with interprofessional care being at least the emergent if not the predominant model of care provision (Xyrichis & Lowton, 2008) many health professionals will need to lead multidisciplinary teams for practice or research. When you are on clinical placement as a later-year student, you may be asked to lead a multidisciplinary team discussion if your particular area of expertise is most beneficial for the patient or situation. So you need to be well prepared to participate and take the lead, if required, for the patient's benefit, while still being comfortable to acknowledge limitations in your knowledge and clinical decision-making.

Some individual health professionals have innate skills and dispositions that help them to cope and thrive in this arena, but many do not, and need to work to develop and utilise this expertise. The sorts of dispositional characteristics that are valued in healthcare include courtesy, cooperation, tolerance, respect, resilience, endurance and empathy. Skills such as excellent time management, effective prioritisation, broad, deep research skills, and conflict management and resolution are greatly appreciated. In the sections that follow, we shall see that these skills and characteristics are also those required within the emerging paradigm of leadership in healthcare. Health professionals in the twenty-first century need to be able to focus not only on patient care but also on the process of healthcare delivery.

/ DISTRIBUTED
LEADERSHIP /
Distributed leadership is characterised by interdependence among members of the team or organisation, with overlapping responsibilities and empowerment of every member of the team or organisation.

/ ENGAGING
LEADERSHIP /
Engaging leadership is grounded in a genuine respect for others, with integrity, transparency and inclusiveness.

Leadership styles

Leadership styles have changed significantly over the past century. In the twenty-first century, two related leadership models are proposed as representative of the emerging trends: **distributed leadership** and **engaging leadership**. Distributed leadership is characterised by interdependence among members of the team or organisation, with overlapping responsibilities and empowerment of every member of the team or organisation. Values such as respect, and behaviours such as cooperation and trust are crucial to this style. Leadership is shared, dispersed or distributed; hence the terminology. Engaging leadership is grounded in a genuine respect for others, with integrity, transparency and inclusiveness central to the style (Alban-Metcalfe, Alban-Metcalfe, & Alimo-Metcalfe, 2009; Alimo-Metcalfe, Alban-Metcalfe, Bradley, Mariathasan, & Samele, 2008). Leaders with an engaging style are able to unite groups, forming a team that develops a shared vision, with a preference for a critically evaluative approach to issues and change. It is proposed that the success of engaging leadership can be judged by the amount of discretionary effort that employees contribute to their work and to the team (Alimo-Metcalfe et al., 2008). Since these two leadership styles are similar, only engaging leadership is discussed further.

Health professionals who successfully adopt an engaging leadership style can anticipate leading productive, happy and healthy teams towards desired patient and organisational outcomes, through a shared vision for success that is well known, understood and communicated (Alban-Metcalfe & Alimo-Metcalfe, 2009). Although most health professionals will not start their careers leading a team of health professionals, almost every health professional will lead productive patient-centred care discussions with a patient, or a patient and family or carer, to achieve mutually agreed health goals, demonstrating and honing the skills necessary for effective engaged leadership.

With new and emerging visions of leadership, such as those outlined above, it is important to be clear as to the essential differences between a manager and a leader, and to know why healthcare professionals should aspire to effective leadership. They need to do so to ensure optimal patient outcomes. Good leaders are characterised by the possession of common sense, organisational knowledge and skills, an ability to see the 'big picture', excellent communication skills and people skills (Al-Ani, Horspool, & Bligh, 2011). Managers, in contrast, are individuals who are in charge of a group or a team with a project or service provision in which to achieve desired outcomes within resource constraints.

Managing expectations and conflict

Conflict results when there is an inconsistency between two or more people, opinions or interests. Conflict is not necessarily good or bad—it can lead to successful change, though it may become divisive and lead to the breakdown of the team. Sources of conflict are many, and can include differences in personality, or differences in individual, group or organisational characteristics. Healthcare environments are potentially conflict-laden environments because of the high demand and work stress that falls on every member of the healthcare team.

Managing the expectations of each member of a patient healthcare team and resolving conflict are crucial to effective healthcare. Five styles of **conflict management** are commonly identified. These are: competitive, collaborative, compromising, avoidant and accommodating (Sportsman & Hamilton, 2007). Some of these styles are more successful than others, though each may have a role to play in different situations. Successful matching of the style to the situation can enable a healthcare professional to demonstrate effective leadership, and may achieve patient safety and desired health outcomes.

/ CONFLICT MANAGEMENT /
Five styles of conflict management are: competitive, collaborative, compromising, avoidant and accommodating.

The first style, the *competitive* strategy, is sometimes considered a strategy of domination, as one group or person remains focused on just a single acceptable outcome. That strategy might not build good relationships in the short term, and will leave sole accountability for outcome with the person or team who becomes dominant. There are circumstances, however—perhaps where patient advocacy is required—when that may be the only ethical stance. This is an important point to appreciate. Remember that patient advocacy is not aggressive nor conflict-laden, but rather assertive, inclusive and patient-focused.

To give just a few examples from practice, let us consider a speech pathologist who is concerned about a patient's inability to swallow tablets due to disease, but who also wishes to ensure that the patient receives medication in a form that will be effective. The speech pathologist may choose to partner with the ward pharmacist to ensure that medicines which should not simply be crushed for administration (perhaps because of controlled release formulation) are safely prepared or alternative medicines sourced. Similarly, a physiotherapist may need to advocate for a patient who has a falls risk, who is recovering from a surgical procedure, and who lives alone and is without family support. It may be quite inappropriate to adhere to the standard care plan of an overnight stay, but rather to delay discharge until community healthcare workers and organisations are alerted, and able to contribute to the patient's care once discharged.

In contrast, the second conflict-management approach, the *collaborative* approach, attempts to achieve mutual agreement and understanding between all conflicting parties. This approach can result in a successful outcome, while reinforcing personal relationships. Unfortunately, this strategy is often the lengthiest resolution to a conflict and may be inefficient when time is the determining factor in decision-making.

A *compromising* approach attempts to achieve a mutually acceptable solution that is expedient. This approach assumes that there is no solution able to be achieved that will yield complete satisfaction for all participants in a limited timeframe, but there is one that is appropriate and suitable.

Avoidance as a conflict-management strategy may be utilised by individuals who do not have enough invested in the issue to see value in the conflict, or there may be an attempt at diplomatically avoiding conflict at a time when another person or group is strongly affected by the issue—this allows a 'cooling-off' period and time to reconsider one's position.

Last, the *accommodating* strategy means yielding to the view of others or following an order or direction when one might prefer not to do so. On minor issues, this approach can be very diplomatic and may build trust and reciprocity. On more serious issues, however, this approach can compromise good patient outcomes. Patients may receive sub-optimal care because a student or an early career health professional did not communicate concern. So, instead of accommodating when an issue is at least serious, how can a younger or more junior person start the conversation about their concern?

First, it is not necessary to fight a battle to protect every patient. A graded assertiveness approach is usually most effective, as the patient is always the focus and the reason (Curtis, Tzannes, & Rudge, 2011). To remember the graded assertiveness 'plan', you need only to recall the acronym *PACE*. This is a memory prompt for **p**robing, **a**lerting, **c**larifying, and **e**mergency. A probing statement is designed to allow you to find out more. An example might be, 'I'm concerned about this patient's slower recovery'. This may be all that is required for the other person to reflect and re-assess. If not, then an alerting statement effectively moves your communication about concern up a level. It might be a statement such as, 'This approach might aggravate his diabetes, is there another therapeutic option?'. If no action is taken after your probing or alerting statements, it may be necessary to raise the level of concern communicated another notch to that of a clarifying statement. At this stage you are increasingly certain that a proposed course of action may potentially harm the patient. A clarifying statement could be, 'I need some clarity please. It seems we are going to perform a procedure on the right knee but the chart notes the left knee'. Finally, if you feel you need to stop something potentially harmful or dangerous, and the lower levels of concern have gone unheeded, then it is appropriate to use an emergency warning. This might sound like: 'Please stop immediately—his chart says he is seriously allergic to sulphonamides'. Always remember to use graded assertiveness with tact and not aggression (Curtis et al., 2011).

No one approach used consistently will always resolve conflict—in some cases it may inflame the situation, so effective conflict management needs flexibility in the application of these approaches (Sportsman & Hamilton, 2007). With experience and wisdom, your leadership skills should develop so that you can use each of the conflict-management strategies for greatest benefit.

SAFETY, QUALITY AND LEADERSHIP

To discover those activities, behaviours and actions that are important in Australian healthcare, please visit the Australian Commission on Safety and Quality in Health Care website http://www.safetyandquality.gov.au/. Knowing how to contribute to patient safety and healthcare quality will help you to demonstrate leadership during workplace learning and future practice. ●

Meetings

As we have seen, communication between and within teams is essential for successful operation, and achievement of goals and objectives. Although face-to-face communication may be sufficient in small teams, meetings are the more usual venue for communication in larger teams and/or those that are widely dispersed. The outcomes expected of different types of meetings vary, but most if not all meetings need a chairperson. Health professionals usually develop the skills of chairing or coordinating while still at university, as part of group projects, such as developing a patient education program and resources.

Depending on the future profession and the structure of the course of study, students may also participate in research projects during workplace learning in a real or simulated worksite such as a clinic or student-led clinic. Most research projects, except for very small ones such as an audit of a particular procedure or medicine, need several participants to complete the task and to report the results of the research.

Later, in practice, health professionals may lead meetings of patients with a common condition, such as those living with Parkinson's disease or type 2 diabetes mellitus. There are many issues that concern patients, and most patient education sessions will benefit from participation of a broad range of health professionals, including physiotherapists, occupational therapists, speech pathologists, pharmacists, and disease-specific educators such as asthma educators, dieticians, psychologists, social workers, podiatrists and, potentially, many others relevant to a particular disease state.

As health professionals assume more responsibilities, education of colleagues such as in-service presentations or provision of sessions of continuing professional development may become another opportunity to organise a meeting, albeit a 'special' one.

SUCCEEDING IN MEETINGS

Before you attend your first meeting, do a quick assessment of areas that may need review. For example, do you know confidently the purpose of an agenda and of minutes? Very simply, agendas announce the date and time of the meeting, the attendance and the proposed issues for discussion and/or action. Minutes provide a record of date, venue, attendance, discussion (topics) and agreed action or outcomes—these may generate an action sheet.

Chairing a meeting

As we have seen earlier, different types of meetings have different purposes and different processes. Chairing a meeting or a session at a conference is an opportunity to demonstrate leadership and effective role-modelling. The chairperson has a responsibility to keep the meeting running to time, and has the pleasant duty of introducing the items of business or the topics and speakers, providing a brief outline of the speakers' expertise and practice. Although meeting types differ, all have common features of a purpose for being held, a venue, date and time, expected outcomes, and records of the outcomes or actions.

conclusion

It is becoming evident that health professionals of the twenty-first century will face challenges and experiences different from those of the past. There are changing demographics of current and future patients and of healthcare providers, changing models of practice, a focus on evidence-based practice, changing workforce participation and mobility, a focus on patient safety and a reduced funding base (Gilmore, Morris, Murphy, Grimmer-Somers, & Kumar, 2011). With its focus on integrity, transparency, inclusiveness and engagement of employees, engaged leadership as opposed to team management is seen as an effective strategy for navigating the changing healthcare environment.

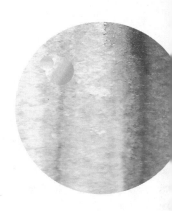

references

Al-Ani, B., Horspool, A., & Bligh, M. C. (2011). Collaborating with 'virtual strangers': Towards developing a framework for leadership in distributed teams. *Leadership, 7*(3), 219–49.

Alban-Metcalfe, J., Alban-Metcalfe, J., & Alimo-Metcalfe, B. (2009). Engaging leadership part two: An integrated model of leadership development. *The International Journal of Leadership in Public Services, 5*(2), 5–13.

Alban-Metcalfe, J., & Alimo-Metcalfe, B. (2009). Engaging leadership part one: Competencies are like Brighton Pier. *The International Journal of Leadership in Public Services, 5*(1), 10–18.

Alimo-Metcalfe, B., Alban-Metcalfe, J., Bradley, M., Mariathasan, J., & Samele, C. (2008). The impact of engaging leadership on performance, attitudes to work and wellbeing at work: A longitudinal study. *Journal of Health Organization and Management, 22*(6), 586–98.

Curtis, K., Tzannes, A., & Rudge, T. (2011). How to talk to doctors—a guide for effective communication. *International Nursing Review, 58*, 13–20.

Gilmore, L. G., Morris, J. H., Murphy, K., Grimmer-Somers, K., & Kumar, S. (2011). Skills escalator in allied health: A time for reflection and refocus. *Journal of Healthcare Leadership, 3*, 53–8.

Sportsman, S., & Hamilton, P. (2007). Conflict management styles in the health professions. *Journal of Professional Nursing, 23*(3), 157–66.

Xyrichis, A., & Lowton, K. (2008). What fosters or prevents interprofessional teamworking in primary and community care? A literature review. *International Journal of Nursing Studies, 45*(1), 140–53.

further reading

Gilmore, L. G., Morris, J. H., Murphy, K., Grimmer-Somers, K., & Kumar, S. (2011). (See above.) This free open access article discusses the healthcare workforce of the future and the challenges for Allied Healthcare professionals that may be required to adequately cope with the future needs driven by changing patient and provider demographics.

useful web resources

For a useful overview on key dispositional characteristics that make individuals effective team members, see www.dummies.com/how-to/content/ten-qualities-of-an-effective-team-player.html

For free templates to record team meeting minutes and action sheets, whether formal or informal, or for specific situations such as an annual general meeting, see office.microsoft.com/en-au/templates/CL102227824.aspx

acknowledgments

We acknowledge Joy Higgs and Mary Jane Mahony, who authored the chapter on this topic in the second edition of this book. Our chapter has revised and updated this earlier version.

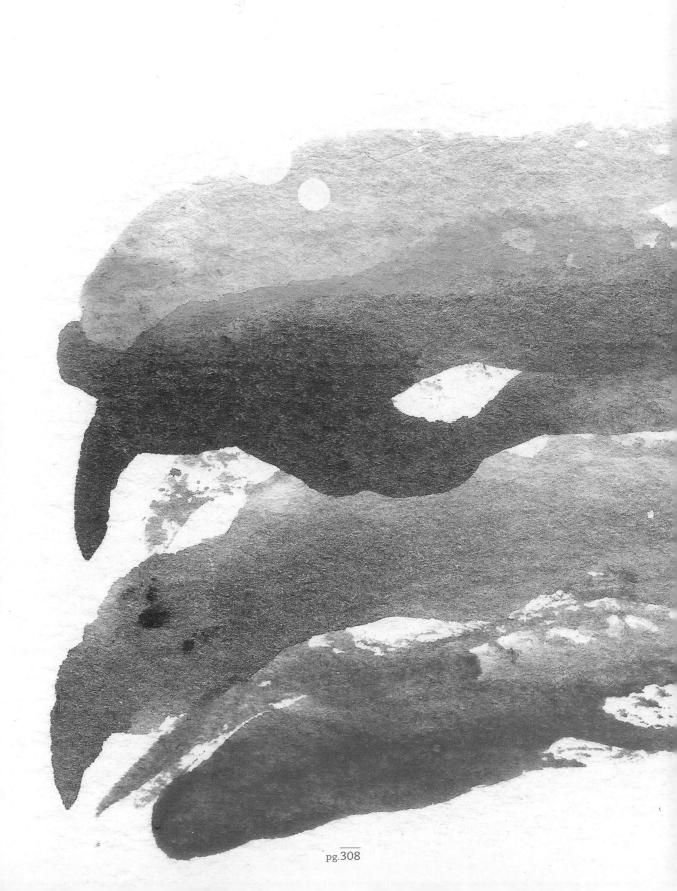

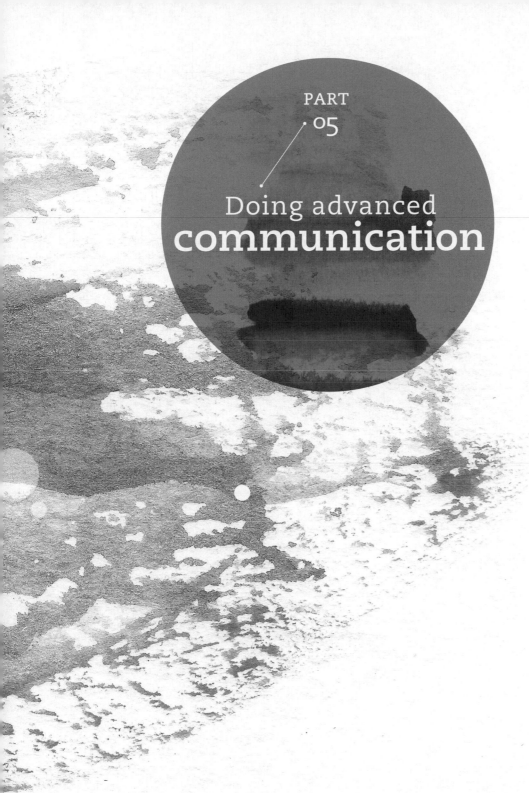

Doing advanced
communication

CHAPTER
31 / Thesis writing

Joy **HIGGS** | Annette **STREET**

key topics

This chapter covers the following topics:

• what is a thesis?

• what makes a good thesis?

• how to craft and structure a thesis

key terms

THESES

PARADIGM

STRUCTURE

Introduction

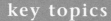

/ **THESES** /
The term thesis refers to the argument presented in the report.

Theses, or dissertations, are major written works that require a special approach to scholarly writing, considering such factors as context, genre, audience and research **paradigm**. They commonly take the form of research reports, but they may be extensive literature reviews or a collection of the author's published research papers. This (last) type of thesis is becoming increasingly widespread and comprises a cohesive series of papers that is accompanied and framed by an analytical commentary. See Chapter 32 for further information on writing papers.

What makes a good thesis?

The term *thesis* refers to the argument presented in the report. A well-written thesis is an argument that is articulated clearly, based on appropriate, well-conducted research that is substantiated by the data collected, and derived logically from a sound process of data analysis and knowledge generation. The thesis should have a **structure**, style and quality appropriate to your university, discipline and level of study. At undergraduate honours level, the purpose of the program is generally for students to learn about well-conducted research and to develop skills in writing a thesis. At masters level, a greater degree of independence is expected of students. At doctoral level, students are expected to contribute to the knowledge in their field, to conduct a substantial review of the relevant literature, and demonstrate sound understanding and use of the relevant research methods. Some students enrol in practice-orientated professional doctorate programs, comprising coursework and research. Expectations of the length of a thesis vary. See Table 31.1 for a guide.

/ STRUCTURE /
The thesis structure is how the sections are organised to make the argument clear and credible.

TABLE 31.1 | LENGTH OF THESES: GUIDELINES ONLY

LEVEL	WORDS (MINIMUM/MAXIMUM)
Undergraduate honours	12,000–15,000, or publishable paper
Research masters	40,000–60,000
Professional doctorate	40,000–60,000
PhD	50,000–100,000

A key feature that examiners look for in every thesis is congruence: do the research questions match the research **paradigm**, discipline genre and expectations, research methods, style of writing, and format and product of the thesis? For example, an experimental study in a department of physiology would be conducted in a different style from an ethnographic study in a school of occupational therapy or an action research project in a school of nursing. Table 31.2 briefly summarises different research paradigms, or frameworks for research. Refer to the 'Further reading' section at the end of this chapter for more information on research paradigms and approaches.

You may find it helpful to read some of the high-quality theses produced by past students in your department. Look at the style, the norms and expectations, the length and the format. Find out from your supervisor if there are any particular rules you must follow, regarding, for example, the use of 'I' or an impersonal style in writing, the type of referencing, headings, length, format and layout.

/ PARADIGMS /
Paradigms are frameworks for research.

An important part of reading is understanding the research genre, and then writing in a way that is consistent with that genre (see Table 31.2). Read relevant books and articles about research methodology to learn how best to conduct your research and to justify your research strategy in your written thesis. See the 'Further reading' section at the end of this chapter for more information on research design and methodology.

TABLE 31.2 | RESEARCH PARADIGMS (BASED ON HIGGS, 2001)

RESEARCH PARADIGM	KEY RESEARCH GOALS	RESEARCH APPROACH(ES) (EXAMPLES)	RESEARCH METHODS: DATA COLLECTION	RESEARCH METHODS: DATA ANALYSIS
Empirico-analytical paradigm	Test hypotheses Identify cause–effect relationships	Experimental method Randomised controlled trials	Controlled trials Interviews Questionnaires	Statistical analysis
Interpretive paradigm	Understand Interpret Seek meaning	Phenomenology Narrative inquiry Arts-based inquiry	Interviews Case studies Storytelling	Repeated return to data Extraction of themes Theorisation
Critical paradigm	Improve Empower Change reality or situation	Action research Collaborative research Feminist research	Interviews Case studies Critical debate	Reflection upon data collected Action and outcomes Review by stakeholders

How to structure a thesis

Structuring a thesis is like writing a non-fiction narrative: the argument is built over an extended work involving several (typically between five and ten) chapters. Unlike a story, however, you are not seeking to create suspense. Instead, you are presenting a clear, credible argument that is substantiated by sound evidence and data analysis procedures. Structure your thesis so that your argument flows and the sections are presented in a credible manner. In the first chapter, you should inform your reader of what is covered in the other chapters. Your thesis is likely to be read in parts because it is a long document; so, at the beginning of each chapter, you should outline briefly the purpose the chapter, and explain how it builds on previous chapters. You may also need to provide cross-references to other parts of the thesis.

Crafting the argument takes a considerable amount of work. You need to examine the literature and create a discussion that is structured in readable sections, while building up the argument in a coherent manner. Link the points within your sentences, paragraphs and chapters clearly so that the argument within and between the chapters flows logically. If there are data, information, explanations and definitions that the reader needs in order to understand your argument, include them in the text where necessary. Information that is not necessary for the argument (such as ethics documents and extensive data sets) is best placed in appendices, with reference made to them in the main body of the thesis, so that the flow of your argument is not disrupted. Similarly, do not use a lot of lists in the text. They break up the flow, and make the reader search for the point you are trying to make.

When structuring the thesis and building your argument, think of your writing as a structured set of sections that follow each other in a meaningful sequence, and an extended argument organised under these headings. In writing a thesis you need to:

- introduce the purpose, significance and context of your research
- list your research questions and describe and justify your research method so that readers can judge its appropriateness and whether it justifies your findings
- describe, analyse and critique your findings
- draw your findings together into a conclusion, summary, model or set of themes that answer your research question and relate your findings to the knowledge of the field.

Table 31.3 illustrates a typical thesis structure, and some alternative headings that might be more applicable to qualitative research studies.

TABLE 31.3 | THESIS STRUCTURE

TYPICAL THESIS HEADINGS	ALTERNATIVE HEADINGS FOR SOME QUALITATIVE RESEARCH STUDIES
Front pages[1]	Front pages[1]
Abstract	Abstract
Introduction	Introduction
Literature review	Theoretical framework
Research methods[2]	Research strategy[3]
Study 1	Research findings and discussion 1 (e.g. the participants' stories)
Study 2 (etc.)[4]	Research findings and discussion 2 (e.g. a model or theory)

< cont. >

< *cont.* >

TYPICAL THESIS HEADINGS	ALTERNATIVE HEADINGS FOR SOME QUALITATIVE RESEARCH STUDIES
Results Discussion	This is covered under findings and discussion
Conclusion	Conclusion
References	References
Appendices	Appendices

[1] Includes title page, statement of authorship (generally), acknowledgments (optional), abstract, list of figures, list of tables, glossary (optional), table of contents, including list of appendices.

[2] Includes aims of the studies, ethics procedures, research design. This information may be incorporated into the individual studies chapters.

[3] Includes, aims, research framework, methods for data collection and analysis, ethics procedures.

[4] Postgraduate theses may include several studies that are commonly reported in full, in sequence.

Matching the research and writing style to the audience, genre and paradigm

You should match your writing style to the context of the work, field of study, discipline (such as physiology, nursing or medicine) and intended audience. Your thesis must first pass the scrutiny of your *examiners*. They will judge your work, including the credibility of your research and the scholarship of your writing. Next, there are countless others (e.g. students and researchers) who may read your thesis or publications arising from it. Consider the needs of this potential audience and how best to communicate to them.

As well, consider which writing and organisation style or genre is typical or expected of the research paradigm you have chosen. For example, experimental research is commonly written in the third person, with the actions of the researcher reported in the passive voice, and using the headings shown in the first column of Table 31.3. Qualitative research takes many forms. In some situations, a particular style of writing is expected from researchers. For instance, the writing of phenomenologists usually demonstrates 'thick description' (evocative and rich descriptions of the human experiences). In all research styles, writing should be scholarly.

TABLE 31.4 | LAYOUT AND PRESENTATION OF THESES (GUIDELINES)

Layout: paragraphs	1.5 spacing of lines (may need to be double-spaced)
	Left justification or double justification
	Leave one blank line between paragraphs

< *cont.* >

< cont. >

Layout: pages	Clear, scholarly presentation
	A4 page size
	One side of paper
	2.5 cm margins, except left margin, 3 cm for binding
	Avoid *widows* and *orphans* (a few lines of text at top or bottom of page)
Binding and paper	Often use soft ('perfect') binding for examination copy
	Use hard (cloth) binding for final copy
	Use acid-free paper for final copy
	Use locally required lettering for thesis spine
Tables and figures	Numbered as per chapter, e.g. Table 3.1, Figure 3.1
Appendices	Tables and figures smaller than half a page may be on a page with text
	Place larger tables or figures on a separate page
	Include clear, meaningful titles for tables, figures, appendices
	All figures and tables must be mentioned in the text
Footnotes	Use sparingly, e.g. for definition of jargon terms or abbreviations

Technical aspects of theses

Refer to Chapter 6 to refresh yourself as to what is expected of your academic writing in terms of grammar, language, presentation and style. Remember that you need to impress your examiners with your research, but the quality of the research can be tarnished by poor technical presentation and writing. Spelling mistakes, poor grammar (especially incomplete sentences), inconsistencies, poor layout or positioning of tables and graphics, and other technical errors are not acceptable. Referencing must be meticulous.

In light of the importance of these technical aspects of presentation, it is helpful to be aware that theses generally have layout requirements (see Tables 31.4 and 31.5 for guidelines). Check your local rules. See Chapter 14 for advice on tables and graphics.

TABLE 31.5 | PROPOSED HEADING STYLES FOR THESIS

LEVEL	FORMAT	FONT	SPACING
HEADING 1	CHAPTER ONE or INTRODUCTION	Capitals, bold, large, for example, 18 point	Centred, space above and below
HEADING 2	1.1 SECTION ONE	Capitals, bold	LHS*, space above
HEADING 3	1.1.1 Sub-Section One	Title case, bold	LHS*
HEADING 4	A Subheading	Sentence case, bold	LHS*
HEADING 5	1 Subheading next	Sentence case, italics	LHS*

* LHS = Left-hand side justified.

The writing task

The task of writing (along with doing your research) includes four phases: preparation, writing, reflection and critique, and proofing and printing.

Preparation involves:

- keeping track of the literature and references you collect
- choosing a referencing system (see Chapter 9)
- developing a style sheet and a 'custom dictionary'. These may be electronically linked to your chapter files
- organising access to good computer hardware and software.

In the *writing phase*:

- plan your argument and develop a plan for writing
- organise your literature and data into a sequence for writing
- create one file per chapter (avoid large files, because you can lose a lot of work and time if a file becomes corrupted)
- back up electronic files regularly, and store back-up copies in more than one place for safety.

Strategies you can use to help with your writing (particularly with a large and complex document like a thesis) include:

- brainstorm (collect all your ideas on the topic)
- develop a flowchart or concept map to organise your thoughts
- create a draft table of contents and write under these headings
- write down your broad ideas on the topic and progressively refine them, to develop an argument, and then structure the information to support and present this argument
- write in 'bite-sized' sections
- just write!—do not worry if it is not good enough the first time. Once you start writing, you will have something to refine and polish later.

Writing the *literature review* poses some particular challenges. Burnard (1996, p. 101) offers these suggestions:

When you write up your research review, try to avoid the rather dull listing of everything you have read. The aim of a literature review is not only to identify what you have read, but for you to offer a critical review of what you have read … comment on the findings that you report. Offer a critique (of the research method) … Indicate in what ways [other] researchers' findings fit in with your study.

In the *reflection and critique phase*:

- put your writing aside for a while then look at it again with a fresh, critical mind
- read your work aloud so that you can see where it does not make sense, where more clarity is needed, and where you have made grammatical errors (such as incomplete sentences)
- ask someone else (a 'critical friend') to read your work and give you feedback
- check that your thesis is well argued, grounded in data and well referenced.

In the *proofing and printing phase*:

- proofread your work; spell-check it (but remember that the computer cannot tell you if you have confused words such as 'were' and 'where')
- format your work consistently
- decide which printer, computer and software you will use to print your final copy (different printers paginate differently, so if you plan your layout for one printer and then print on another, your page breaks might not coincide with those of the new printer)
- paginate your work, ensuring that figures and tables are placed appropriately and pages are numbered sequentially, checking that the page numbers of pages set out in 'landscape' format are positioned appropriately.
- check the printout during printing for layout and page numbering.

Making the most of your supervisor

Your supervisor has five key roles in relation to your research program. He or she:

- knows how the administrative system works, and can help with such tasks as enrolment, meeting the deadlines and requirements of the program, keeping on target with specific tasks, getting ethics approval, finding appropriate examiners and preparing your thesis for examination
- helps you get access to research infrastructure (e.g. resources, funding, scholarships and resource people)
- has knowledge in your topic area and/or knows people who can help you learn more about your topic
- knows how to do research, and is a guide and role model for you
- provides feedback on your work; on your research design and activities, your findings and how you are interpreting them, and your writing.

handy hint 31.1

WORKING WITH YOUR RESEARCH SUPERVISOR

- Remember your supervisor is there to help you; ask for help whenever you need it.
- Take an agenda or a list of questions to your meetings with your supervisor. It helps to be organised.
- Negotiate dates with your supervisor for handing in your writing and getting feedback about your work.
- Ask your supervisor for help or advice about accessing resources, funding and finding resource people. Your supervisor knows how the system works.

Where to from here?

Research can be rewarding and also challenging. Spend some time thinking about your tasks and the people who can help you. Train yourself to balance learning about research (such as reading and attending training sessions) with getting on with it. As you approach your submission deadline, you want to complete your work in a timely fashion, rather than be overloaded with tasks such as writing-up or data processing. Writing a thesis is a major task in itself, alongside and as part of your research. It needs planning, structuring and rigour, as well as style.

references

Burnard, P. (1996). *Writing for health professionals: A manual for writers* (2nd edn). London: Chapman & Hall.

Higgs, J. (2001). Charting standpoints in qualitative research. In H. Byrne-Armstrong, J. Higgs & D. Horsfall (Eds.), *Critical moments in qualitative research* (pp. 44–67). Oxford: Butterworth-Heinemann.

further reading

Allison, B. (2004). *The student's guide to preparing dissertations and theses* (2nd edn). London: RoutledgeFalmer.

Becker, H. S., & Richards, P. (2007). *Writing for social scientists: How to start and finish your thesis, book or article* (2nd edn). Chicago: The University of Chicago Press.

Davies, M. B. (2007). *Doing a successful research project: Using qualitative or quantitative methods*. New York: Palgrave Macmillan.

Denzin, N. K., & Lincoln, Y. S. (Eds.) (2011). *Handbook of qualitative research* (4th edn). Thousand Oaks, CA: Sage.

Glatthorn, A. A., & Joyner, R. L. (2005). *Writing the winning dissertation: A step-by-step guide* (2nd edn). Thousand Oaks, CA: Corwin Press.

Garson, G. D. (2002). *Guide to writing empirical papers, theses and dissertations*. New York: Marcel Dekker.

Hammell, K. W., Carpenter, C., & Dyck, I. (Eds.) (2000). *Using qualitative research: A practical introduction for occupational and physical therapists*. London: Churchill Livingstone.

Heppner, P. P., & Heppner, M. J. (2003). *Writing and publishing your thesis, dissertation and research: A guide for students in the helping professions*. Minnesota: Brooks Cole.

MacArthur, C. A., Graham, S., & Fitzgerald, J. (Eds.) (2006). *Handbook of writing research*. New York: The Guildford Press.

Mauch, J. E. (2003). *Guide to the successful thesis and dissertation: A handbook for students and faculty* (5th edn). New York: Dekker.

Minichiello, V., Sullivan, G., Greenwood, K., & Axford, R. (Eds.) (2004). *Handbook of research methods in health sciences* (2nd edn). Sydney: Addison-Wesley.

Palmer, W. (2012). *Discovering arguments: An introduction to critical thinking, writing, and style* (4th edn). Boston: Prentice Hall.

Polgar, S., & Thomas, S. A. (2007). *Introduction to research in the health sciences.* (5th edn). Edinburgh: Churchill Livingstone.

Terryberry, K. J. (2004). *Writing for the health professions (Applied English).* Clifton Park, NY: Delmar Cengage Learning.

Thomas, R. M. (2003). *Blending qualitative and quantitative research methods in theses and dissertations.* Thousand Oaks, CA: Corwin Press.

Thomas, S. (2000). *How to write health science papers, dissertations and theses.* New York: Churchill Livingstone.

Thomas, R. M., & Brubaker, D. L. (2007). *Theses and dissertations: A guide to planning, research and writing.* Westport, CT: Bergin & Garvey.

Turabian, K. L., Booth, W. C., Colomb, G. G., & Williams, J. M. (2007). *A manual for writers of research papers, theses, and dissertations* (7th edn). Chicago: The University of Chicago Press.

White, B. (2011). *Mapping your thesis: The comprehensive manual of theory and techniques for master and doctoral research.* Camberwell, VIC: ACER Press.

Writing papers for journals

Annette STREET | Joy HIGGS

key topics

This chapter covers the following topics:

- choosing the right journal
- writing a plan
- designing the paper

key terms

HIGH-IMPACT JOURNALS

PEER-REVIEWED JOURNAL

WRITING PLAN

LITERATURE REVIEW

Introduction

A journal article is the most common form of international communication about scholarly work in the health sciences. Articles take a variety of forms and cover a range of interests, from editorials, opinion pieces, research papers, debates and systematic reviews to papers describing health and practice innovations. Journals are targeted to selected audiences and have specific presentation conventions. Choosing the right journal and preparing your article to be acceptable to that journal are important skills. You will usually have a supervisor, mentor or other member of staff who can offer advice (and who may be a co-author).

Choosing the right journal

It is a waste of time to write an article and *then* try to find a journal that will accept it. As soon as you have a draft of your ideas, begin to search for the right journal. Ask yourself the following questions: What is the purpose of this paper? What type of message or research am I writing about? Who is my audience? There needs to be a clear match between the audience of the journal and your paper (Wachs, Williamson, Moore, Roy, & Childre, 2010). If your topic is specific to a select audience, compile a list of journals that publish in that area. A paper entitled 'Sharing responsibility in home birth' would fit in midwifery, health sociology or women's health journals.

Once you have considered the potential audience for your article and matched it to a list of possible journals, do your homework on the journals. **High-impact journals** are those whose articles tend to receive many citations, indicating that they have a wide and prestigious readership. They enable your article to reach a larger audience and have your work cited, which will gain you credit in research performance indicator systems. Check measurable features such as 'impact factor' and citations indexes on journal home pages, or online in university library databases such as Web of Science. However, you need to balance your goal of reaching a particular audience with these measures; sometimes the best journal for your audience may not be a high-impact journal.

If the editor of a **peer-reviewed journal** considers your article fits with the journal's aims and is of sufficient quality it will be sent to peer review. The review process ensures that every published article has been critiqued by experts before it is published. Read carefully the information to contributors provided by the journal (usually inside the cover or on the journal's website). Also read the tables of contents of some past issues to find out what has been published recently. If you are not sure whether the journal will be interested in your topic or method, you can email the editor to ask if a submission on your topic or method would be considered. Doing homework in advance can save you a great deal of time preparing and formatting the paper for a journal and waiting, possibly for many months, to receive advice that the paper does not suit the journal.

/ **HIGH-IMPACT JOURNALS** /

High-impact journals are those whose articles tend to receive many citations, indicating that they have a wide and prestigious readership.

/ **PEER-REVIEWED JOURNAL** /

If the editor of a peer-reviewed journal considers your article fits with the journal's aims and is of sufficient quality, it will be sent to peer review. The review process ensures that every published article has been critiqued by experts before it is published.

CHOOSING A JOURNAL

- Does my paper fit the journal's aims and scope?
- What types of articles are published in this journal?
- Who is the main journal audience?
- Is the journal published internationally?
- What is the status and impact factor of the journal?
- How long are the articles in the journal?
- What referencing style does this journal use?

It is also helpful to look at the style of writing that is accepted by the proposed journal. Some journals provide clear instructions on how to write different kinds of papers (e.g. *Journal of Advanced Nursing*). Find out whether your preferred style of writing (such as first person or a narrative style) is accepted, or whether more technical or scientific language is required. If your paper is a **literature review**, make sure the selected journal accepts literature reviews for publication. Look to see if a journal predominantly publishes research papers, and whether they include qualitative or quantitative research, or both. Remember that different research approaches are written up quite differently (e.g. see Peat, Elliott, Baur, & Keenan, 2002).

Take into account whether the journal's articles have a separate introduction, background and literature review, or whether these sections are combined or not required. See if the journal allows you enough words for the style of research or paper you want to write. Look at the number of words generally allocated to each section, to guide the structure of your paper. Never include unnecessary tables, figures or inserts; reviewers will reject them (McConnell, 2004).

/ **LITERATURE REVIEW** /
The literature review needs to provide sufficient background to locate your work in its context.

Writing plan

Once you have chosen your journal it is a good idea to start with a **writing plan** (Perneger & Hudelson, 2004). Collect a couple of articles structured like the one you are planning to write (not necessarily on the same topic) to use as models for your own paper. Are you gathering material to synthesise for a literature review or conceptual paper? If you have conducted a research project, then you need to find a paper that matches the style of research that you have done (see Peat et al., 2002). Plan the sequence of sections and determine how detailed or how long each needs to be. The plan should reflect the interests of the journal, whether it be a science, social science and humanities or education journal. Handy Hint 32.2 provides a sample plan for an article of 3000 words.

/ **WRITING PLAN** /
A writing plan should reflect the interests of the journal, whether it be a science, social science and humanities or education journal.

Writing with colleagues

It is a common practice in the health sciences to write with one's colleagues, particularly when writing up collaborative research or a joint theoretical paper. Collaborative writing has the potential to produce a richer paper, on the principle that two or more heads are better than one. It does, however, add to the preparation time, as it requires ongoing negotiation to work well. If you are planning a joint paper, you need to be clear at the outset about what contribution each person will make to the paper. One person might contribute expertise in the methods; another might have specific professional knowledge. Some journals ask for a percentage weighting for the contribution of each person when you submit a joint paper. This requirement is also frequently used in university reporting of publications to national funding bodies. You must be clear about authorship. Decide who will be first-listed, who the subsequent authors will be, and who will take responsibility for ensuring that the paper meets the standards of the target journal and for submitting the final agreed version. This latter person will usually be the contact person, whose institutional address appears with the paper and who will deal with correspondence with the journal editor. Deciding on these matters at the start often saves hassles later on.

SAMPLE WRITING PLAN

Deciding on authorship

See section 5 on Authorship in the *Australian code for the responsible conduct of research*, http://www.nhmrc.gov.au/_files_nhmrc/publications/attachments/r39.pdf

Journal paper

- Total words allowed: 3000
- Title (no more than 10 words)
- Abstract (no more than 200 words)
- Keywords (up to 5)
- Reference style: Vancouver

Body of paper

- *Introduction* **(about 500 words): includes rationale**, study aims and key literature; justifies the need for and explains the scope of the paper
- *Method* **(about 500 words): includes sample/participants**, data-collection methods, data-analysis strategies and ethics
- *Results and findings* **(750 words**, and up to four tables or figures): answers the research question or provides the evidence supporting your argument
- *Discussion* **(800–900 words): analyses the findings in relation to the topic and the supporting literature**
- *Conclusion, limitations, recommendations:* reiterates new knowledge, outlines limitations of the paper, and makes recommendations for further action ◗

Designing the paper

When you choose a title, make sure that it contains relevant keywords so that others will be able to find your article quickly in searches (Hays, 2010). Creative, eye-catching titles need a subtitle that clarifies the topic and method. Sometimes a well-crafted abstract will be the guide for the paper, but always return to it at the end of writing the paper to ensure that it reflects the content and logic of the final draft. When *keywords* are requested, it is important to choose words that fit with the choices in major search engines. You can find these in online databases such as Medline, CINAHL and Sociofile.

When you begin to plan the body of the paper, remember that journals are interested in new information. Do not try to write everything you know. Organise your material to focus on the knowledge you are adding to what is known, rather than trying to cover everything that can be said on the topic. Select and order your material to develop a strong argument. It is often helpful to develop a framework or outline to indicate the logic of your argument and the flow of the paper (Driscoll & Aquilina, 2011).

Keep accurate records of sources as you write. Decide which sources you will quote from directly and which ideas you will paraphrase; both types of inclusion in the text need to be referenced. Limit the use of direct quotations, and summarise key conclusions that you want to support or refute. Remember it is *your* work you are presenting; do not just regurgitate other people's work. Make sure you understand exactly what constitutes plagiarism, and avoid deliberately or accidentally plagiarising the work of others. Set up your referencing system. See Chapters 9 and 17 for more information about plagiarism and referencing. It is usually considered good scholarship to acknowledge the first author(s) who generated a new idea or conclusion. Otherwise, use up-to-date references unless you have a good reason for citing earlier work. Explain why you are drawing on earlier work. Choose the information (such as quotes, tables and graphics) to include to support your argument or explain your findings, and consider the best format for presentation.

Then write a draft of the whole paper. Make sure that you discuss its scope and limitations, so that readers know what to expect as they read it. Remember to review critically, not just retell the literature.

Good writing is clear, and logical and concise. Do not use technical jargon unnecessarily. Always introduce and define complex or technical language that would not be familiar to your readers. This will depend on whether you have chosen a specialist journal or a more general one. You may be able to use commonly accepted acronyms (such as 'WHO' for the World Health Organization—check the journal style). Write out other acronyms in full the first time they appear, with the acronym in brackets. When defining jargon terms or spelling out acronyms, it is normally best to do it in the text. Occasionally, an expanded explanation is required that would break up the flow of the text. You may use footnotes if they are accepted by the journal. Many journals will not accept footnotes for such added material, but will allow a limited number of endnotes (notes at the end of the paper). Check journal policy.

A useful strategy to determine whether your argument makes sense is to write a summary sentence for each paragraph and read these sentences in sequence. In this way you can make sure that your paper has a logical flow that matches (or even improves on) your initial writing plan. Check that you have emphasised what is new or special about the contribution your paper makes to the field. In other words, sell your 'take-home' message.

Editing and revising

Editing your work is always a challenge. It is easy to see the mistakes in the work of others but difficult to find them in your own. The tendency is to read what you think is there, rather than what actually *is* there. Reading your work aloud slowly often shows up grammar and logic errors. Reduce all long sentences. Check your spelling and grammar. Often, your computer will provide spelling and grammatical suggestions and alert you to errors. Be careful, though, to set the spell-checker to the language of the journal. English spelling differs between the United Kingdom, the United States and Australia, for example.

Ask friends or colleagues to read your paper and give you feedback. Ask them to highlight any confusing sentences and indicate where more explanation or linking is needed. Listen to what they say without becoming defensive. Revise your work so that it becomes clearer.

Preparation for submission

By now you should be satisfied with your paper, but there is still work to be done before it is ready to send to the journal (Dixon, 2001). Re-read the journal's information for contributors, including its guidelines for online submission. Check carefully that your paper meets all the criteria (length, form of presentation, style and number of copies) and that the references are presented in the required format. Make sure you have drafted your letter appropriately (or attached the required form), addressing the journal's requirements about ownership or copyright. If you have used figures or other material copyrighted by another person, you must write to the copyright holder for permission to use the material, and include the copyright holder's response in your submission. Increasingly, journals from the health sciences are asking for proof of ethical clearance for articles reporting research on human subjects or animals. (*Note:* It is essential to obtain this clearance from the relevant committee *before* undertaking research). Ensure that you have made the right number of copies of the manuscript to be submitted and that all your pages are properly linked if you are submitting the manuscript by email or online. This may mean that you have to scan copies of your letter and permissions to send with your paper.

CHECKLIST FOR JOURNAL SUBMISSIONS

- Carefully choose a journal.
- Write a plan.
- Develop an abstract or a summary.
- Write your draft paper.
- Edit and revise.
- Ask a colleague to read it.
- Revise again.
- Prepare your submission carefully.

Responding to reviewers

Responding to reviewers is another skill to learn (Algase, 2008). Peer-reviewed journals send submitted papers to at least two reviewers. This process is usually 'blind'; that is, the reviewers are not given identifying information about you, so that they judge the paper on its merits alone. You will also not know the identity of the reviewers. A good reviewer reads the paper with the intention of helping you to improve it. Try not to be defensive or upset that the reviewers have criticised your work. Some of the changes they suggest may be editorial and will enhance your paper. Others might relate to content; read these carefully and follow the advice given, unless the changes are inconsistent with your data or arguments.

You might discover that one reviewer likes one section of your paper but wants changes made to another section, whereas another reviewer wants changes made to the section reviewed favourably by the first reviewer. Sometimes reviewers can make inappropriate suggestions, such as asking why you did not also interview people with a similar condition to make comparisons, or advising that a different tool or method might be better. If this occurs, do not panic. Write a carefully worded letter to the editor, explaining why you have chosen not to address that issue, or insert a sentence in the paper that explains more clearly why your study was deliberately limited in a particular way. Editors recognise the vagaries of the review process and will understand if you give a well-justified reason for not adopting all the reviewers' suggestions.

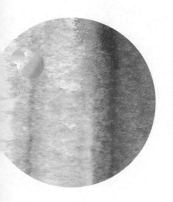

conclusion

Writing for publication can be difficult. It is challenging to get your ideas down on paper and to receive feedback on your work. Remember that your first paper may well be the hardest to write and have published, as you are learning many new skills in the process. Nevertheless, writing can be stimulating and rewarding, as you craft your ideas into a cohesive and well-substantiated argument and then see your name in print.

references

Algase, D. L. (2008). Responding to peer reviews: Pointers that authors don't learn in school. *Research and theory for nursing practice, 22*(4), 219–21.

Dixon, N. (2001). Writing for publication: A guide for new authors. *International Journal for Quality in Health Care, 13*(5), 417–21.

Driscoll, J., & Aquilina, R. (2011). Writing for publication: A practical six step approach. *International Journal of Orthopaedic and Trauma Nursing, 15*(1), 41–8.

Hays, J. C. (2010). Eight recommendations for writing titles of scientific manuscripts. *Public Health Nursing, 27*(2), 101–103.

McConnell, C. R. (2004). Getting your ideas into print: Writing for a professional journal. *The health care manager, 23*(4), 355–67.

Peat, J., Elliott, E., Baur, L., & Keenan, V. (2002). *Scientific writing: Easy when you know how*. Sydney: BMJ Books.

Perneger, T. V., & Hudelson, P. M. (2004). Writing a research article: Advice to beginners. *International Journal for Quality in Health Care, 16*(3), 191–92.

Wachs, J. E., Williamson, G., Moore, P. V., Roy, D., & Childre, F. (2010). It starts with an idea! *AAOHN journal: Official journal of the American Association of Occupational Health Nurses, 58*(5), 177–81.

further reading

Garrard, J. (2011). *Health sciences literature review made easy: The matrix method* (3rd edn). Sudbury, MA: Jones & Bartlett Learning.

Johnstone, M. (2004). *Effective writing for health professionals: A practical guide to getting published*. Crows Nest, NSW: Allen & Unwin.

Moos, D. D. (2011). Novice authors ... What you need to know to make writing for publication smooth. *Journal of Perianesthesia Nursing, 26*(5), 352–6.

Preparing posters

Tony **MCKENZIE** | Stephanie **SEDDON** | Iain **HAY** |
Ann **SEFTON**

key topics

This chapter covers the following topics:

- creating posters

- deciding on content

- presentation and layout

key terms

TEXT STYLE

MEDIA

DESIGN

Introduction

Posters are a useful way of presenting the results of research and other information to your peers and to scholarly and public audiences. You need a combination of graphic and written skills to ensure your posters achieve their potential and communicate with power and simplicity. Posters are an increasingly common and important form of communication at scientific and professional conferences (MacIntosh-Murray, 2007). At conferences, posters may be on display without the authors being present. Sometimes, however, the authors may be asked to attend poster sessions to answer questions and discuss the material (such as research) contained in the poster, or to give a short talk (perhaps 5 minutes) on the research, to foster discussion.

Creating posters

/ DESIGN /

Design is the way the work is planned and presented, often based on key goals, principles or disciplinary styles/genre.

The key to an effective poster is combining simplicity with good **design**. There must be a balance between the artistic and technical aspects of the poster, as this combination appeals to the way our brains process information; that is, both the logical and analytical left side of the brain and the creative and visually oriented right side of the brain (Ellerbee, 2006).

Traditionally, academic posters are presented on paper or card, but 'electronic posters' are also becoming common, as poster presenters and conference organisers increasingly recognise the communicative capabilities of electronic media.

/ MEDIA /

In communication, media refers to either the physical or digital/electronic means of conveying information/messages.

One of the early decisions you should make is what **media** you will use. Check with the organisers of the event whether paper or electronic posters are options. Some of the factors to consider when choosing your presentation media are listed in Table 33.1. Also check the conference poster guidelines for any limitations on the size of the poster and any other requirements.

TABLE 33.1 | SOME CONSIDERATIONS WHEN CHOOSING YOUR PRESENTATION MEDIA

PAPER-MEDIATED POSTER	ELECTRONIC POSTER
Choose between a single large sheet or multiple smaller sheets that are easier to transport and can be laid out edge-to-edge at the venue	May comprise a single slide but more commonly a multi-slide presentation
Easy to mount	Power and equipment needed
Less affected by ambient light	Can be affected by ambient light (LCD monitors are hard to read in certain light conditions)
Can be left unattended	Consider security of equipment
Relies on your poster composition skills for its effectiveness	Relies on your projected presentation or web design skills for its effectiveness
Appeals to visitors accustomed to poster presentations	Appeals to visitors accustomed to dynamic content
Consider providing a complementary handout	Consider incorporating live internet feeds if web access is available

If you are to be present at a scheduled poster session, how will you and your poster interact with visitors and vice versa? You need to think about this when choosing the media for your poster. If you are thinking of creating an electronic poster, we suggest you also read Chapter 13, *Projected presentations*. In the present chapter we largely focus on paper-based posters.

All communicators stand to gain something from understanding and considering the strengths and limitations of their chosen medium of communication. As the creator of an academic poster, you would do well to consider some of the ground rules of graphic design. We will highlight some of the relevant principles in the poster-creation process.

Deciding on content

Your poster needs to present a clear message, regardless of the complexity of the project or work it presents. Whether you are collaborating with others or creating a poster by yourself, there is value at the outset in seeking out your elegant, simple, take-home message. Spend some time considering how that message can be best conveyed in terms of suitability for the audience or conference; for example, making the poster memorable. Can you capture the key in the poster title, a prominent quotation, or a vivid image and caption?

THE KEY MESSAGE

The more effectively you can identify the significance of your project, the more elegant and striking your poster can be. There are two prized capabilities here:

- the ability to reach a simple distillation of your argument
- the ability to convey this powerfully to your audience through striking language and presentation.

The information you are presenting must be accurate and informative. Aim to deliver the essential ideas and data in a way that informs and engages your audience. Keep the text concise and minimise visual clutter, to help focus and hold viewers' attention. There is no need to give all the details of the project or topic your poster is reporting on; people who are especially interested in the topic can contact you or consult some of the literature in the reference list. You might like to consider producing a handout to accompany your poster so that people can read it later and contact you with further enquiries. This could be an A4 version of your poster with additional details and technical information.

Text

Consider the appropriate **text style** for your poster text. Your poster's text should follow the conventions of academic writing in your field. Certain devices such

/ TEXT STYLE /
Text style includes the general genre (e.g. casual, scholarly) as well as the choice of font (typeface, e.g. Arial; and size, e.g. 10 pt).

as bullet lists are effective in condensing and visually arranging related ideas in a concise way. Matthews (1990) gives some helpful guidance for condensing research text, then grouping and displaying this condensed information in ways that facilitate reading and comprehension. The text for an academic research poster is typically set out in clear sections. The *IMRAD* structure (introduction, method, results and discussion) commonly used in research papers is also used for posters, and may be required at some conferences. A professional research poster would typically include six sections.

1. The *title* (and any *subheadings*) must be succinct. The title is probably the most important single element of a poster, because it influences people's decision whether to examine the rest of the poster, so think about it carefully. It also helps if the title is memorable and effectively summarises the subject, so that your poster will attract the right audience. Immediately beneath the title, present your name and your professional affiliation (or your class, group or university) and, if appropriate, your contact details (such as an email address).

2. An *abstract* is a short, written statement summarising the key points of the poster. This usually appears immediately after the title and your name. Not all posters need an abstract, but it is usually expected of posters presented at professional conferences.

3. An *introduction* gives the context and background for the work and makes a clear statement about the aims of the project. Explain what is already known about the topic (referring to the work of others) and how your work contributes to the field. If your work has experimental hypotheses, state them in this section.

4. The poster then includes several key sections in which the topic or report is presented. It could include the following sections if the poster is reporting on research:

   • A *materials and methods* section explains the research techniques you used.

   • The *results* are a key part of the poster. Readers want to see compelling evidence in this section if they are to believe your conclusions. Set out the primary data on which your conclusions are based.

   • A *discussion* section tells readers how you interpreted the data. It also refers back to information from the introduction to remind readers about the data's disciplinary and social significance, and it may set out your plans for future work in the area.

5. A final section, such as a *conclusion*, *summary* or *reflection*, sums up the main messages in the poster.

6. *References* to all work cited in the poster should also be set out, usually in the lower right-hand corner.

Graphics

Images are another important part of a good poster. The images you use might include a variety of graphics, such as diagrams, cartoons, bar charts, pie diagrams, graphs, flow charts and photographs. Photographs could be used, for example, to compare a healthy mole with a melanoma, and an accompanying diagram could depict some of the abnormal cell growth associated with a melanoma. Figure 33.1 shows an example of a poster.

FIGURE 33.1 | POSTER EXAMPLE

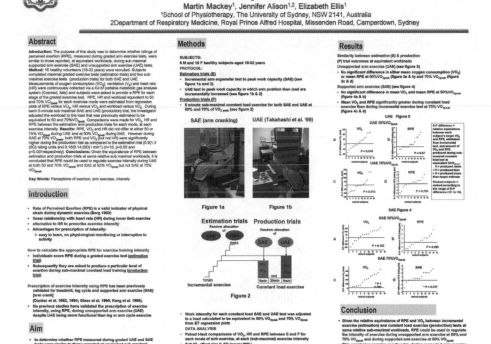

Source: M. Mackey (reproduced with permission)

If you use photographs in your poster, ensure that they are in focus, have sharp contrast, and are sufficiently large to be interpreted from at least 1.5 metres. A caption should make the photograph's subject clear and, if relevant, should indicate such elements as the degree of magnification used. Any images you use in a poster should be of high quality and must be relevant. Do not make the mistake of littering your poster with unnecessary and poor quality graphs and photographs. Make sure you obtain permission to use the photograph (from the subject and/or the photographer).

Presentation and layout

Good layout is vital to effective graphic communication. Posters need not be set up in a linear form, with readers moving from top left to bottom right. Various alternatives exist, including cyclical diagrams and spider diagrams. A couple of examples are shown in Figure 33.2. Just as you should prepare an essay plan before writing it, it is a good idea to produce sketch diagrams or mock-ups of your poster before you begin. Experiment with different layouts, and discuss them with friends and tutors; but whatever design you choose, it is essential that the reader has a clear sense of direction through the poster. Numbers, arrows or headings that reflect well-known procedural sequences (such as Introduction, methods and results) may be helpful. Keep each section consistent in style.

FIGURE 33.2 | TWO FORMS OF POSTER LAYOUT

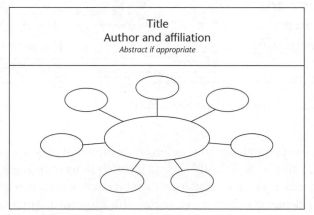

Source: Adapted from Hay and Thomas (1999)

A poster layout can be analysed in terms of three fundamental elements of graphic design: text, graphics and *white space*. Text includes both headings and body text (the main discourse). Graphic elements comprise images (as described previously) and also lines and borders. *White space* is the term used for open space, whether the poster background is white or coloured.

These same three elements can be considered as essential ingredients in the design process. Therefore, as your starting point, consider adopting the goal of *an attractive and meaningful arrangement of all three* in your design.

WHITE SPACE

Consider the importance of including adequate white space in your design. Here is a short exercise. First, visit and absorb the design of these posters on the web: http://www.cs.colostate.edu/~anderson/res/rl/rlTurbinePoster2010.pdf and http://www.waspacegrant.org/for_students/student_internships/wsgc_internships/img/Translife.jpg.

Consider the space allocated in these posters respectively to text, to graphics and white space. As contrast, consider these posters: http://erl.wustl.edu/documents/posters/spie-2007-mi.pdf and http://erl.wustl.edu/documents/posters/mcim2007-pids.pdf.

Did you notice the different spatial ratios between text, graphics and white space in these posters? Which of these posters do you find more inviting? How important is white space to the overall design of the poster? (If you can't view these examples simply imagine two posters—one with generous white space, the other with minimal margins and space surrounding text and graphics.)

We have already referred to the challenge of achieving a dynamic, simple, take-home message. Simplicity and elegance are qualities that are achieved in part by choosing not to include too much detail in your poster. Sometimes this is difficult, because the poster will also be judged by the scholarly rigour of its content. If your poster is going to give an account of a complex research project, ask yourself: what is sufficient information and what is too little? Resolving *this* question is a key to good academic poster design.

Headings and fonts

Headings and text should be large enough to read by someone standing at a distance of 1–1.5 metres from your poster. Generally, headings should be at least 36-point type or more, and text at least 14 points (see Table 33.2). Try printing out sample combinations of different fonts for headings, and test their effectiveness and impact. Basically, heading size should reflect the logic of your heading structure. For example, level 1 headings are first-order ideas; level 2 headings portray ideas that are nested within the parent level 1 headings, and so on. The size and impact of headings should visually suggest the hierarchical structure of the set. Bear in mind that body text should employ both upper- and lower-case letters (this is called 'sentence case'), *not* all capitals, WHICH ARE A LOT MORE DIFFICULT TO READ. (Sometimes all upper case is used in headings.)

Typeface is an important aspect of poster design, especially in relation to selection of particular fonts for headings. The body of the text needs to be clear and simple, and should be all in the same font, but extra graphic character and meaning can be added to the poster through the choice of a suitably evocative typeface. For example, Bookman Old Style might be appropriate for a poster considering historical aspects of a nation's healthcare conditions, and Comic Sans MS might add a 'zest for living' feel to a poster about children's exercise. With the smorgasbord of fonts available, however, please avoid the temptation go too far with complex or highly decorative fonts such as Old English Text MT and Vivaldi; they just make reading your poster hard work! Apart from typeface, you can also vary the appearance of your poster text by changing type weight, style and size, as shown in Table 33.2. See also Forsyth and Waller (1995) for a more detailed discussion of choice of fonts and use of typographical techniques to enhance visual literacy.

TABLE 33.2 | FONTS FOR POSTERS

ASPECT OF FONT	DESCRIPTION AND SUGGESTIONS
Typeface	The particular character of the letter forms. There are thousands of typefaces to choose from (such as Courier, *Balzano* and **Impact**)
Type weight	The thickness of the letter stroke (such as Regular and **Bold**)
Type style	This includes *Italic*, Condensed and Extended
Type size	Main headings: 96–180 point (27–48.5 mm)
	Secondary headings: 48–84 point (12.9–25.4 mm)
	Section headings: 24–36 point (5.9–8.7 mm)
	Text and captions: 14–18 point (3.2–4.6 mm)

Colour

Colour is a vital part of a poster, either adding to or detracting from the overall impact of the project. It can command attention, bring pleasure, and clarify a point. Use a small selection of colours to minimise confusion, and give some consideration to colour combinations. Ellerbee (2006) suggests using a colour wheel to help with colour combinations; for example, choosing colours adjacent to each other for a harmonious effect (e.g. blue–green) or colours that are directly opposite each other (complementary colours) to attract attention (e.g. yellow and violet). It is a good idea, however, to avoid using the complementary colours red and green together, as some people have trouble differentiating them. When choosing combinations of text and background colours, take care to ensure that the text contrasts with the background for easier reading. For example, black text on a white background is much easier to read than orange on yellow.

Colour, like typeface, can evoke an atmosphere suited to the theme of a poster. A poster on the physiological consequences of heart surgery might effectively employ the colour red to highlight the nature and intensity of the treatment method. Particular colours are often associated with specific cultures and nations, and they can be useful if you are discussing an issue that is specific to that group; for example, red, yellow and black are now often associated with the Indigenous populations of Australia.

conclusion

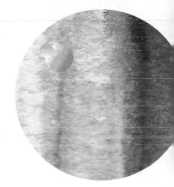

The academic, research or conference poster could be considered an art form. Your audience will expect you to demonstrate academic rigour in the project you are reporting on. For that reason you might assume that viewers will make allowances for 'content heaviness' at the expense of white space. But that should not dissuade you from considering the visual appeal of the poster. By including a handout in your communication strategy, you can take the pressure off the poster to tell the whole story by itself.

references

Ellerbee, S. M. (2006). Posters with an artistic flair. *Nurse Educator*, *31*(4), 166–9.

Forsyth, R., & Waller, A. (1995). Making your point: Principles of visual design for computer aided slide and poster production. *Archives of Disease in Childhood*, *72*, 80–84.

Hay, I., & Thomas, S. (1999). Making sense with posters in biological science education. *Journal of Biological Education*, *33*(4), 209–14.

MacIntosh-Murray, A. (2007). Poster presentations as a genre in knowledge communication: A case study of forms, norms and values. *Science Communication*, *28*(3), 347–76.

Matthews, D. L. (1990). The scientific poster: Guidelines for effective visual communication. *Technical Communication*, *3*, 225–32.

further reading

Block, S. M. (1996). Do's and don't's of poster presentation. *Biophysical Journal*, *71*, 3527–9.

Miller, J. E. (2007). Preparing and presenting effective research posters. *Health Services Research, 42*(1 Pt 1), 311–28. doi: 10.1111/j.1475-6773.2006.00588.x. Available http://www.ncbi.nlm.nih.gov/pmc/articles/PMC1955747/ These articles offer advice to researchers on what not to do when creating posters for professional conferences.

useful web resources

QUT Printing Services. *Develop great research posters using Microsoft PowerPoint®: A step-by-step guide*. Available at http://www.qps.qut.edu.au/pdf/students/ qps_createaposter.pdf. This step-by-step guide helps you to understand the purpose and aesthetics of a research poster and instructs you on how to develop your own research poster using Microsoft PowerPoint.

NASA, The basics of poster design: www.waspacegrant.org/for_students/student_ internships/wsgc_internships/posterdesign.html. This site uses an example poster to guide you through the design issues in poster design.

To learn poster creation with PowerPoint visit http://www.qps.qut.edu.au/pdf/ students/qps_createaposter.pdf

To learn poster creation via an example see www.waspacegrant.org/for_students/ student_internships/wsgc_internships/posterdesign.html

CHAPTER

34

Presenting talks at conferences

Rola **AJJAWI** | Annette **STREET** | Iain **HAY**

key topics

This chapter covers the following topics:

- reasons for speaking at a conference

- characteristics of an effective presentation

- strategies for preparation and presentation

- using visual aids

- managing questions

key terms

CONFERENCE

ABSTRACT

Introduction

Speaking at a **conference** is a vital way of summarising your work for others, positioning yourself in a particular field, and receiving collegial feedback. Although your education provides experience of speaking in class to fellow students (see Chapter 12), it is important to also be able to present your work effectively to professional peers and to respond confidently to their questions and comments.

/ CONFERENCE /
A conference or professional seminar is one of the best places to hear about cutting-edge advances in your field and to present your ideas.

Speaking at conferences

A conference or professional seminar is one of the best places to hear about cutting-edge advances in your field and to present your ideas. It can be daunting to stand up and talk about your work to an audience of strangers, but public speaking in various forms is part of the role of professionals. Educating others about our work and ideas is an essential component of our professional responsibility to develop our disciplines (see Schmoll, 2002). Likewise, keeping abreast in your field, networking with others, responding to questions and using feedback constructively are vital to professional development. These skills are valued highly in all the health professions and are best learned early.

Before you make a decision to attend and to present your work, find out as much as you can about the conference and the likely audience for your work. You may decide to prepare and present a poster (see Chapter 33) or present a paper. Many conferences encourage students to present their work; some even have a student prize. Some professional associations have student subgroups that conduct student conferences. If it is your first presentation, you should look out for a conference that has a student focus or encourages practitioners or novice researchers to present. You will find a more supportive environment, receive helpful feedback, meet others with similar interests, and establish networks with current and future leaders in your specialty.

Many conferences focus on a major theme, but they invariably have a variety of subthemes and/or discipline groups, to allow people with shared interests to network. Professional conferences and scientific meetings commonly feature keynote papers or symposia, as well as many short papers or posters reporting technical findings and practice advances, presented in concurrent sessions. Larger scientific meetings can have a huge number of papers, workshops, poster displays, showcases of technical equipment and discipline-specific meetings happening concurrently, and the audience at each of these sessions could be small. Some conferences have longer discursive papers, with more time allocated for discussion.

Your winning abstract

The selection of presentations for conferences commonly occurs via a competitive, peer-reviewed process. Once you have decided which conference you want to attend, the next task is to write a winning **abstract** so that you are given the opportunity to deliver an oral presentation or present a poster. This requires you to clarify the main arguments and/or research findings you will present, and the mode of delivery of your presentation. Read any requirements for abstracts carefully (including the deadline for abstract submission). Your abstract should be matched by an arresting presentation title that reflects the conference theme.

/ ABSTRACT /
An abstract is a short précis of all the key elements in your paper or poster.

You can be imaginative with your presentation titles, but you should not promise more than the actual presentation will deliver.

An abstract is a short précis of all the key elements in your paper or poster. Writing a good abstract is essential on three counts. First, the abstract can determine whether your paper is accepted for the conference. It can also influence whether you are asked to deliver a long paper, a short paper or a poster. Second, potential members of the audience may base their decision on whether to come to your presentation entirely on the impression conveyed by your abstract. Third, abstracts of accepted papers are often reproduced in a book of abstracts called conference proceedings that is published or distributed to colleagues interested in your work. Make sure that your abstract covers the main points of your message and that your talk can deliver what you promise. It is not usual to submit an abstract before results and conclusions are available. Only do so if the abstract is required well before the conference and you are confident that your analyses will be completed in time. Withdrawal of an abstract reflects poorly on the writer.

handy hint 34.1

GETTING STARTED PREPARING A TALK

- Do your homework on the conference.
- Develop a catchy title for your paper.
- Write a winning abstract, following guidelines closely.
- Research your target audience.
- Consider the amount of time you have been allocated and what you can achieve in that time.
- Examine the content of papers grouped with yours.
- Check out the **venue** and audiovisual arrangements.

Preliminary preparation

Your well-prepared abstract has been accepted for a conference. What happens next? The first rule is that you can never be too prepared. No matter how experienced you are, preparation is required for an excellent presentation (Tyler, Kossen, & Ryan, 2005). Start planning early. Decide on manageable steps, and begin work on one or more steps as soon as you receive confirmation from the conference organisers. Consider the factors listed below.

The target audience

Think carefully about the characteristics of your potential audience. What will these people want to know about your work? Estimate their level of knowledge, to help you target your paper. Unlike a classroom presentation, in which the audience probably shares your knowledge base, a conference brings people together with a wide variety of interests and levels of knowledge. You can deliberately narrow your audience by adding a subtitle, such as 'Implications for speech pathology', which should encourage specialists in your area of expertise to attend (and may discourage others).

The amount of time you have been allocated

Conferences have different lengths of time available for presentations. Find out if the time allocated to you allows for questions from the audience, or whether these are to be handled at the end of a series of papers. Managing time is a crucial skill. Audiences appreciate a well-timed presentation, especially if they want to move to attend another session after yours. It is also embarrassing and frustrating if you have to be stopped talking before you have concluded, or if people stand up and leave the room before you have finished.

The content of papers grouped with yours

Conference organisers usually try to create themes in concurrent sessions, and group papers that address similar topics or use similar methods. Before you finalise your paper, examine the conference program and read the abstracts of other papers in your session. Consider if papers grouped with yours can assist your selection of material to include, emphasise or ignore. A paper exploring women's experiences of breast cancer could be grouped with papers on body image or breast cancer treatments. The grouping may affect the audience for a series of papers in the session, and will alert you to their probable interests and expectations. Likewise, if papers preceding yours seem likely to deal with something replicated in your paper, you may choose not to emphasise that area in your discussion.

The venue and audiovisual arrangements

Conference facilities and audiovisual support vary. Conference organisers will either ask you to inform them of your needs or tell you the range of audiovisual equipment available in the room where you will be presenting. They may insist on a particular format for presentation (such as PowerPoint, on a memory stick). Sometimes organisers will send you a plan and information about the seating capacity of your allocated venue. This can help you to decide which audiovisual support you will use. You may also be asked to forward your presentation file in advance to the conference organisers to be uploaded.

Developing an effective presentation

You have an attention-grabbing title and an idea of the audience's characteristics. Now you must maintain their interest. Draw on the conference theme, and introduce your paper with a short narrative, arresting statistics, thought-provoking quotes, interesting visuals, or a cartoon. Do not attempt to tell a joke unless you have a real gift for humour that is regularly affirmed by others. However, *do* think about boring and irritating talks you have attended, and avoid duplicating poor practices (Smith, 2000; Gruhn, 2001). Some examples include: having too many slides with lots of information and a small font that is difficult to read, lack of eye contact with the audience, mumbling, fidgeting and reading from the notes.

Prepare for the ear and the eye

Different health and social science disciplines have different presentation styles at conferences. Health science presenters rarely read a paper. Usually, they talk from the points on slides or PowerPoint presentations. In contrast, a policy analyst presenting a critical history of aged-care reform may present a prepared paper. Whatever the tradition of your field, as a novice you would be wise to prepare speaking notes and practise aloud, preferably in front of an audience of friends or colleagues. Remember that oral presentations are not essays read aloud (Bly, 2003). Oral presentations are specially structured to present information in a way that anticipates and answers the questions in the minds of the audience. To do this, you need to ask yourself what your audience will want to know at various points during the talk, in order to maintain their interest and aid understanding. Use short sentences without complex jargon; do not assume that your audience is familiar with your technical language. Give brief explanations of terms that are to be used throughout the talk (Lunemann, 2001). Use visual aids to illustrate your points but do not overload them with text. It is recommended that you plan your talk first (including content and flow) before turning to PowerPoint or designing your visual aids (Harden, 2008). According to Harden, starting with PowerPoint can lead to focusing on the format rather than the content; planning your talk first enables you to use the visual aids appropriately to tell your story.

Some basic guidelines for structuring a presentation are shown in Table 34.1. Remember that you will need to tailor your talk to the time available. Note that while the guidelines in Table 34.1 seem to advocate repetition, you are not repeating the same words but rather highlighting the key message differently to introduce, detail and conclude your topic.

TABLE 34.1 | STRUCTURING A PRESENTATION

TASK	DESCRIPTION
Tell them what you are going to tell them	Introduce the topic
	State the aims or purpose
	Define the scope and limitations
	Provide an outline of the presentation and the availability of handouts
Tell them	Present the key content of your paper in three or four main points
	Use evidence from a variety of appropriate sources to defend each point
	Illustrate each point with examples
	Reiterate and restate the points and the links between them
Tell them what you told them	Summarise your presentation as a take-home message
	Provide direction for the audience on how to follow up or use your work

Introduction

Be clear about the goals of your talk at the outset. Let your audience know about the structure of your talk. Consider doing this with an opening visual that you discuss briefly. You should also define the scope of the presentation. For example, if you were using Figure 34.1 as your opening visual, you could alert the audience to the fact that although data are available on maternal satisfaction with Australian home births, because of your time constraints only data on health outcomes will be presented.

FIGURE 34.1 | EXAMPLE OF AN OUTLINE VISUAL

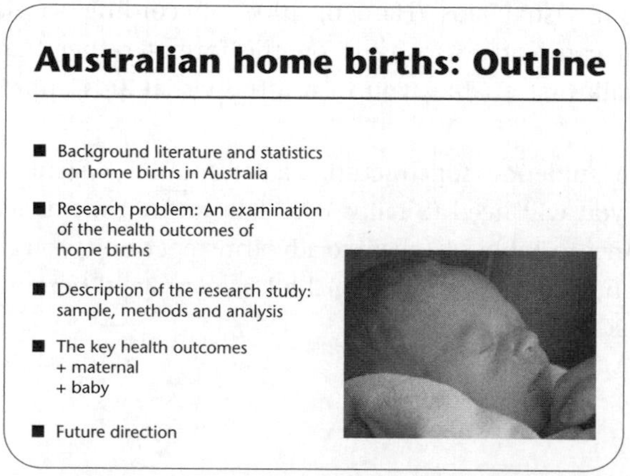

Australian home births: Outline

- Background literature and statistics on home births in Australia

- Research problem: An examination of the health outcomes of home births

- Description of the research study: sample, methods and analysis

- The key health outcomes
  + maternal
  + baby

- Future direction

Explain the choices you have made about the content you will cover, and direct the audience to other sources of information about your work. If you have handouts available, alert the audience to that at the start of your talk, so they can listen without needing to take notes.

Body of the talk

The body of the session should construct a convincing argument, supported by examples from your research or practice. Possibilities for practice-based papers vary across disciplines, from accounts of policy development, educational programs and resources and practice guidelines or protocols, to demonstrations of practice interventions and uses of specialist equipment. At intervals, remind your audience of what they have heard and tell them what is coming next; for example: 'I have just listed the physiological challenges identified by people in cardiac rehabilitation programs. Now I want to detail the use of different physical therapies by this group'. Presenters of poorly thought-out talks sometimes find themselves responding to interrupting questions about things they are planning to cover later or not at all.

The conclusion is the take-home message. It should not introduce anything new, but should reiterate what has been covered and offer the audience a way to move forward with further reading, following up on your research or taking action. The goal is to send your audience away with a clear message. Do not forget that yours is only one of many presentations that audience members will listen to in the day. You want it to be memorable for the right reasons.

Visual support

Choosing the right form of visual support is essential. In Table 34.2 we have adapted a list of different forms of visual support from Bly (2003) for you to consider. Make sure you are confident in your choice of visual support. If you are told that you must use PowerPoint and you are not familiar with it, then learn it, and practise using it before the conference. Harden (2008, p. 833) cautions against an 'unending stream of slides with bullet lists, animations that obscure rather than clarify the point and cartoons that distract rather than convey the message'. For more information about how to create a PowerPoint presentation see Chapter 13. Alternative open source software such as Prezi (www.prezi.com) will enable you to create less linear presentations and embed a variety of media into your presentation. If using such software, the same principles apply— but beware of making the audience feel motion sick with too much zooming in and out!

TABLE 34.2 | THE USE OF VISUAL SUPPORTS

VISUAL	WHAT THIS VISUAL SHOWS
Photograph or drawing	What something looks like
Map	Where something is located
Diagram or concept map	How something works or is organised
Graph	How much there is of something
Pie chart	Proportions and percentages
Bar chart	Comparisons among quantities
Table	A related body of data
Numbered list	A sequential list of data

Rehearsing

People are not 'born public speakers'. Public speaking skills can be learned, but they take preparation and practice. The key difficulties for novice speakers include 'speed talking' as a result of nerves, trouble timing their talk to allow listeners to hear and retain the main points, and problems using the audiovisual equipment. You can take steps to overcome these difficulties, either through practice and feedback from peers or through professional help. If you are concerned that you will become nervous during presentations, seek help regarding management strategies.

Rehearsing your talk aloud, with your visual aids, is sensible for a number of reasons:

- it enables you to practise pacing and timing
- it allows you to hear if you sound stilted, boring or pompous when moving from the written word to oral speech (you could tape your talk and listen to see if you need to change the style of presentation or content)
- it helps you become competent at managing the material and the audiovisual supports within the set time.

When you arrive at the conference

As a priority, check the venue in which you will be speaking. Examine the setup carefully. How crowded is the room? How flexible is the space? How close is it to distracting noises? Check how much lighting will be available for you to read your notes when the lights are dimmed. What is the audiovisual setup? Can you reach the computer mouse or the overhead projector easily? Will you need to dim or increase the lighting?

Sit in a few chairs around the room to get an idea of how you will look to audience members. If possible, attend an earlier presentation in the same room and see how others cope with the space. Where did the session convenor sit? Did the presenters sit on the stage or in the audience before the presentation? Is water provided, or will you need to take a bottle with you? Is there a clock in view, or will you need to put your watch in a visible spot? Is there a microphone, and does that mean you need to stay in one place?

Organise a time to conduct any audiovisual checks with a technician before your presentation. Check the lectern and any control buttons. If you are showing scientific or clinical images, will you need a pointer to indicate the key elements? Practise using the remote pointer and slide changer if available.

PRESENTING CONFIDENTLY

- Think about your appearance: make it appropriate for the audience.
- Relax, engage with the audience, do not talk to your notes.
- Be enthusiastic about your topic.
- Speak firmly and clearly into the microphone.
- Avoid long, complex sentences.
- Avoid reading only the same words as are on the slide; slides should be integrated with your commentary (Harden, 2008).
- Be aware of the non-verbal messages you convey; for example, through distracting movements of your laser pointer (Munter & Russell, 2003).
- Pace your presentation: keep an eye on the time you have left.
- Watch for nods of understanding. If some in your audience look puzzled, be prepared to reiterate your point or rephrase it.
- Conclude strongly and clearly.

Delivering your talk

Two related keys to effective presentation are: to be convincing and to sell your message (Parvis, 2001). People go to conferences to discover what is new in the field, to be inspired and to be challenged to think differently. After all your preparation, this is the time to relax as much as possible and deliver the talk as you have practised it.

Answering questions

Managing question time is an integral part of every session. Normally, there is a chairperson who moderates questions, and makes sure that they are taken in order and that no one dominates the occasion with his or her own interests or concerns.

DEALING WITH QUESTION TIME

- Maintain good eye contact with all members of the audience.
- If you do not understand a question, ask for clarification.
- Repeat a question briefly if it is likely that part of the audience could not hear it.
- Provide brief, clear answers; do not start another lecture.
- Direct your answer to the whole audience, not just the questioner.
- If people make a comment and do not ask a question, thank them for their comment.
- Offer to follow up individually if someone has a complex question or an emotional issue they want discussed.
- Do not bluff if you do not know the answer; admit you have not considered the issue.
- Allow other experts in the audience to offer ideas or opinions.

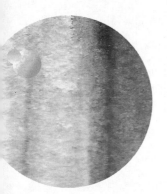

conclusion

Giving a talk at a conference can be a challenging experience, but with good material and careful preparation it can also be tremendously rewarding, both personally and professionally. If you take the time to practise, if you watch other speakers to learn what to do and what not to do, and if you regard your audience with respect but not apprehension, you will be well on the way to giving a first-class conference presentation.

references

Bly, R. W. (2003). Give memorable presentations. *Chemical Engineering Progress*, *99*(1), 84–7.

Gruhn, P. (2001). Terrified of public speaking? Not anymore …. *In Tech*, *48*(5), 84.

Harden, R. M. (2008). Death by PowerPoint—the need for a 'fidget index'. *Medical Teacher, 30*(9–10), 833–5.

Lunemann, R. (2001). Oral presentations for technical communication. *Technical Communication, 48*(3), 328–9.

Munter, M., & Russell, L. (2003). *Guide to presentations*. Upper Saddle River, NJ: Prentice Hall.

Parvis, L. F. (2001). The importance of communication and public speaking. *Environmental Health, 63*(9), 44.

Schmoll, B. J. (2002). Writing, speaking, and communication skills for health professionals. *Physical Therapy, 82*(5), 524–5.

Smith, R. (2000). How not to give a presentation. *British Medical Journal, 321*, 570–1.

Tyler, S., Kossen, C., & Ryan, C. (2005). *Communication: A foundation course* (2nd edn). Frenchs Forest, NSW: Pearson Education.

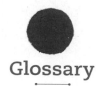

Glossary

ABSTRACT
An abstract is a short précis of all the key elements in your paper or poster.

ACADEMIC HONESTY
The term academic integrity encompasses academic honesty, ethical communication and other values. It is one of the core qualities required for good scholarship.

ACADEMIC INTEGRITY
The term academic integrity encompasses academic honesty, ethical communication and other values. It is one of the core qualities required for good scholarship.

ACADEMIC WRITING
Academic writing presents a scholarly argument clearly.

ACCOUNTABLE
Being held accountable involves taking personal responsibility.

ACTIVE LISTENING
Active listening involves combined communication strategies that help you to listen and respond to another person to better understand them.

ADVOCACY
Advocacy is presenting the cause of another individual or group. Clients may need advocacy of a political, social, legal, personal or health nature.

AGGRESSIVE BEHAVIOUR
Aggressive behaviour is taking physical, mental or verbal action to increase your own dominance.

ASSERTIVE BEHAVIOUR
Assertive behaviour is taking actions that ensure that your rights and responsibilities, and those of others, are respected and honoured.

ASYNCHRONOUS COMMUNICATION
Asynchronous communication means 'not at the same time', where participants communicate or engage in collaborative project work separated by time, space or both.

AUGMENTATIVE COMMUNICATION
Augmentative communication involves combined approaches and devices to improve the communication of people who cannot speak or be understood.

BIBLIOGRAPHIC DATABASE
A bibliographic database is an organised collection of references to published works, including journal articles, newspaper articles and conference proceedings, but usually not monographs.

CASE CONFERENCE

A case conference is a meeting of healthcare professionals to make decisions about patient management.

CASE PRESENTATION

A case presentation is an interview and/or clinical assessment to provide information for the case conference.

CASE STUDY PRESENTATION

Case study presentations involve you being able to briefly describe your client's progress to date, treatment interventions, response to treatment, anticipated timeframes and future recommendations.

CLIENT

The term client in this book refers to all people receiving team services—including consumers, patients, communities and populations.

CLINICAL REASONING

Clinical reasoning is a broad term denoting the thinking, judgments and decision-making involved in clinical practice.

CLINICAL REPORTS

Clinical reports have a number of different purposes in patient care, including keeping records and handing over client information.

COMMUNICATING

Communicating can be defined as the actions and processes of sharing information and ideas; a core component for working together in teams.

COMMUNICATION

Communication is conferring through speech, writing or non-verbal means (including body language) to create a shared meaning. It is a two-way process: whereas talking, listening, writing and reading can be one-sided; communicating involves two or more people sharing information.

COMMUNITY

A community is a group of people who share many aspects of life (e.g. location, culture) and usually see themselves as belonging together.

COMMUNITY DEVELOPMENT

Community development is a form of community organisation that also aims to empower the community.

COMMUNITY ENGAGEMENT

Community engagement is the communication, cooperation and collaboration with a community undertaken by health professionals to improve or maintain that community's health.

COMMUNITY HEALTH

Community health services focus more on promoting and maintaining the health of people living within their communities.

COMMUNITY PROFILE

A community profile helps you determine and describe: the demographic and social issues shaping the community; the values, health needs, resources, potential project partnerships within the community; and the power and leadership within the community.

CONCEPT MAP

A concept map is a diagram of the relationships between each concept or element of an idea or theory.

CONFERENCE

A conference, or professional seminar, is one of the best places to hear about cutting-edge advances in your field and to present your ideas.

CONFIDENCE

Confidence is a state of being certain that one's prediction or action is the best.

CONFIDENTIALITY

Confidentiality entails that we keep information about clients private. To safeguard clients' confidentiality, share information only with those authorised to access it.

CONFLICT MANAGEMENT

Five styles of conflict management are: competitive, collaborative, compromising, avoidant and accommodating.

CONSULTING

Consulting with other professionals means seeking their advice or information, and exchanging opinions.

COPYRIGHT

Copyright means something may not be reproduced except with the author's permission.

CULTURAL COMPETENCE

Cultural competence is the ability to engage appropriately and effectively with people across different cultures.

DESIGN

Design is the way the work is planned and presented, often based on key goals, principles or disciplinary styles/genre.

DIALOGUES

A dialogue, or conversation, is where the interviewer and interviewee jointly construct a story about the interviewee's health.

DIFFICULT CONVERSATIONS

We have a duty to confront our colleagues, clients and family members if their behaviour is impeding learning, quality care or professional relationships.

DIGITAL COMMUNICATION

Explore digital communication alternatives and select those that work best for you and thus build your personal learning environment (PLE).

DISTRIBUTED LEADERSHIP

Distributed leadership is characterised by interdependence among members of the team or organisation, with overlapping responsibilities and empowerment of every member of the team or organisation.

DUTY OF CARE

Duty of care is a professional's responsibility to take reasonable care and ensure no harm is done to patients and clients.

ELECTRONIC COMMUNICATION DEVICES

Electronic communication devices are tools such as telephones that are used for multiple forms of verbal and written communication. They create a 'networked world'.

EMOTIONAL INTELLIGENCE

Emotional intelligence is the ability to identify, assess and respond to the emotions of yourself and others.

ENGAGING LEADERSHIP

Engaging leadership is grounded in a genuine respect for others, with integrity, transparency and inclusiveness.

EPORTFOLIO

Using an electronic portfolio (eportfolio) you can create evidence to support your learning and invite others to view your work.

ETHICAL RESEARCH

Integrity and the five values it encompasses are central features of ethical research. For research to be ethical there are also related principles, including respecting the privacy and confidentiality of participants and others involved, which researchers must follow.

FACILITATE

To facilitate, the tutor uses questions to explore and stimulate student thinking, and helps the group set standards for depth and breadth of knowledge, develop reasoning ability and enhance communication skills.

FEEDBACK

Feedback includes 'information about a person's performance of a task which is used as a basis for improvement'. It is based on observation and is formative.

FIGURES

Tables are characterised by horizontal rows and related vertical columns. All other forms of graphics, including diagrams, charts, photographs, pictures, maps, icons, graphic organisers and drawings are called figures.

FUNDING PROPOSAL

Funding proposals must be written to finance the design, development, delivery and evaluation of new community services and health promotion projects.

GRAMMAR

Grammar refers to the structural rules of language.

GREY LITERATURE

Grey literature is written work that is not published in easily accessible journals and may not be found in databases or through web searches.

HEALTH COMMUNICATION

Health communication utilises a variety of carefully developed communication strategies to improve or maintain the health of individuals, communities and populations.

HEALTH SCIENCES

The term health sciences refers to the variety of professional groups that provide healthcare services to people in community settings or healthcare facilities. These professions include medicine, dentistry, nursing, physiotherapy, occupational therapy, radiography, speech pathology, dietetics, emergency care work, podiatry, pharmacy, health education and public health.

HEALTH TEAM

A health team is a team of practitioners who work together to prevent health problems or disability, maintain good health, improve health and/or maximise ability.

HEURISTICS

Heuristics include maxims (sayings) that remind the interviewer to be aware of some of the dangers that await the inexperienced.

HIGH-IMPACT JOURNALS

High-impact journals are those whose articles tend to receive many citations, indicating that they have a wide and prestigious readership.

HONESTY

Honesty is about being truthful (a positive element) and not being deceitful by, for example, telling lies or omitting relevant information (negative elements).

INTELLECTUAL PROPERTY

Intellectual property is the 'research, words and ideas generated by an author'.

INTERCULTURAL COMMUNICATION

Intercultural communication involves working effectively and relating appropriately to others in diverse cultural contexts.

LIBRARY CATALOGUE

A library catalogue is an index of items held by a library, including books, journals and audiovisual material.

LITERATURE REVIEW

The literature review needs to provide sufficient background to locate your work in its context.

MEDIA

In communication, media refers to either the physical or digital/electronic means of conveying information/messages.

MEDIATION

Mediation involves an independent party seeking to resolve disagreements or disputes between people.

MEDICO-LEGAL REPORTS

Medico-legal reports may be requested by insurers, courts (by subpoena) or government departments to provide independent assessment of a person's current and potential future capacity, or professional judgment of another professional's work.

MNEMONICS

Mnemonics help a person to recall things.

MOBILE LEARNING

Mobile learning uses mobile devices such as smart phones and tablet devices for communication and accessing information for learning purposes.

MULTIMEDIA PRESENTATION

A multimedia presentation is a combination of multiple forms of media, including more than one of the following: text, graphics, pictures, audio, animation, video and others.

NEEDS ASSESSMENT

A needs assessment assesses and describes the needs of the community of interest.

NEGOTIATION

Negotiation involves seeking agreement about matters people are concerned about or interested in changing.

NON-VERBAL COMMUNICATION

Non-verbal communication includes aspects such as eye contact, posture, facial expression, fine and gross movements, and artefacts such as clothing.

PARADIGM

Paradigms are frameworks for research.

PARALANGUAGE

Paralanguage includes communicative aspects such as speed, tone, volume, pitch and intonation of the voice.

PATIENT RECORDS

Patient records record results of daily, weekly or intermittent treatment sessions; may form part of the main medical record or patient file, centrally located but accessible to all service providers so that all providers are kept up to date and can coordinate care.

PEER-REVIEWED JOURNAL

If the editor of a peer-reviewed journal considers your article fits with the journal's aims and is of sufficient quality, it will be sent to peer review. The review process ensures that every published article has been critiqued by experts before it is published.

PERSONAL LEARNING ENVIRONMENT (PLE)

Explore digital communication alternatives and select those that work best for you and thus build your personal learning environment (PLE).

PLAGIARISM

Plagiarism contains two parts: theft (of a thought or words) and fraud (presenting them as our own).

PLAGIARISM DETECTION SOFTWARE

Plagiarism detection software compares the text with online material and the institution's own database of previously submitted student assignments.

PRESENTATION SKILLS

Effective presentation skills form a significant component of the raft of communication skills integral to successful health professional practice.

PRIMARY SOURCE

A primary source is a work that gives you direct or primary knowledge of an event, period, original thought or research findings.

PROBLEM-BASED LEARNING

Problem-based learning (PBL) is one particular method of case-based, active learning which has been growing in popularity in higher education for many years.

PROFESSIONALISM

Professional behaviour (or professionalism) comprises those actions, standards and considerations of ethical and humanistic conduct expected by society and by professional associations from members of professions.

PROOFREADING

Proofreading is a process that involves a detailed review of the grammar, spelling, punctuation and mechanics of style of your submission.

PROTOCOLS

Protocols break the interview process up into a series of stages.

RAPPORT

Rapport is a close and harmonious relationship in which there is common understanding.

REFERENCE MANAGEMENT SOFTWARE

Reference management software helps you to manage bibliographies and references.

REFERENCES

References acknowledge the sources of the ideas, information, data and arguments you present in your work.

REFERRALS

Referrals are written to another professional to request assessment and recommendations for management of client, or request a second opinion.

ROLE-PLAY

Role-play involves students acting out a clinical scenario in front of fellow students.

SEARCH ENGINES

Search engines are computer programs that search documents based on given key words or phrases.

SECONDARY SOURCE

A secondary source provides commentary written about a primary source.

SELF-DIRECTED LEARNING

Students are encouraged to assume responsibility for their self-directed learning by identifying knowledge gaps, then finding and appraising information to close those gaps, and following up any learning issues pertinent to the case. Identifying knowledge gaps is an important part of PBL.

SOCIAL MARKETING

Social marketing is the application of commercial marketing communication techniques (e.g. advertising, sponsorship) to promote health and other socially desirable outcomes.

STORYBOARD

A storyboard is a sequence of images and text used to plan a presentation.

STRUCTURE OF AN ESSAY

The structure of an essay has three main parts: the introduction, body and conclusion.

STRUCTURE

The thesis structure is how the sections are organised to make the argument clear and credible.

STYLE

When we apply a style to a word or sentence in Word we can change an entire set of characteristics at once. Styles enable you to format different types of text consistently. Styles give structure to your document.

SYNCHRONOUS COMMUNICATION

Communicating in real time is called synchronous communication.

SYSTEMATIC REVIEW

A systematic review is a literature review involving rigorous critical assessment and synthesis of all research and evidence relating to a particular question/clinical issue.

TABLES

Tables are characterised by horizontal rows and related vertical columns. All other forms of graphics, including diagrams, charts, photographs, pictures, maps, icons, graphic organisers and drawings are called figures.

TASK MANAGEMENT
Task management involves understanding the job, planning what to do, getting it done, evaluating the outcome, then asking 'what now?'.

TEAM MEMBERS
Team members are participants in collective action, predominantly based on the nature of their professional socialisation and on their personal and professional experiences.

TEMPLATE
A template is a pre-formatted page layout in presentation software that assists in the creation of slides that all have a similar design.

TEXT STYLE
Text style includes the general genre (e.g. casual, scholarly) as well as the choice of font (typeface, e.g. Arial; and size, e.g. 10 pt).

THESES
The term thesis refers to the argument presented in the report.

TIME BUDGET
Your estimate of time to be allocated to your various study tasks. The way you apportion your total study time for optimal results.

TRANSACTIONAL MODEL OF COMMUNICATION
The transactional model of communication suggests that communication is a dynamic process in which individuals receive and send information simultaneously.

WORK–LIFE BALANCE
Taking care of yourself by seeking to balance the important parts of your day.

WRITING PLAN
A writing plan should reflect the interests of the journal, whether it be a science, social science and humanities or education journal.

Index